Antimicrobial Drug Resistance: Clinical Aspects

Antimicrobial Drug Resistance: Clinical Aspects

Editor: Armando Guerrero

AMERICAN
MEDICAL PUBLISHERS
www.americanmedicalpublishers.com

AMERICAN
MEDICAL PUBLISHERS
www.americanmedicalpublishers.com

Cataloging-in-Publication Data

Antimicrobial drug resistance : clinical aspects / edited by Armando Guerrero.
p. cm.
Includes bibliographical references and index.
ISBN 978-1-63927-217-4
1. Drug resistance in microorganisms. 2. Anti-infective agents. 3. Microorganisms--Effect of drugs on.
4. Drug resistance. I. Guerrero, Armando.
QR177 .A58 2022
616.904 1--dc23

American Medical Publishers,
41 Flatbush Avenue,
1st Floor, New York,
NY 11217, USA

ISBN 978-1-63927-217-4 (Hardback)

Contents

Preface

Antimicrobial drug resistance is defined as the ability to resist the effects of medication by a microbe. Resistance can be developed through three mechanisms. These are natural resistance, genetic mutation and acquired resistance. Such resistance can be developed by all classes of microbes. These classes include bacteria, fungi, virus and protozoa. Bacteria develop antibiotic resistance, fungi develop antifungal resistance, viruses develop antiviral resistance, and protozoa develop antiprotozoal resistance. Growing resistance is mainly caused by the excessive use of antimicrobials by humans and animals. Its preventive measures have been undergoing through further research. These researches include alternating therapy, phage therapy, new drug development and use of vaccines. This book presents the clinical aspects of antimicrobial drug resistance in the most comprehensible and easy to understand language. It consists of contributions made by international experts. The book will serve as a valuable source of reference for graduate and postgraduate students.

This book unites the global concepts and researches in an organized manner for a comprehensive understanding of the subject. It is a ripe text for all researchers, students, scientists or anyone else who is interested in acquiring a better knowledge of this dynamic field.

I extend my sincere thanks to the contributors for such eloquent research chapters. Finally, I thank my family for being a source of support and help.

Editor

1

Shiga (Vero)-toxin producing *Escherichia coli* isolated from the hospital foods; virulence factors, o-serogroups and antimicrobial resistance properties

Reza Ranjbar[1], Mojtaba Masoudimanesh[2], Farhad Safarpoor Dehkordi[3], Nematollah Jonaidi-Jafari[4*] and Ebrahim Rahimi[5]

Abstract

Background: According to the presence of the weak, diabetic and immunosuppressive patients in hospitals, hospital foods should have a high quality and safety. Cooking a lot of foods higher than daily requirement, storage of cooked foods in an inappropriate condition and presence of nurses and servants in distribution of food to patients are the main reasons caused contamination of hospital foods. Shiga toxigenic *Escherichia coli* is one of the common cause of food poisoning in hospitals. The present research was carried out to study the distribution of virulence factors, O-serogroups and antibiotic resistance properties in STEC strains recovered from Iranian hospital food samples.

Methods: Five-hundred and eighty raw and cooked food samples were collected and immediately transferred to the laboratory. *E. coli*-positive strains were subjected to PCR and disk diffusion method.

Results: Thirty-nine out of 580 (6.72%) hospital food samples were contaminated with *E. coli*. Raw (20%) and cooked meat (6%) were the most commonly contaminated samples. Raw samples had the higher prevalence of *E. coli* (*P* <0.01). Samples which were collected in the summer season had the highest prevalence of bacteria (64.10%). Significant difference was seen between the prevalence of EHEC and AEEC subtypes (*P* <0.01). The most commonly detected virulence factors in both EHEC and AEEC subtypes were stx*1* and *eae*. The most commonly detected serogroups were O26 (43.75%) and O157 (25%) and there were no positive results for O103, O145, O91, O113 and O128 serogroups. *Aac* (3)-*IV* (100%), *CITM* (100%) and *tetA* (62.50%) were the most commonly detected antibiotic resistance genes. STEC strains harbored the highest levels of resistance against ampicillin (93.75%), gentamycin (93.75%), tetracycline (87.50%) and ciprofloxacin (81.25%). All of the STEC strains were resistant to at least 3 antibiotics, while the prevalence of resistance against more than 12 antibiotics were 12.50%.

Conclusions: High presence of O157 serogroups, EHEC strains and animal-based antibiotics in cooked foods showed insufficiency of cooking time and temperature in the kitchens of hospitals. Judicious prescription of antibiotics and attentions to the principles of food safety can reduce the risk of resistant and virulent strains of STEC in hospital foods.

Keywords: Shiga-toxin producing *escherichia coli*, Virulence factors, O-serogroups, Antibiotic resistance properties, Hospital foods, Iran

* Correspondence: Jonaidi2000@yahoo.com
[4]Health Research Center, Baqiyatallah University of Medical Sciences, Tehran, Iran
Full list of author information is available at the end of the article

Background

Access to adequate amounts of safe and healthy foods is key to supporting life and promoting good health of people. Insecure food containing pathogenic bacteria, viruses, parasites or harmful chemical elements, causes more than two-hundred diseases and disorders – ranging from diarrhea to cancers [1, 2]. Foodborne diseases cause approximately 76 million illnesses, 325,000 hospitalizations, and 5,000 deaths in the United States each year [2–4]. Observation of basic principles of food hygiene can control and eliminate the distribution of foodborne diseases. Attention to the principles of food hygiene is more urgent especially in public places such as hospitals, restaurants, kindergartens, prisons, barracks, elderly care centers and asylums.

Using from regular, nutritious, safe and accurate food diet based on the characters of patients is one of the main aspects of treatment in hospitals. Due to the general weakness and suppression of the immune system of majority of patients in hospitals, hospitals foods should have good sanitary quality. Among all pathogenic agents causing food-borne diseases and food poisoning in hospitals, *Escherichia coli* (*E. coli*) had a had a significant importance [5–8].

E. coli is a gram-negative, non-sporulating, flagellated, rod-shaped and facultative anaerobic bacterium which belongs to *Enterobacteriaceae* family. Shiga (vero) toxin (*Stx*)-producing *E. coli* (STEC) is a subdivision of an important pathogenic group of this bacterium named enterohemorrhagic *E. coli* (EHEC) [9–11]. STEC strains are responsible for intensive clinical syndromes like lethal hemolytic uremic syndrome (HUS), bloody and non-bloody diarrhea, thrombotic thrombocytopenic purpura (TTP) and hemorrhagic colitis (HC) [9–11]. *E. coli* strains that cause HC and HUS in humans, express high levels of Shiga toxins (stx), cause attaching-effacing (A/E) lesions in intestinal epithelial cells, and possess a specific 60-MDa EHEC plasmid are known as EHEC [9–11]. One feature EHEC and Enteropathogenic *E. coli* (EPEC) have in common is the causation of intestinal epithelial lesions known as attaching and effacing (A/E). Attaching-effacing *E coli* (AEEC) is a designation for those *E. coli* strains known to cause A/E lesions or at least carry the genes for this trait, and therefore include organisms that fall into either the EHEC or EPEC classes [9–11].

Outbreak of food poisoning, foodborne diseases, HUS, TTP and HC are associated with certain STEC O-serogroups mainly including O157, O26, O91, O103, O121, O113, O111, O145, O45 and O128 as well as untypeable groups [9–11]. Presence of latent virulence factors including Shiga toxins (*stx1* and *stx2*), intimin (*eaeA*) and hemolysin (*hlyA*) which are responsible for adhesion, colonization and invasion of bacterial cells into the intestinal walls is another factor for outbreak of foodborne diseases and disorders [9–11].

High levels of resistance in STEC strains is another important factor which increase the pathogenicity of bacteria. Unfortunately, STEC strains recovered from food stuffs and also cases of diarrhea and food poisoning harbored the high levels of resistance against commonly used groups of antibiotics including quinolones, aminoglycosides, macrolides, cephalosporins, sulfonamides, fluoroquinolones and tetracycline [9–15]. In the other hands, STEC strains of food poisoning show a high incidence of resistance (85-100%) against commonly used antimicrobial agents [9, 10, 12–14, 16, 17]. Molecular epidemiological researches showed that presence of certain antibiotic resistance genes including the genes that encode resistance against fluoroquinolone (*qnr*), trimethoprim (*dfrA1*), cephalothin (*blaSHV*), tetracycline (*tetA* and *tetB*), ampicillin (*CITM*), gentamicin (*aac (3)-IV*), sulfonamide (*sul1*), chloramphenicol (*cat1* and *cmlA*), aminoglycosides (*aadA1*), and erythromycin (*ereA*) is the most important reason for occurrence of antibiotic resistance in STEC strains [9–14, 16, 18].

According to the uncertain role of STEC strains in hospital foods and lack of epidemiological investigations in this field in Iran, the present research was carried out to study the distribution of virulence factors, O-serogroups, antibiotic resistance genes and antibiotic resistance pattern of STEC strains isolated from various types of raw and cooked hospital food samples.

Methods

Samples and *E. coli* isolation

From September 2013 to September 2014, a total of 580 various types of raw and cooked hospital foods including raw meat ($n = 60$), raw chicken ($n = 60$) and raw fish ($n = 70$) and cooked meat ($n = 100$), cooked chicken ($n = 100$), cooked fish ($n = 110$), and soup ($n = 80$) were randomly collected and immediately transferred to the Food Hygiene Research Center of the Islamic Azad University of Shahrekord in cooler with ice-packs. Samples were collected from the various hospitals in Isfahan province, Iran. All food samples showed normal physical characters including odor, color and consolidation. All samples were collected through 4 different seasons of the year including summer ($n = 120$), autumn ($n = 150$), winter ($n = 160$) and spring ($n = 150$).

Totally, 10-g of crushed food samples were homogenized for 2 min in 90 ml of Peptone Water (PW, Merck, Germany). Then the samples were cultured on 5% sheep blood and MacConkey agar (Merck, Germany) and incubated for 18 to 24 h at 37 °C. Colonies with the typical color and appearance of *E. coli* were picked and streaked again on blood agar plates and re-streaked on EMB agar

(Merck, Germany). All plates were further incubated for 24 h at 37 °C. The green metallic sheen colonies were considered as *E. coli*. The presumptive colonies were biochemically tested for growth on triple sugar iron agar (TSI) and lysine iron agar (LIA), oxidative/fermentative degradation of glucose, citrate utilization, urease production, indol fermentation, tryptophan degradation, glucose degradation (methyl red test) and motility.

PCR confirmation of *E. coli* strains

The colonies were further confirmed using the *16S rRNA*-based Polymerase Chain Reaction (PCR) based on the method previously described [19]. Bacterial strains were subcultured overnight in Luria-Bertani broth (Merck, Germany) and further incubated for 48 h at 37 °C. Genomic DNA was extracted from bacterial colonies using the DNA extraction kit (Fermentas, Germany) according to manufacturer's instruction. The 10 ml bacterial DNA extract and controls were amplified with 0.5 mM primers (Forward: 5'-AGTTTGATCCTGGCTCAG-3' and Reverse: 5'-AGGCCCGGGAACGTATTCAC-3') (1343 bp) [19], 200 mM of each dNTP (Fermentas, Germany), 2 mM MgCl2, 10 mM KCl PCR buffer and 1.0 U Taq polymerase (Fermentas, Germany). The DNA was amplified in a programmable thermal cycler (Eppendorf, Mastercycler® 5330, Eppendorf-Netheler-Hinz GmbH, Hamburg, Germany) PCR device using the following protocol: 94 °C for 5 min, 40 cycles of 94 °C for 1 min, 55 °C for 1 min, 72 °C for 2 min, and final 72 °C for 5 min.

PCR amplification of virulence factors, O-serogroups and antibiotic resistance genes

Table 1 shows the list of primers as well as program and condition of each reaction used for detection of O-serogroups, virulence genes and antimicrobial resistant genes [11, 20]. Programmable DNA thermo-cycler (Eppendorf Flexrcycler^2, Germany) was used in all PCR reactions. The PCR amplification products (15 μl) were subjected to electrophoresis in a 1.5% agarose gel in 1× TBE buffer at 80 V for 30 min, stained with SYBR Green (Fermentas, Germany). All runs included a negative DNA control consisting of PCR grade water and strains of *E. coli* O157:K88ac:H19, CAPM 5933 and *E. coli* O159:H20, CAPM 6006 were used as positive controls.

Antimicrobial susceptibility testing

Pattern of antimicrobial resistance was studied using the simple disk diffusion technique. The Mueller–Hinton agar (Merck, Germany) medium was used for this purpose. Antibiotic resistance of *E. coli* strains against 23 commonly used antibiotics was determined using the instruction of Clinical and Laboratory Standards Institute guidelines [21]. Susceptibility of *E. coli* strains were tested against tetracycline (30 u/disk), mezlocillin (30 u/disk), ampicillin (10 u/disk), cefotaxime (30 μg/disk), gentamycin (10 μg/disk), ciprofloxacin (5 μg/disk), amikacin (30 u/disk), ceftazidime (30 μg/disk), imipenem (30 u/disk), cotrimoxazole (30 μg/disk), meropenem (10 μg/disk), enrofloxacin (5 μg/disk), sulfamethoxazole (25 μg/disk), trimethoprim (5 μg/disk), levofloxacillin (5 μg/disk), cefipime (30 μg/disk), streptomycin (10 μg/disk), polymyxin B (300 U/disk), vancomycine (5 μg/disk), and chloramphenicol (30 μg/disk) antibiotic agents (Oxoid, UK). All of the inoculated plates were aerobically incubated at 37 °C for 18-24 h in an aerobic atmosphere. Results were interpreted based on the instruction provided by CLSI (2014) [21]. *E. coli* ATCC 25922 was used as quality control organisms in antimicrobial susceptibility determination.

Statistical analysis

Statistical analysis was performed using SPSS/16.0 software for significant relationships. The incidences of serogroups, virulence factors, O-serogroups and antibiotics resistance properties of *E. coli* isolated from various types of hospital food samples were statistically analyzed. Statistical significance was regarded at a P value < 0.05.

Results

Table 2 represents the total distribution of *E. coli* in various types of hospital food samples. Thirty-nine out of 580 (6.72%) hospital food samples were contaminated with *E. coli* strains. Raw meat (20%), raw chicken (16.66%) and cooked meat (6%) had the highest prevalence of *E. coli*. Statistically significant difference was seen for the prevalence of *E. coli* between raw and cooked hospital food samples (P <0.01). Figure 1 shows the total distribution of *E. c*oli strains in various seasons of the year based on the total numbers of 39 *E. coli* isolated. We found that hospital food samples of summer season had the highest prevalence of *E. coli* (25/39: 64.10%), while those of winter had the lowest (3/39: 7.69%). In the other hand, 25 out of 120 samples collected in summer (20.83%), 5 out of 150 samples collected in autumn (3.33%), 3 out of 160 samples collected in winter (1.87%) and 6 out of 150 samples collected in spring (4%) were positive for *E. coli*. Statistically significant difference was seen for the prevalence of *E. coli* between warm and cold season of the year (P <0.05).

Table 3 represents the distribution of virulence factors in *E. coli* subtypes isolated from hospital food samples. Prevalence of EHEC and AEEC subtypes in the raw meat, raw chicken, cooked meat, cooked chicken, cooked fish and soup samples were 16.66% and 50%, 20% and 60%, 25% and 50%, 0% and 33.33%,0% and 50% and finally 33.33% and 66.66%, respectively. All of the

Table 1 The oligonucleotide primers and the PCR programs used for amplification of O-serogroups, virulence factors and antibiotic resistance genes of *Escherichia coli* isolates of hospital foods

Target gene	Primer sequence (5′–3′)	PCR product (bp)	PCR programs	PCR Volume (50 μL)
O157	F: CGGACATCCATGTGATATGG R: TTGCCTATGTACAGCTAATCC	259	1 cycle: 95 °C — 3 min. 30 cycle: 95 °C — 20 s 58 °C — 40 s 72 °C — 30 s 1 cycle: 72 °C — 8 min	5 μL PCR buffer 10× 2 mM $Mgcl_2$ 150 μM dNTP (Fermentas) 0.75 μM of each primers F & R 1.5 U Taq DNA polymerase (Fermentas) 3 μL DNA template
O145	F: CCATCAACAGATTTAGGAGTG R: TTTCTACCGCGAATCTATC	609		
O103	F: TTGGAGCGTTAACTGGACCT R: GCTCCCGAGCACGTATAAG	321		
O26	F: CAGAATGGTTATGCTACTGT R: CTTACATTTGTTTTCGGCATC	423		
O111	F: TAGAGAAATTATCAAGTTAGTTCC R: ATAGTTATGAACATCTTGTTTAGC	406		
O91	F: GCTGACCTTCATGATCTGTTGA R: TAATTTAACCCGTAGAATCGCTGC	291	1 cycle: 94 °C — 6 min. 34 cycle: 95 °C — 50 s 58 °C — 70 s 72 °C — 55 s 1 cycle: 72 °C — 10 min	5 μL PCR buffer 10× 2 mM $Mgcl_2$ 150 μM dNTP (Fermentas) 0.75 μM of each primers F & R 1.5 U Taq DNA polymerase (Fermentas) 3 μL DNA template
O128	F: GCTTTCTGCCGATATTTGGC R: CCGACGGACTGATGCCGGTGATT	289		
O121	F: TGGCTAGTGGCATTCTGATG R: TGATACTTTAGCCGCCCTTG	322		
O113	F: GGGTTAGATGGAGCGCTATTGAGA R: AGGTCACCCTCTGAATTATGGCAG	771		
O45	F: CCGGGTTTCGATTTGTGAAGGTTG R: CACAACAGCCACTACTAGGCAGAA	527		
stx1	F: AAATCGCCATTCGTTGACTACTTCT R: TGCCATTCTGGCAACTCGCGATGCA	366	1 cycle: 95 °C — 3 min. 34 cycle: 94 °C — 60 s 56 °C — 45 s 72 °C — 60 s 1 cycle: 72 °C — 10 min	5 μL PCR buffer 10× 2 mM $Mgcl_2$ 150 μM dNTP (Fermentas) 0.75 μM of each primers F & R 1.5 U Taq DNA polymerase (Fermentas) 3 μL DNA template
stx2	F: CGATCGTCACTCACTGGTTTCATCA R: GGATATTCTCCCCACTCTGACACC	282		
eaeA	F: TGCGGCACAACAGGCGGCGA R: CGGTCGCCGCACCAGGATTC	629		
ehly	F: CAATGCAGATGCAGATACCG R: CAGAGATGTCGTTGCAGCAG	432		
aadA1	F: TATCCAGCTAAGCGCGAACT R: ATTTGCCGACTACCTTGGTC	447	1 cycle: 94 °C — 8 min. 32 cycle: 95 °C — 60 s 55 °C — 70 s 72 °C — 2 min 1 cycle: 72 °C — 8 min	5 μL PCR buffer 10× 2 mM $Mgcl_2$ 150 μM dNTP (Fermentas) 0.75 μM of each primers F & R 1.5 U Taq DNA polymerase (Fermentas) 3 μL DNA template
tetA	F: GGTTCACTCGAACGACGTCA R: CTGTCCGACAAGTTGCATGA	577		
tetB	F: CCTCAGCTTCTCAACGCGTG R: GCACCTTGCTGATGACTCTT	634		
dfrA1	F: GGAGTGCCAAAGGTGAACAGC R: GAGGCGAAGTCTTGGGTAAAAAC	367		
qnr	F: GGGTATGGATATTATTGATAAAG R: CTAATCCGGCAGCACTATTTA	670		
aac (3)-IV	F: CTTCAGGATGGCAAGTTGGT R: TCATCTCGTTCTCCGCTCAT	286		
sul1	F: TTCGGCATTCTGAATCTCAC R: ATGATCTAACCCTCGGTCTC	822		
blaSHV	F: TCGCCTGTGTATTATCTCCC R: CGCAGATAAATCACCACAATG	768		
CITM	F: TGGCCAGAACTGACAGGCAAA R: TTTCTCCTGAACGTGGCTGGC	462		
cat1	F: AGTTGCTCAATGTACCTATAACC R: TTGTAATTCATTAAGCATTCTGCC	547		
cmlA	F: CCGCCACGGTGTTGTTGTTATC R: CACCTTGCCTGCCCATCATTAG	698		

Table 2 Total prevalence of *Escherichia coli* in various types of hospital food samples

Types of samples	No. samples collected	No positive strains (%)	PCR confirmation (%)
Raw meat	60	12 (20)	12 (20)
Raw chicken	60	10 (16.66)	10 (16.66)
Raw fish	70	1 (1.42)	1 (1.42)
Cooked meat	100	6 (6)	6 (6)
Cooked chicken	100	3 (3)	3 (3)
Cooked fish	110	3 (2.72)	3 (2.72)
Soup	80	4 (5)	4 (5)
Total	580	39 (6.72)	39 (6.72)

EHEC strains harbored all three *stx1*, *eae* and *ehly* genes together (100%), while AEEC strains harbored variable percent of each gene. Statistically significant difference was seen between the prevalence of EHEC and AEEC subtypes ($P < 0.01$). We found that from a total of 39 *E. coli* strains isolated from samples, 16 strains (41.02%) were positive for AEEC and EHEC subtypes which were considered as STEC strains. Raw fish samples had no positive strains for the EHEC and AEEC subtypes. EHEC strains which harbored all three *stx1*, *eae* and *ehly* genes together were considered as a O157 serogroup.

Table 4 shows the total distribution of O-serogroups in the STEC strains isolated from various types of hospital food samples. We found that O26 (43.75%) and O157 (25%) were the most commonly detected serogroups in the STEC strains of hospital food samples. There were no positive results for the O103, O145, O91, O113 and O128 serogroups. Statistically significant differences were seen for the prevalence of STEC O-serogroups between various types of samples ($P < 0.05$). Totally, raw chicken and soup samples harbored the most variable types of O-serogroups.

Total distribution of antibiotic resistance genes in the STEC strains isolated from various types of hospital food samples is shown in Table 5. We found that *aac (3)-IV* (100%), *CITM* (100%), *tetA* (62.50%), *dfrA1* (56.25%) and *sul1* (56.25%) were the most commonly detected antibiotic resistance genes. The less commonly detected antibiotic resistance genes were *cmlA* (12.50%), *cat1* (25%) and *tetB* (31.25%). Statistically significant differences were seen for the prevalence of antibiotic resistance genes between various types of samples ($P < 0.05$).

Table 6 indicates the antibiotic resistance pattern of the STEC strains of various types of hospital food samples. STEC strains of our investigation harbored the highest levels of resistance against ampicillin (93.75%), gentamycin (93.75%), tetracycline (87.50%), ciprofloxacin (81.25%) and amikacin (75%). Resistance of STEC strains of cooked samples against human-based antibiotics was entirely higher than animal-based antibiotics. Statistically significant differences were seen for the prevalence of antibiotic resistance between various types of samples ($P < 0.05$). Figure 2 represents the prevalence of multi-drug resistance in the STEC strains of hospital food samples. We found that all of the STEC strains of our investigation were resistant to at least 3 antibiotics, while prevalence of resistance against ten, eleven, twelve and more than twelve antibiotics were 37.50%, 25%, 18.75% and 12.50%, respectively.

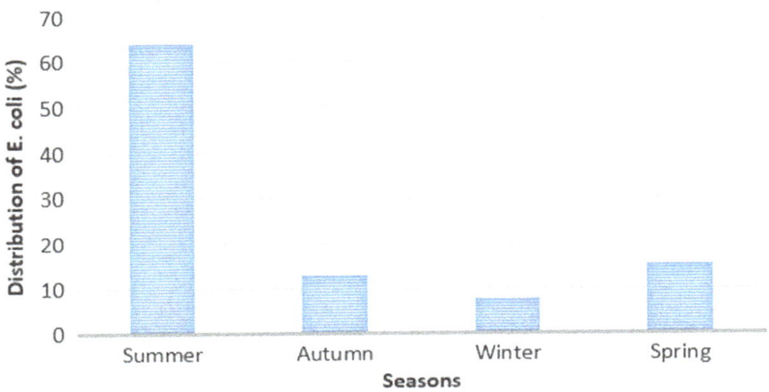

Fig. 1 Seasonal distribution of *Escherichia coli* in the hospital food samples

Table 3 Distribution of virulence factors in *Escherichia coli* subtypes isolated from hospital food samples

Samples (No. positive)	Subtypes	No. positive samples	Virulence genes
Raw meat (12)	Non detected	2 (33.33)	-
	EHEC	1 (16.66)	*stx1*, eae, ehly: 1 (100)
	AEEC	3 (50)	stx1: 3 (100) stx2: 1 (33.33) eaeA: 3 (100) stx1, eaeA: 1 (33.33) stx2, eaeA: 1 (33.33) stx1, stx2, eaeA: 1 (33.33)
	Total	6 (50)	
Raw chicken (10)	Non detected	1 (20)	-
	EHEC	1 (20)	stx1, eae, ehly: 1 (100)
	AEEC	3 (60)	stx1: 3 (100) stx2: 1 (33.33) eaeA: 3 (100) stx1, eaeA: 1 (33.33) stx2, eaeA: 1 (33.33) stx1, stx2, eaeA: 1 (33.33)
	Total	5 (50)	-
Raw fish (1)	Non detected	1 (100)	-
	EHEC	-	-
	AEEC	-	stx1: - stx2: - eaeA: - stx1, eaeA: - stx2, eaeA: - stx1, stx2, eaeA: -
	Total	1 (100)	-
Cooked meat (6)	Non detected	1 (25)	-
	EHEC	1 (25)	stx1, eae, ehly: 1 (100)
	AEEC	2 (50)	stx1: 2 (100) stx2: 1 (50) eaeA: 2 (100) stx1, eaeA: 1 (50) stx2, eaeA: 1 (50) stx1, stx2, eaeA: 1 (50)
	Total	4 (66.66)	-
Cooked chicken (3)	Non detected	1 (33.33)	-
	EHEC	-	-
	AEEC	1 (33.33)	stx1: 1 (100) stx2: - eaeA: 1 (100) stx1, eaeA: 1 (100) stx2, eaeA: - stx1, stx2, eaeA: -
	Total	2 (66.66)	-
Cooked fish (3)	Non detected	1 (50)	-
	EHEC	-	-
	AEEC	1 (50)	stx1: 1 (100) stx2: - eaeA: 1 (100) stx1, eaeA: 1 (100) stx2, eaeA: - stx1, stx2, eaeA: -
	Total	2 (66.66)	-
Soup (4)	Non detected	-	-
	EHEC	1 (33.33)	stx1, eae, ehly: 1 (100)
	AEEC	2 (66.66)	stx1: 2 (100) stx2: 1 (50) eaeA: 2 (100) stx1, eaeA: 1 (50) stx2, eaeA: 1 (50) stx1, stx2, eaeA: 1 (50)
	Total	3 (50)	-

Discussion

As far as we know the present investigation is the first prevalence report of the isolation of *E. coli* strains from raw and cocked hospital foods as well as molecular characterization and antimicrobial resistance properties of their STEC strains in the world. We found that 6.72% of hospital food samples were contaminated with *E. coli* strains and the prevalence of STEC strains were 41.02% which was considerable high. Gram-negative bacteria like *E.* coli are responsible for 30-70% of hospitalization in developed countries and *E. coli* was the most common etiologic gram-negative organism in the hospital environment [22, 23].

There were some probable reasons for the high prevalence of *E. coli* and also STEC strains in the hospital food samples. At first. high-volume food production and long process of catering caused several problems such as lack of adequate precision and accuracy in the preparation and washing of raw materials and even their well cooking, lack of enough time and even temperature for cooking of raw materials, cooling of foods during processing, lack of reaching of sufficient heat to the center of meat and other food materials, lack of enough time to withdraw meat from the frozen state and finally cooking of meat and its products more than the daily requirement and then their storage at improper temperature and conditions. These mentioned circumstances maybe lead to survival and even growth of pathogenic microorganisms in food stuffs. At second, using from unsanitary and also contaminated equipment and dishes for production of

Table 4 Total distribution of O-serogroups in the Shiga toxigenic Escherichia coli strains isolated from various types of hospital food samples

Samples (No. STEC strains)	Distribution of O-serogroups (%)									
	O157	O26	O103	O111	O145	O45	O91	O113	O121	O128
Raw meat (4)	1 (25)	2 (50)	-	1 (25)	-	-	-	-	-	-
Raw chicken (4)	1 (25)	1 (25)	-	1 (25)	-	-	-	-	1 (25)	-
Cooked meat (3)	1 (33.33)	1 (33.33)	-	-	-	1 (33.33)	-	-	-	-
Cooked chicken (1)	-	1 (100)	-	-	-	-	-	-	-	-
Cooked fish (1)	-	1 (100)	-	-	-	-	-	-	-	-
Soup (3)	1 (33.33)	1 (33.33)	-	-	-	-	-	-	1 (33.33)	-
Total (16)	4 (25)	7 (43.75)	-	2 (12.50)	-	1 (6.25)	-	-	2 (12.50)	-

foods in hospitals. At third, presence of nurses and servants, which maybe the sources of dangerous pathogenic agents, in the distribution of food to patients. Prevalence of *E. coli* in raw and cooked fish samples were 1.42% and 2.72%, respectively. Presence of powerful competitor microflora in raw fish and also their destruction and addition of *E. coli* strains derived from contaminated staffs of the hospital's kitchen are two main reasons for above findings. Because the large numbers of *E. coli* isolates recovered from raw meat, proper preparation of the raw meat can eliminate the distribution of bacteria. Unfortunately, basic principles of meat inspections were not observed in Iranian slaughterhouses. Therefore, close contact of animal carcasses with each other and even slaughterhouse floor, blood, content of the digestive tract and wool and skin of slaughtered animal caused transmission and distribution of pathogenic agents like *E. coli* to meat of slaughtered animals. Besides, the role of possible colonizers such as meat inspectors, butchers and miscellaneous people which mainly have come into the slaughterhouse for buying of meat and finally animals like rats, cats and birds which have been entered from outside the slaughterhouse as a sources of pathogenic *E. coli* should not be overlooked. Survival of STEC strains of raw food samples even after cooking procedure and occurrence of cross contamination after cooking procedure are two important routes of hospital foods contamination.

We found marked seasonality in distribution of *E. coli* strains in hospital food samples. High incidence of *E. coli* strains in summer season (64.10%) could be related to the low levels of individual hygiene in this season. The higher prevalence of STEC strains may be related to higher growth of them in hot seasons of the year. Of studies that have been conducted in this field [24–26], all have shown a seasonal distribution for *E. coli* with a higher prevalence of strains in warmer months of the year [24–26].

The results of the current study showed that resistant and virulence STEC strains had the high prevalence in the hospital food samples. Limit studies have been conducted in this field. Ifeadike et al., [27] revealed that the prevalence of *E. coli* strains in food handlers of Nigerian hospitals were 1.8% which was lower than our findings in hospital foods. They concluded that poor and faulty food-handling practices have been identified as the leading cause of the majority of food-borne disease in hospitals. Ha et al., [7] in a research which was conducted in order to study the contamination rate of raw foods in schools, factories, and hospitals of Vietnam reported that the prevalence of *E. coli* in raw poultry, meat, fish and vegetable samples were 45, 21.3, 6.6 and 18.5%, respectively which all were higher than our results.

STEC strains of our investigation harbored resistance against multiple antibiotics. The results of disk diffusion

Table 5 Total distribution of antibiotic resistance genes in the Shiga toxigenic Escherichia coli strains isolated from various types of hospital food samples

Samples (No. STEC strains)	Distribution of antibiotic resistance genes (%)										
	aadA1	tetA	tetB	dfrA1	qnr	aac (3)-IV	sul1	blaSHV	CITM	cat1	cmlA
Raw meat (4)	1 (25)	1 (25)	-	1 (25)	1 (25)	4 (100)	2 (50)	1 (25)	4 (100)	1 (25)	-
Raw chicken (4)	2 (50)	2 (50)	1 (25)	2 (50)	1 (25)	4 (100)	4 (100)	2 (50)	4 (100)	3 (75)	2 (50)
Cooked meat (3)	1 (33.33)	3 (100)	2 (66.66)	2 (66.66)	2 (66.66)	3 (100)	1 (33.33)	1 (33.33)	3 (100)	-	-
Cooked chicken (1)	-	1 (100)	1 (100)	1 (100)	1 (100)	1 (100)	1 (100)	-	1 (100)	-	-
Cooked fish (1)	-	1 (100)	-	1 (100)	-	1 (100)	-	-	1 (100)	-	-
Soup (3)	1 (33.33)	2 (66.66)	1 (33.33)	2 (66.66)	1 (33.33)	3 (100)	1 (33.33)	1 (33.33)	3 (100)	-	-
Total (16)	5 (31.25)	10 (62.50)	5 (31.25)	9 (56.25)	6 (37.50)	16 (100)	9 (56.25)	5 (31.25)	16 (100)	4 (25)	2 (12.50)

Table 6 Antibiotic resistance pattern of Shiga toxigenic *Escherichia coli* strains isolated from various types of hospital food samples

Antibiotic resistance	Samples (No. STEC strains)						
	Raw meat (4)	Raw chicken (4)	Cooked meat (3)	Cooked chicken (1)	Cooked fish (1)	Soup (3)	Total (16)
Tetracycline	4 (100)	4 (100)	2 (66.66)	1 (100)	1 (100)	2 (66.66)	14 (87.50)
Ampicillin	4 (100)	4 (100)	3 (100)	1 (100)	1 (100)	2 (66.66)	15 (93.75)
Gentamycin	4 (100)	4 (100)	2 (66.66)	1 (100)	1 (100)	3 (100)	15 (93.75)
Amikacin	2 (50)	3 (75)	2 (66.66)	1 (100)	1 (100)	3 (100)	12 (75)
Imipenem	-	-	-	1 (100)	-	1 (33.33)	2 (12.5)
Meropenem	-	-	-	-	-	1 (33.33)	1 (6.25)
Mezlocillin	-	-	1 (33.33)	1 (100)	1 (100)	1 (33.33)	4 (25)
Sulfamethoxazole	1 (25)	3 (75)	1 (33.33)	1 (100)	1 (100)	2 (66.66)	9 (56.25)
Cefotaxime	-	-	-	1 (100)	-	2 (66.66)	3 (18.75)
Ciprofloxacin	2 (50)	3 (75)	3 (100)	1 (100)	1 (100)	3 (100)	13 (81.25)
Enrofloxacin	2 (50)	4 (100)	-	-	-	1 (33.33)	7 (43.75)
Cotrimoxazole	-	-	2 (66.66)	1 (100)	1 (100)	2 (66.66)	6 (37.50)
Ceftazidime	-	-	1 (33.33)	1 (100)	1 (100)	2 (66.66)	5 (31.25)
Trimethoprim	1 (25)	2 (50)	2 (66.66)	1 (100)	1 (100)	1 (33.33)	8 (50)
Cefipime	-	-	2 (66.66)	1 (100)	1 (100)	2 (66.66)	6 (37.50)
Levofloxacillin	-	-	2 (66.66)	1 (100)	1 (100)	3 (100)	7 (43.75)
Streptomycin	1 (25)	2 (50)	-	-	-	-	3 (18.75)
Vancomycine	-	-	1 (33.33)	1 (100)	1 (100)	2 (66.66)	5 (31.25)
Polymyxin B	-	-	1 (33.33)	1 (100)	1 (100)	1 (33.33)	4 (25)
Chloramphenicol	1 (25)	2 (50)	-	-	-	-	3 (18.75)

method obtained from STEC strains of our investigation were also confirmed by the presence of specific antibiotic resistance genes encode resistance against determined antibiotics. Stewardson et al., [5] reported that 92% of all food samples which were collected from hospitals in Switzerland were positive for Extended-Spectrum-Beta-lactamase-producing-Enterobacteriaceae (ESBL-PE). ESBL-producing *E. coli* was the most commonly detected (44.77%). They showed 6.45% of eligible food handlers were positive for ESBL-PE and prevalence of *E. coli* strains among ESBL-PE strains were 83.33%. ESBL-PE strains were generally not multidrug resistant, with 100, 90, 87, 79, and 98% of strains susceptible to meropenem, gentamicin, ciprofloxacin, cotrimoxazole, and fosfomycin, respectively. Antibiotic resistance-based finding of Stewardson et al., [5] study was in contrast with our results which showed the high prevalence of resistance and also antibiotic resistance genes. This part of our study was similar

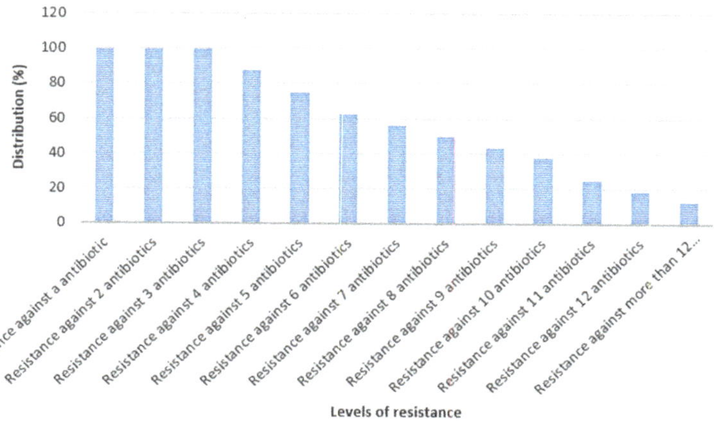

Fig. 2 Prevalence of multi-drug resistant strains of Shiga toxigenic *Escherichia coli* isolated from hospital food samples

with those of India [28] (high prevalence of resistance against erythromycin, cephalothin, amikacin, kanamycin and gentamicin antibiotics), South Africa [29] (high presence of *CITM*, *blaSHV* and *tetA* antibiotic resistance genes), Korea [30] (high prevalence of resistance against ampicillin, tetracycline, streptomycin and amikacin antibiotics) and Mexico [31] (high presence of *tet*, *blaSHV*, *qnr* and *aac (3)-IV* antibiotic resistance genes and also high prevalence of resistance against ampicillin, trimethoprim-sulfamethoxazole, chloramphenicol and cephalotine antibiotics). Momtaz et al., [20] reported that *aac (3)-IV* (68.03%), *sul1* (82.78%), *blaSHV* (56.55%), *aadA1* (60.65%) and *tetA* (51.63%) and also resistance against tetracycline (86.88%), penicillin (100%), gentamycin (62.29%) and streptomycin (54.91%) were the most commonly reported antibiotic resistance-based finding of STEC strains of diarrheic patients which was similar to our results.

STEC strains of hospital food samples and especially cooked samples harbored the high levels of resistance against human-based antibiotics such as meropenem, levofloxacillin, mezlocillin, cefipime, polymyxin B, cefotaxime, ciprofloxacin, cotrimoxazole, ceftazidime and imipenem which can indirectly confirm their anthropogenic origin of these strains. The prevalence of antibiotic resistance genes and especially those that were encode resistance against human-based antibiotics were also high among STEC strains recovered from cooked hospital food samples which also can indirectly approved the transmission of anthropogenic STEC strains probably from staffs of hospital kitchens to foods after cooking process. Prevalence of resistance against chloramphenicol antibiotic in the STEC strains of meat and chicken samples of our investigation were 25 and 50%, respectively. There were no positive results in other raw and also all of the cooked food samples. The Iranian Food and Drug Administration (FDA) listed chloramphenicol as a forbidden antibiotic for treatment of diseases of animals and poultries. It is because of prescription of this antibiotic may cause dangerous effects on animals and even humans who use from their edible sources like meat and milk. The presence of high chloramphenicol resistance showed its irregular and unauthorized use in veterinary treatment and especially field of poultry in Iran. Veterinary practitioners of the field of poultry use from this antibiotic as a primary choice for treatment of diseases. Therefore, in a very short period of time, antibiotic resistance appears. Similar results have been reported by Momtaz and Jamshidi [32], Ranjbar et al., [33] and Colello et al., [34]. Momtaz and Jamshidi [32] reported that 73.17% of STEC strains recovered from poultry meat samples were resistant against chloramphenicol which was higher than our findings. Ranjbar et al., [33] found that the prevalence of resistance against chloramphenicol in the STEC strains recovered from various types of food samples were 21.95% which was considerable. Colello et al. [34] showed that majority of STEC strains in the Argentina harboured the gene that encodes resistance against chloramphenicol.

The most commonly detected serogroups in the STEC strains of hospital food samples of our study were O26 and O157. Presence of O157 serogroup showed that some of our strains had animal-based origin. O157 serogroup is predominant in foods with animal origin. STEC strains of raw foods with animal origins like those of meat and chicken were remained even after cooking of foods. Presence of this serogroup. High prevalence of O157 and O26 serogroups have been reported previously from Iran (Hemmatinezhad et al., [35]), Nigeria (Mamza et al., [36]), Canada (Neher et al., [37]) and Turkey (Avaz et al., [38]). Dehkordi et al., [11] reported similar profile for distribution of STEC O-serogroups. They showed that total prevalence of O157, O145, O128, O121, O113, O111, O103, O91, O45 and O26 serogroups in the STEC strains of food stuffs were 26, 6, 8, 4, 6, 6, 6, 4, 4 and 12%, respectively, which was similar to our findings.

Another part of our investigation focused on the distribution of *stx1*, *stx2*, *eaeA* and *ehly* virulence factors in the *E. coli* strains of hospital foods. High presence of these factors in EHEC and AEEC subtypes showed their high pathogenicity for human and especially patients. Simultaneous presence of *stx1* and *eaeA* and *stx2* and *eaeA* virulence factors in some strains of *E. coli* of hospital foods indicated the important public health problem facing Iranian hospitals and health centers which can attributed to occurrence of dangerous food poisoning and STEC-based food-borne diseases in hospitals. Simultaneous presence of *stx1* and *eaeA* and *stx2* and *eaeA* virulence factors have been reported previously [39–41]. In a study which was conducted by Momtaz et al., [42] the prevalence of EHEC and AEEC subtypes in *E. coli* strains of food samples were 15.06 and 49.31%, respectively. They showed that all of the EHEC strains were positive for all stx*1*, *eaeA* and *ehly* virulence genes, while the prevalence of these genes in AEEC subtypes were 77.77, 13.88 and 55.55%, respectively. Higher prevalence of AEEC subtypes was also reported by various investigations [9–11, 20, 32, 33]. Prevalence of AEEC subtypes in the studies of Momtaz et al., [9] and Dehkordi et al., [11] were 79.41 and 62%, respectively which were higher than EHEC subtype in both studies. Momtaz et al., [10] reported that the prevalence of AEEC subtypes in the *E. coli* strains recovered from the meat samples of beef, sheep, goat and camel species were 45.54, 44.87, 39.02 and 50.00%, respectively which were higher than those of EHEC. Momtaz et al., [20] reported that the prevalence of AEEC subtypes among the *E. coli* strains of Iranian diarrheic patients had a range of 47 to 75% which was entirely high.

Conclusions

In conclusions, we identified a large number of O-serogroups, virulence factors, antibiotic resistance genes and pattern of antibiotic resistance in STEC strains recovered from hospital foods. Raw meat, raw chicken and cooked meat, summer season, *stx1* and *eaeA* virulence factors, AEEC subtype, O26 and O157 serogroups, *aac (3)-IV, CITM, tetA, dfrA1*) and *sul1* antibiotic resistance genes, resistance against ampicillin, gentamycin, tetracycline, ciprofloxacin and amikacin and presence of multi-drug resistant strains were the most commonly detected characters in the STEC strains of hospital foods. Presence of O157 serogroups, EHEC strains, animal-based antibiotics and even antibiotic resistance genes which encode resistance against animal-based antibiotics in cooked foods showed insufficiency of cooking time and temperature in the kitchens of hospitals. It seems that there were no strict supervisions on the principles of food hygiene in Iranian hospitals. Due to the low levels of STEC resistance against imipenem, meropenem, streptomycin and cefotaxim antibiotics, occurrence of food poisonings due to the STEC strains in tested Iranian hospitals can be treated with their regular prescription. Attentions to the results of disk diffusion method and principles of hazard analysis and critical control point (HACCP) system can reduce the risk of STEC strains in hospital food stuffs.

Abbreviations

AEEC: Attaching and effacing E. coli; E. coli: Escherichia coli; Eae: Intimin; EHEC: Enterohemolysin or Enterohaemorrhagic Escherichia coli; Ehly: Hemolysin; HC: Hemorrhagic Colitis; HUS: Hemolytic Uremic Syndrome; PCR: Polymerase Chain Reaction; SPSS: Statistical Package for the Social Sciences; STEC: Shiga toxin producing Escherichia coli; Stx: Shiga toxin

Acknowledgements

The authors would like to thank Prof. Hassan Momtaz at the Department of Microbiology, Islamic Azad University of Shahrekord, Shahrekord Iran and Prof. Afshin Akhondzadeh Basti and Prof. Ali Misaghi at the Department of Food Hygiene and Quality Control, University of Tehran, Tehran, Iran for their important technical support.

Funding

This work was supported by the Baqiyatallah University of Medical Sciences, Tehran, Iran (grant no. 94/5050).

Authors' contributions

RR and MM contributed to study design, culture-based identification, disk diffusion and PCR genetic alignments. ER and MM carried out on samples collection, statistical analysis and DNA extraction. NJJ and FSD wrote and drafted the manuscript. All authors road and approved the final manuscript.

Competing interests

The authors declare that they have no competing interests

Consent for publication

There was no consent for publication.

Author details

[1]Molecular Biology Research Center, Baqiyatallah University of Medical Sciences, Tehran, Iran. [2]Doctor Veterinary Medicine, College of Veterinary Medicine, Islamic Azad University, Shahrekord Branch, Shahrekord, Iran. [3]Young Researchers and Elites Club, Shahrekord Branch, Islamic Azad University, Shahrekord, Iran. [4]Health Research Center, Baqiyatallah University of Medical Sciences, Tehran, Iran. [5]Department of Food Hygiene and Public Health, College of Veterinary Medicine, Shahrekord Branch, Shahrekord, Iran.

References

1. Gould LH, Walsh KA, Vieira AR, Herman K, Williams IT, Hall AJ, Cole D. Surveillance for foodborne disease outbreaks—United States, 1998–2008. MMWR Surveill Summ. 2013;62:1–34.
2. Havelaar AH, Kirk MD, Torgerson PR, Gibb HJ, Hald T, Lake RJ, Praet N, Bellinger DC, De Silva NR, Gargouri N. World Health Organization Global estimates and regional comparisons of the burden of foodborne disease in 2010. PLoS Med. 2015;12:e1001923.
3. Control CD. Prevention. Surveillance for Foodborne Disease Outbreaks, United States, 2013, Annual Report. Atlanta: US Department of Health and Human Services; 2014.
4. Scallan E, Hoekstra RM, Angulo FJ, Tauxe RV, Widdowson M-A, Roy SL, Jones JL, Griffin PM. Foodborne illness acquired in the United States—major pathogens. Emerg Infect Dis. 2011;17:7–15.
5. Stewardson AJ, Renzi G, Maury N, Vaudaux C, Brassier C, Fritsch E, Pittet D, Heck M, van der Zwaluw K, Reuland EA. Extended-Spectrum β-Lactamase–Producing Enterobacteriaceae in Hospital Food: A Risk Assessment. Infect Control Hosp Epidemiol. 2014;35:375–83.
6. Luo Y, Cui S, Li J, Yang J, Lin L, Hu C, Jin S, Ye L, Zhao Q, Ma Y. Characterization of Escherichia coli isolates from healthy food handlers in hospital. Microb Drug Resist. 2011;17:443–8.
7. Anvarinejad M, Farshad SH, Ranjbar R, Giammanco GM, Alborzi A, Japoni A. Genotypic analysis of E. coli strains isolated from patients with cystitis and pyelonephritis. Iran Red Crescent Med J. 2012;14:408–16.
8. Cooke EM, Kumar P, Shooter R, Rousseau S, Foulkes A. Hospital food as a possible source of Escherichia coli in patients. Lancet. 1970;295:436–7.
9. Momtaz H, Farzan R, Rahimi E, Safarpoor Dehkordi F, Souod N. Molecular characterization of Shiga toxin-producing Escherichia coli isolated from ruminant and donkey raw milk samples and traditional dairy products in Iran. Sci World J. 2012;2012:231342.
10. Momtaz H, Dehkordi FS, Rahimi E, Ezadi H, Arab R. Incidence of Shiga toxin-producing Escherichia coli serogroups in ruminant's meat. Meat Sci. 2013;95:381–8.
11. Dehkordi FS, Yazdani F, Mozafari J, Valizadeh Y. Virulence factors, serogroups and antimicrobial resistance properties of Escherichia coli strains in fermented dairy products. BMC Res Notes. 2014;7:1.
12. Tajbakhsh E, Khamesipour F, Ranjbar R, Ugwu IC. Prevalence of class 1 and 2 integrons in multi-drug resistant Escherichia coli isolated from aquaculture water in Chaharmahal Va Bakhtiari province, Iran. Ann Clin Microbiol Antimicrob. 2015;14:37.
13. Ranjbar R, Karami A, Farshad S, Giammanco GM, Mammina C. Typing methods used in the molecular epidemiology of microbial pathogens: a how-to guide. New Microbiol. 2014;37:1–15.
14. Wang J, Stanford K, McAllister TA, Johnson RP, Chen J, Hou H, Zhang G, Niu YD. Biofilm Formation, Virulence Gene Profiles, and Antimicrobial Resistance of Nine Serogroups of Non-O157 Shiga Toxin–Producing Escherichia coli. Foodborne Pathog Dis. 2016;13:316–24.
15. Farshad S, Ranijbar R, Japoni A, Hosseini M, Anvarinejad M, Mohammadzadegan R. Microbial susceptibility, virulence factors, and plasmid profiles of uropathogenic Escherichia coli strains isolated from children in Jahrom, Iran. Arch Iran Med. 2012;15:312–6.
16. Ranjbar, R, Haghi-Ashtiani, MT, Jafari, NJ, Abedini, M. The prevalence and antimicrobial susceptibility of bacterial uropathogens isolated from pediatric patients. Iran J Publ Health. 2009;38:134–138.
17. Abdi S, Ranjbar R, Vala MH, Jonaidi N, Bejestany OB, Bejestany FB. Frequency of bla TEM, bla SHV, bla CTX-M, and qnrA Among Escherichia coli Isolated From Urinary Tract Infection. Arch Clin Infect Dis. 2014;9:e18690.
18. Momtaz H, Karimian A, Madani M, Dehkordi FS, Ranjbar R, Sarshar M, Souod N. Uropathogenic Escherichia coli in Iran: serogroup distributions, virulence factors and antimicrobial resistance properties. Ann Clin Microbiol Antimicrob. 2013;12:1.

19. Woo PC, Cheung EY, K-w L, K-y Y. Identification by 16S ribosomal RNA gene sequencing of an Enterobacteriaceae species with ambiguous biochemical profile from a renal transplant recipient. Diagn Microbiol Infect Dis. 2001;39:85–93.
20. Momtaz H, Dehkordi FS, Hosseini MJ, Sarshar M, Heidari M. Serogroups, virulence genes and antibiotic resistance in Shiga toxin-producing Escherichia coli isolated from diarrheic and non-diarrheic pediatric patients in Iran. Gut Pathog. 2013;5:1.
21. Wayne P. Clinical and Laboratory Standards Institute (CLSI). Performance standards for antimicrobial susceptibility testing. Twenty-second informational supplement M100-S21. United States, Wayne. 2012.
22. Hidron AI, Edwards JR, Patel J, Horan TC, Sievert DM, Pollock DA, Fridkin SK. Antimicrobial-resistant pathogens associated with healthcare-associated infections: annual summary of data reported to the National Healthcare Safety Network at the Centers for Disease Control and Prevention, 2006–2007. Infect Control Hosp Epidemiol. 2008;29:996–1011.
23. Peleg AY, Hooper DC. Hospital-acquired infections due to gram-negative bacteria. N Engl J Med. 2010;362:1804–13.
24. Alam M, Zurek L. Seasonal prevalence of Escherichia coli O157: H7 in beef cattle feces. J Food Prot. 2006;69:3018–20.
25. Barkocy-Gallagher GA, Arthur TM, Rivera-Betancourt M, Nou X, Shackelford SD, Wheeler TL, Koohmaraie M. Seasonal prevalence of Shiga toxin-producing Escherichia coli, including O157: H7 and non-O157 serotypes, and Salmonella in commercial beef processing plants. J Food Prot. 2003;66:1978–86.
26. Williams MS, Withee JL, Ebel ED, Bauer Jr NE, Schlosser WD, Disney WT, Smith DR, Moxley RA. Determining relationships between the seasonal occurrence of Escherichia coli O157: H7 in live cattle, ground beef, and humans. Foodborne Pathog Dis. 2010;7:1247–54.
27. Ifeadike C, Ironkwe O, Adogu P, Nnebue C, Emelumadu O, Nwabueze S, Ubajaka C. Prevalence and pattern of bacteria and intestinal parasites among food handlers in the Federal Capital Territory of Nigeria. Niger Med J. 2012;53:166–71.
28. Mahanti A, Samanta I, Bandopaddhay S, Joardar SN, Dutta TK, Batabyal S, Sar TK, Isore DP. Isolation, molecular characterization and antibiotic resistance of Shiga Toxin-Producing Escherichia coli (STEC) from buffalo in India. Lett Appl Microbiol. 2013;56:291–8.
29. Iweriebor BC, Iwu CJ, Obi LC, Nwodo UU, Okoh AI. Multiple antibiotic resistances among Shiga toxin producing Escherichia coli O157 in feces of dairy cattle farms in Eastern Cape of South Africa. BMC Microbiol. 2015;15:213.
30. Kang E, Hwang SY, Kwon KH, Kim KY, Kim JH, Park YH. Prevalence and characteristics of Shiga toxin-producing Escherichia coli (STEC) from cattle in Korea between 2010 and 2011. J Vet Sci. 2014;15:369–79.
31. Castillo FYR, González FJA, Garneau P, Díaz FM, Barrera ALG, Harel J. Presence of multi-drug resistant pathogenic Escherichia coli in the San Pedro River located in the State of Aguascalientes, Mexico. Front Microbiol. 2013;4:147.
32. Momtaz H, Jamshidi A. Shiga toxin-producing Escherichia coli isolated from chicken meat in Iran: Serogroups, virulence factors, and antimicrobial resistance properties. Poult Sci. 2013;92:1305–13.
33. Ranjbar R, Sheikhshahrokh A, Jonaidi Jafari N. Shiga (vero) toxin producing *Escherichia coli* in various types of food stuffs; virulence factors, O-serogroups and antimicrobial resistance properties. J food Safety. 2016;1–12.
34. Colello R, Etcheverría AI, Conza JAD, Gutkind GO, Padola NL. Antibiotic resistance and integrons in Shiga toxin-producing Escherichia coli (STEC). Braz J Microbiol. 2015;46:1–5.
35. Hemmatinezhad B, Khamesipour F, Mohammadi M, Safarpoor Dehkordi F, Mashak Z. Microbiological Investigation of O-Serogroups, Virulence Factors and Antimicrobial Resistance Properties of Shiga Toxin-Producing Escherichia Coli Isolated from Ostrich, Turkey and Quail Meats. J Food Saf. 2015;35:491–500.
36. Mamza SA, Egwu GO, Mshelia GD. Antibiotic susceptibility patterns of beta-lactamase-producing Escherichia coli and Staphylococcus aureus isolated from chickens in Maiduguri (Arid zone), Nigeria. Vet Arhiv. 2010;80:283–97.
37. Neher S, Hazarika A, Barkalita L, Borah P, Bora D, Sharma R. Isolation and characterization of Shiga toxigenic Escherichia coli of animal and bird origin by multiplex polymerase chain reaction. Vet World. 2016;9:123.
38. Ayaz ND, Copuroglu G, Ormeci E, Oz B. Presence of Staphylococcus aureus and Shiga Toxigenic Escherichia coli O157: H7 in Raw Meat in Ağrı Turkey. Int J Enteric Pathog. 2016;4:e36523.
39. Franz E, Klerks MM, De Vos OJ, Termorshuizen AJ, van Bruggen AH. Prevalence of Shiga toxin-producing Escherichia coli stx1, stx2, eaeA, and rfbE genes and survival of E. coli O157: H7 in manure from organic and low-input conventional dairy farms. Appl Environ Microbiol. 2007;73:2180–90.
40. Jay-Russell MT, Hake AF, Bengson Y, Thiptara A, Nguyen T. Prevalence and characterization of Escherichia coli and Salmonella strains isolated from stray dog and coyote feces in a major leafy greens production region at the United States-Mexico border. Plos One. 2014;9:e113433.
41. Kabiru LM, Bello M, Kabir J, Grande L, Morabito S. Detection of pathogenic Escherichia coli in samples collected at an Abattoir in Zaria, Nigeria and at different points in the surrounding environment. Int J Environ Res Public Health. 2015;12:679–91.
42. Momtaz H, Safarpoor Dehkordi F, Taktaz T, Rezvani A, Yarali S. Shiga toxin-producing Escherichia coli isolated from bovine mastitic milk: serogroups, virulence factors, and antibiotic resistance properties. Sci World J. 2012;2012:618709.

2

Prospective surveillance of healthcare-associated infections and patterns of antimicrobial resistance of pathogens in an Italian intensive care unit

Aida Bianco, Maria Simona Capano, Valentina Mascaro, Claudia Pileggi and Maria Pavia*

Abstract

Background: The study aimed to evaluate the distribution of healthcare-associated infections (HAIs), the incidence rates and device utilization ratio (DUR) of device-associated infections (DAIs), as well as the distribution and patterns of antimicrobial resistance of the responsible pathogens.

Methods: Eligible patients who were admitted to an adult Intensive Care Unit (ICU) from May 1, 2013 to December 31, 2016 were included in the surveillance. Demographics, intrinsic and extrinsic risk factors, information regarding infection and isolated pathogens with antibiogram results were collected.

Results: One thousand two hundred eighty-three patients were included in the surveillance. One hundred forty-seven HAIs were detected with a cumulative incidence of 9.2 per 100 patients 4-year period and an incidence rate of 17.4 per 1000 patient days. Fifty-six out of 1283 patients were affected by at least one episode of ICU-acquired pneumonia, and 72.7% of these were associated with intubation. ICU-acquired bloodstream infections (BSIs) occurred in 4.4% of patients and 89.5% were catheter-related. ICU-acquired urinary tract infections (UTIs) occurred in 1% of patients, with 84.6% of the episodes being associated with the use of an urinary catheter. The pattern of antimicrobial-resistance in the isolates showed, among the Gram-positive bacteria, that 66.6% and 16.6% of *Staphylococcus epidermidis* were oxacillin and teicoplanin resistant, respectively. Among the Gram-negative bacteria, carbapenem resistance was found in 91. 6% of *Acinetobacter baumannii* and 28.5% of *Klebsiella pneumoniae* isolates.

Conclusions: The majority of HAIs in the ICU studied were associated with the use of invasive devices. Since a significant proportion of these HAIs are considered preventable, reinforcement of the evidence-based preventive procedures are needed.

Keywords: Healthcare-associated infection, Intensive care unit, Italy, Surveillance

Background

Healthcare-associated infections (HAIs) represent a major threat to patient safety, leading to significant mortality and financial losses for health systems worldwide. In high-income countries, for every 100 hospitalized patients, 7 develop at least one HAI and the frequency of HAIs acquired by patients in intensive care units (ICUs) is at least 3 fold higher (approximately 30%) [1].

* Correspondence: pavia@unicz.it
Department of Health Sciences, University of Catanzaro "Magna Græcia", Via T. Campanella, 115, 88100 Catanzaro, Italy

In Europe it is estimated that 4,131,000 patients are affected by HAI and approximately about 4,544,100 episodes occur each year [2]. HAIs cause 16 million extra days of hospital stay and 37,000 attributable deaths. The burden of HAIs in patients admitted to ICUs vary from 9.7–31.8% in Europe [3].

In Italy, a national network for the prospective surveillance of HAIs in all wards is not in place. Continuous multicenter infection surveillance systems have been adopted in ICUs, and reported cumulative incidence range from 9.1 [4] to 15.5 per 100 patients [5].

Table 1 Incidence of device-associated infections (DAIs) by site, 2013–2016

Year	VAP				CLABSI				CAUTI			
	n.	MVdays	Rate[a]	DUR[b]	*n.*	CLdays	Rate[a]	DUR[b]	*n.*	UCdays	Rate[a]	DUR[b]
2013	12	502	23.9	0.32	14	1241	11.2	0.81	0	1224	0[c]	0.80
2014	24	897	26.7	0.34	15	2255	6.6	0.86	2	2258	0.9	0.86
2015	10	915	10.9	0.40	10	1535	6.5	0.67	6	1560	3.8	0.68
2016	10	826	12.1	0.40	12	1528	7.8	0.75	3	1528	1.9	0.75
TOTAL	56	3140	73.6	1.46	51	6559	32.1	3.09	11	6570	6.6	3.09

NOTE. *VAP* ventilator-associated pneumonia, *CLABSI* central line-associated bloodstream infection, *CAUTI* catheter-associated urinary tract infection, *MV* mechanical ventilator , *DUR* device utilization ratio, *CL* central line, *UC* urinary catheter

[a]Device–associated infection rate $= \frac{\text{Number of device–associated infections for an infection site}}{\text{Number of device–days}} \times 1000$

[b]Device utilization ratio (DUR) $= \frac{\text{Number of device–days}}{\text{Number of patient–days}}$

[c]The rate was not calculated since the number of CAUTI in 2013 was 0

In the literature, variable proportions of HAIs, considered to be preventable by intensive hygiene and control programs, have been reported [6, 7]. Among the infection prevention initiatives, surveillance of HAIs is the cornerstone to decrease infection rates in hospitalized patients [8], and it is considered to be the best way to assure patient safety [9]. Continuous monitoring of HAI rates can be used to assess effectiveness of interventions and provides information which may be used for benchmarking comparison [10]. Routine surveillance of HAIs should become an integral part of infection prevention and quality assurance in hospitals [11].

This study reports the results of a 4-year period prospective surveillance in an ICU in an Italian teaching hospital aimed at evaluating: 1) the cumulative incidence and incidence rate of HAIs; 2) the incidence rates of device-associated infections (DAIs); 3) the device utilization ratio (DUR); 4) the distribution of the responsible pathogens; and 5) the patterns of their antimicrobial resistance.

Methods

An HAIs surveillance system based on that of the Centers for Disease Control and Prevention's (CDC) National Healthcare Safety Network (NHSN) [12] was established in 2013 by the Hospital Prevention & Control Group for the prospective surveillance of events and their corresponding denominator data by trained Infection Preventionists in an adult ICU.

Setting and patients

The ICU is an 8-bed unit that is part of a university-affiliated teaching hospital, with two single rooms for isolation. The ICU type was classified according to the NHSN criteria as a medical/surgical unit of a major teaching hospital. It has approximately 382 admissions per year.

All eligible patients admitted from May 1, 2013 to December 31, 2016 have been included in the surveillance. Patients who were transferred to the ICU from an outside hospital are also included. The exclusion criteria were patients with a community acquired infection, ICU stay for less than 48 h and death within 48 h of ICU admission. The follow-up of each patient was continued until discharge, referral, or death.

Data collection

Surveillance data on all ICU-acquired HAIs, both in patients with or without a device, and their causative pathogens were collected prospectively on a specifically designed form (Additional file 1) by the investigators using medical records comprising charts, daily flow sheets, laboratory (eg, complete blood count, serology, microbiology, biochemistry) and radiographic results. The collected data included demographics; intrinsic and extrinsic risk factors for infection; date of infection onset; clinical signs; administered antibiotics; isolated pathogens with antibiogram results; and outcome on discharge from the ICU. The risk factors were evaluated from the time of admission until the onset of HAI. For patients who did not develop HAI, the risk factors were evaluated for their entire ICU stay.

The definitions of HAIs, and DURs are based on those established by the CDC, which are used by the NHSN system [13]. Particular attention is paid to data on DAIs [ventilator-associated pneumonias (VAPs), central line–associated bloodstream infections (CLABSIs), and catheter-associated urinary tract infections (CAUTIs)], and denominator data (patient days and specific device days). An infection is defined as device-associated (i.e., mechanical ventilator (MV), urinary catheter (UC), or central line-associated (CL)) if the corresponding device was in place on the date of infection and within two calendar days prior. Surgical site infections were not monitored because we performed a ward-based surveillance, rather than a procedure-based surveillance.

Global prevalence of the pathogens causing DAIs and antimicrobial resistance rates are also calculated.

Multidrug-resistance (MDR) is defined in accordance with current published interim standard definitions, which are used in the most recent NHSN antimicrobial resistance report [14].

Statistical analysis

Rates and ratios are calculated according to standard methods [12]. Briefly, DUR are calculated as the total number of MV, CL, or UC days, divided by the total number of patient days. The infection frequency is calculated as the number of infections per 100 ICU eligible patients (cumulative incidence) and the number of infections per 1000 patient-days (incidence rate). Rates for DAIs are reported as the number of infections per 1000 device days.

The first part of the analysis examines the entire cohort of patients. Data are summarized using the mean and standard deviation (SD) for continuous variables and frequency and percentage for discrete and nominal variables. Univariate analysis was tentatively used to compare variables for the outcome groups of interest (HAIs versus no HAIs), and all tests of significance were two tailed. The T test was used for comparing continuous variables, while the χ^2-statistic or Fisher-exact test was used for discrete and nominal variables. All statistical analyses were performed using the Stata software program, version 14 (Stata).

Results

During the 4 year study period, 1283 patients were included in the surveillance. The population mean age was 66 (±12) years and 841 (66%) were males. Overall, 147 ICU-acquired HAIs were detected with a cumulative incidence of 9.2 per 100 patients 4-year period and an incidence rate of 17.4 per 1000 patient days. A total of 118 DAIs were found, of which 38.1% were VAPs, 34.7% CLABSIs and 7.5% CAUTIs.

In the population, 56 out of 1283 patients (6%) were affected by at least one episode of ICU-acquired pneumonia, and 72.7% of these were VAPs. The incidence rate of ICU-acquired pneumonia was 9 episodes per 1000 patient-days and VAP incidence rate was 17.8 per 1000 MV days (> 90th percentile).

On average, ICU-acquired BSIs occurred in 4.4% of patients staying in an ICU for more than 2 days. The incidence rate was 6.8 BSI episodes per 1000 patient-days. 89.5% of cases were CLABSIs with an incidence rate of 7.7 per 1000CL days (> 90thpercentile).

On average, ICU-acquired urinary tract infections (UTIs) occurred in 1% of patients staying in an ICU for more than 2 days, with 84.6% of UTI episodes being associated with the use of a UC The incidence rate per ICU was 1.5 UTI episodes per 1000 patient-days and a mean device-adjusted rate of 1.6 CAUTI episodes per 1000 UC -days (25th- 50th percentile).

The trend during the surveillance period showed that the rate of VAP considerably decreased from 23.9 in 2013 to 12.1 in 2016 per 1000 MV days; CLABSI reduced from 11.2 in 2013 to 7.8 in 2016 per 1000 CL days. The incidence rate of CAUTI had been constantly contained during the surveillance period, ranging from 0 in 2013 to 3.8 in 2015, while in 2016 it was found to be 1.9 per 1000 UC days (Table 1).

Among Gram-negative bacteria, the most common isolated pathogens were *Klebsiella pneumoniae* (17.8%), *Acinetobacter baumannii* (10.2%), *Escherichia coli* (8. 5%), *Pseudomonas aeruginosa* (5%); among Gram-positive bacteria *Staphylococcus epidermidis* (10%) was the most common. All yeasts found were classified as *Candida species.* Throughout the surveillance period, *Klebsiella pneumoniae* was the most frequent pathogen associated with VAPs (n = 12) followed by *Acinetobacter baumannii* (n = 6), *Escherichia coli* (n = 6) and *Pseudomonas aeruginosa* (n = 6). Thirteen VAP episodes were non-microbiologically confirmed. The most frequently isolated microorganisms in ICU-acquired CLABSI episodes were coagulase-negative staphylococci (n = 21) and of these 11 were *Staphylococcus epidermidis*; among Gram-negative bacteria *Klebsiella pneumoniae* (n = 7) and *Acinetobacter baumannii* (n = 5) were the most frequent isolates. *Candida species* (45.4%) and *Klebsiella pneumoniae* (18.1%) were the most frequently isolated microorganisms in CAUTI episodes.

The antimicrobial-resistance in the isolates associated with ICU-acquired DAIs showed, among the Gram-positive bacteria, that 66.6% and 16.6% of *Staphylococcus epidermidis* isolates were β-lactam (oxacillin) - and glycopeptide (teicoplanin) - resistant, respectively. Among the Gram-negative bacteria third-generation cephalosporins (cefotaxime or ceftazidime) resistance was found in 52.3% of *Klebsiella pneumoniae* and 30% of *Escherichia coli* isolates; and carbapenem (imipenem, meropenem, ertapenem) resistance in 91.6% of *Acinetobacter baumannii* and 28.5% of *Klebsiella pneumoniae* isolates. MDR phenotypes were reported in all *Pseudomonas aeruginosa,* in *Acinetobacter baumannii* (91.6%), *Escherichia coli* (40%) and *Klebsiella pneumoniae* (52.3%) isolates. Resistance to colistin, an antibiotic from the polymyxin group, was observed in 4% of the *Klebsiella pneumoniae* isolates.

Results of univariate analysis showed that no statistically significant difference between infection and the independent covariates was found (data not shown).

Discussion

The cumulative incidence of HAIs in ICU wards varies widely among countries (5%–38.9%) [15], and the detected rate in the present surveillance (9.2%) was in the range of values specified in other studies. Data reported by The European Surveillance System showed that, in 2014, 8% of the patients staying in the ICU for more than 2 days presented at least one HAI [16]. The HAI incidence rate of 17.4 per 1000 patient days was slightly higher than that noticed in the study from the USA where the rate of HAI in an adult ICU was shown to be 16.2 per 1000 patient days[17]. The majority of HAIs in ICUs are associated with the use of invasive devices. Therefore, our surveillance system paid particular attention to DAIs, since a significant proportion of these HAIs are considered preventable. The findings showed that the most common DAI was VAP (47.5%), consistent with the reported literature. Globally, the VAP rate we observed (17.8/1000 MV days) was higher than the surveillance data from Germany (5.4/1000 MV days) [18] and from the United States where the VAP incidence rate was 2.1 per 1000 device days in medical/surgical major teaching ICUs [19]. A more pertinent benchmarking information could be obtained on a national scale. The cumulative incidence of the ICU-acquired HAIs (9.2%) is very similar to that reported in a continuous multicenter infection surveillance program (9.1%) involving 125 Italian ICUs promoted by the Italian Group for the Evaluation of Interventions in Intensive Care Medicine [4]. Similarly, VAP was the most frequently diagnosed, but the incidence rate was lower than that reported in the present surveillance program (8.9/1000 vs 17.8/1000 MV days) [4]. However, the Italian Nosocomial Infections Surveillance in ICUs network, SPIN-UTI, reported surveillance data from a 6-year period (2006–2011), with a third survey showing a more similar VAP incidence rate (17.3 per 1000 MV days) [20], while the VAP incidence rate was higher in a surveillance program organized in an Italian single-centre 12-bed ICU (23.14/1000 MV days) [21].

The CLABSI incidence rate (7.7 per 1000 CL days) we observed was much lower than that reported from limited-resource countries [22, 23], but higher than 1.1 per 1000 CL days reported in the medical/surgical major teaching ICUs in the healthcare facilities adhering to NHSN surveillance [19]. In the SPIN-UTI, in the 2010–2011 survey, and in the GiViTi projects the CLABSI incidence rate was 1.8 and 1.9 per 1000 CVC days, respectively [20, 4]. The higher rate in the present surveillance could be explained by a high CL utilization ratio, exceeding the 90th percentile of the NHSN distribution for medical/surgical major teaching ICUs. Intravascular devices remain an essential component of ICU care, but many studies recognize CL duration as a risk factor for CLABSI [24, 25].

The reasons for lower CAUTI rates observed in the present study compared with other studies may be related to the effectiveness of the interventions implemented in our setting. They included educational strategies, UC avoidance, policies for UC insertion, daily necessity review and limiting catheter days that have been proven to decrease CAUTI events [26].

In the present study Gram-negative bacteria were the most common causal pathogens, in agreement with several surveillance studies in the United States [27], Europe [28], Saudi Arabia [29] and Brazil [30]. Among these Gram-negative bacteria, *Klebsiella pneumoniae* (17.8%) and *Acinetobacter baumannii* (10.2%) were the most frequently reported. This finding is of particular concern, since these organisms are often involved in outbreaks that require the activation of an organizational response until the outbreak is under control [31].

In the present study, the high level of resistance to multiple antibiotics is of great concern, especially since resistance to colistin was also reported. This condition represents an indication of seriously limited options for the treatment of patients infected with those microorganisms.

A variability in DAI rates across the surveillance period can be observed. Part of this variability can be attributed to the small number of episodes, and characteristics of the patient population, such as clinical severity and infection control practices that had been reinforced during surveillance. Over the 4 year study several infection control practices, such as the active surveillance cultures to detect asymptomatic colonization and preemptive contact isolation of patients were implemented.

The strengths of the study lie in the prospective nature, and application of NHSN methodology. It is well known that indicators of HAIs provided by surveillance activities require comparison with adequate reference data to stimulate further infection control actions and to enhance quality of care [32]. The NHSN methodology has proven to be adaptable in our context and useful as benchmark.

This study had a couple of limitations. An HAI incidence study should preferably be performed on large cohorts, taken from a national ICU sample. The consequence of a small population size is the low probability of detecting an important effect, since the analysis is underpowered. For this reason, we did not show the results of the univariate analysis. The present surveillance was conducted in one adult ICU in Southern Italy, and the results cannot be generalized to all public Italian hospital settings. It is reasonable to suppose that an analogous context may be referred to the Southern part of our country.

Conclusion

Given the limitations cited above, the authors believe that to have more insight into HAI indicators as measured by a surveillance system, it is crucial to estimate the burden of HAIs and to compare the performance to that of other contexts, as well as to evaluate new preventive procedures.

Acknowledgements
Not applicable

Funding
No external funding for this manuscript.

Authors' contributions
AB made substantial contributions to the conception and design of the study, to analysis and interpretation of the data and wrote the paper. MSC, VM and CP collected the data, contributed to analysis of the data and drafting of the paper. MP made substantial contributions in the design of the study, was responsible for analysis of the data and revising the paper critically for important intellectual content. All authors approved the final paper as submitted, and agree to be accountable for all aspects of the work in ensuring that questions related to the accuracy or integrity of any part of the work are appropriately investigated and resolved. AB and MP are guarantors for the study.

Consent for publication
Not applicable

Competing interests
The authors declare that they have no competing interests.

References

1. World Health Organization. Healthcare-associated infections: fact sheet; 2014. Available at http://www.who.int/gpsc/country_work/gpsc_ccisc_fact_sheet_en.pdf. Accessed 4 May 2017.
2. World Health Organization. The Burden of Health Care-Associated Infection Worldwide. A Summary; 2010. Available at http://www.who.int/gpsc/country_work/summary_20100430_en.pdf. Accessed 10 Feb 2017.
3. Vincent JL, Bihari DJ, Suter PM, Bruining HA, White J, Nicolas-Chanoin MH, et al. The prevalence of nosocomial infection in intensive care units in Europe. Results of the European prevalence of infection in intensive care (EPIC) study. EPIC international advisory committee. JAMA. 1995;274:639–44.
4. Malacarne P, Boccalatte D, Acquarolo A, Agostini F, Anghileri A, Giardino M, et al. Epidemiology of nosocomial infection in 125 Italian intensive care units. Minerva Anestesiol. 2010;76:13–23.
5. Masia MD, Barchitta M, Liperi G, Cantu AP, Alliata E. Validation of intensive care unit-acquired infection surveillance in the Italian SPIN-UTI network. J Hosp Infect. 2010;76:139–42.
6. Brown J, Doloresco FIII, Mylotte JM. "Never events": not every hospital-acquired infection is preventable. Clin Infect Dis. 2009;49:743–6.
7. Harbarth S, Sax H, Gastmeier P. The preventable proportion of nosocomial infections: an overview of published reports. J Hosp Infect. 2003;54:258–66.
8. O'Neill E, Humphreys H. Use of surveillance data for prevention of healthcare-associated infection: risk adjustment and reporting dilemmas. Curr Opin Infect Dis. 2009;22:359–63.
9. Van Bunnik BA, Ciccolini M, Gibbons CL, Edwards G, Fitzgerald R, McAdam PR, et al. Efficient national surveillance for health-care-associated infections. BMC Public Health. 2015;15:832.
10. Mitchell BG, Russo PL. Preventing healthcare-associated infections: the role of surveillance. Nurs Stand. 2015:2952–8.
11. Gastmeier P, Geffers C, Brandt C, Zuschneid I, Sohr D, Schwab F, et al. Effectiveness of a nationwide nosocomial infection surveillance system for reducing nosocomial infections. J Hosp Infect. 2006;64:16–22.
12. Dudeck MA, Horan TC, Peterson KD, Allen-Bridson K, Morrell G, Anttila A, et al. National Healthcare Safety Network report, data summary for 2011, device-associated module. Am J Infect Control. 2013;41:286–300.
13. Horan TC, Andrus M, Dudeck MA. CDC/NHSN surveillance definition of health care-associated infection and criteria for specific types of infections in the acute care setting. Am J Infect Control. 2008;36:309–32.
14. Magiorakos AP, Srinivasan A, Carey RB, Carmeli Y, Falagas ME, Giske CG, et al. Multidrug-resistant, extensively drug-resistant and pandrug-resistant bacteria: an international expert proposal for interim standard definitions for acquired resistance. Clin Microbiol Infect. 2012;18:268–81.
15. World Health Organization. Education sessions for trainers, observers and health-care workers. 2009. Available at https://www.ntuh.gov.tw/ifc/hhc/HandHygiene/Education%20Sessions%20for%20Trainers%20and%20Observers%20and%20Health-care%20Workers.pdf Accessed 02 Sept 2017.
16. Center for Disease Control and Prevention. Healthcare-associated infections acquired in intensive care units. 2016. Available at https://ecdc.europa.eu/en/publications-data/healthcare-associated-infections-acquired-intensive-care-units-annual Accessed 28 Sept 2017.
17. Richards MJ, Edwards JR, Culver DH, Gaynes RP. Nosocomial infections in combined medical-surgical intensive care units in the United States. Infect Control Hosp Epidemiol. 2000;21:510–5.
18. Kohlenberg A, Schwab F, Behnke M, Geffers C, Gastmeier P. Pneumonia associated with invasive and noninvasive ventilation: an analysis of the German nosocomial infection surveillance system database. Intensive Care Med. 2010;36:971–8.
19. Dudeck MA, Edwards JR, Allen-Bridson K, Gross C, Malpiedi PJ, Peterson KD, et al. National Healthcare Safety Network report, data summary for 2013, device-associated module. Am J Infect Control. 2015;43:206–21.
20. Agodi A, Auxilia F, Barchitta M, Brusaferro S, D'Alessandro D, Grillo OC, et al. GISIO-SITI. Trends, risk factors and outcomes of healthcare-associated infections within the Italian network SPIN-UTI. J Hosp Infect. 2013;84:52–8.
21. Boncagni F, Francolini R, Nataloni S, Skrami E, Gesuita R, Donati A, et al. Epidemiology and clinical outcome of healthcare-associated infections: a 4- year experience of an Italian ICU. Minerva Anestesiol. 2015;81:765–75.
22. Talaat M, El-Shokry M, El-Kholy J, Ismail G, Kotb S, Hafez S, et al. National surveillance of health care–associated infections in Egypt: developing a sustainable program in a resource-limited country. Am J Infect Control. 2016;44:1296–301.
23. Dereli N, Ozayar E, Degerli S, Sahin S, Koç F. Three-year evaluation of nosocomial infection rates of the ICU. Braz J Anesthesiol. 2013;63:73–8.
24. Mer M, Duse AG, Galpin JS, Richards GA. Central venous catheterization: a prospective, randomized, double-blind study. Clin Appl Thromb Hemost. 2009;15:19–26.
25. Sheridan RL, Weber JM. Mechanical and infectious complications of central venous cannulation in children: lessons learned from a 10-year experience placing more than 1000 catheters. J Burn Care Res. 2006;27:713–8.
26. Galiczewski JM. Interventions for the prevention of catheter associated urinary tract infections in intensive care units: an integrative review. Intensive Crit Care Nurs. 2016;32:1–11.
27. Weiner LM, Webb AK, Limbago B, Dudeck MA, Patel J, Kallen AJ, et al. Antimicrobial-resistant pathogens associated with healthcare-associated infections: summary of data reported to the National Healthcare Safety Network at the Centers for Disease Control and Prevention, 2009-2010. Infect Control Hosp Epidemiol. 2013;34:1–14.
28. Vincent JL. Nosocomial infections in adult intensive care units. Lancet. 2003; 361:2068–77.
29. Khan MA. Bacterial spectrum and susceptibility patterns of pathogens in ICU and IMCU of a secondary care hospital in Kingdom of Saudi Arabia. Int J Pathol. 2012;10:64–70.
30. Rubio FG, Oliveira VD, Rangel RM, Nogueira MC, Almeida MT. Trends in bacterial resistance in a tertiary university hospital over one decade. Braz J Infect Dis. 2013;17:480–2.
31. Bianco A, Quirino A, Giordano M, Marano V, Rizzo C, Liberto MC, et al. Control of carbapenem-resistant *Acinetobacter baumannii* outbreak in an intensive care unit of a teaching hospital in southern Italy. BMC Infect Dis. 2016;16:747.
32. Center for Disease Control and Prevention. Surveillance of healthcare-associated infections and prevention indicators in European intensive care units. 2017. Availdable at https://ecdc.europa.eu/sites/portal/files/documents/HAI-Net-ICU-protocol-v2.2_0.pdf. Accessed 10 July 2017.

3

Antibiotic resistance and biofilm formation among coagulase-negative staphylococci isolated from clinical samples at a tertiary care hospital of eastern Nepal

Lok Bahadur Shrestha*, Narayan Raj Bhattarai and Basudha Khanal

Abstract

Background: Coagulase negative staphylococci were long regarded non-pathogenic as they are the commensals of human skin and mucosa but the recent changes in the medical practice and changes in underlying host populations, they are being considered significant pathogens associated with number of nosocomial infections. The objective of the study was to determine the species, antimicrobial susceptibility pattern, biofilm forming ability of the clinically significant CoNS isolates and to compare the different methods for the detection of biofilm formation.

Methods: A total of 52 clinically significant CoNS isolates obtained from different units during a year period were studied. Characterization was done using standard microbiological guidelines and antimicrobial susceptibility was done following CLSI guidelines. Biofilm formation was detected by using three methods i.e. tissue culture plate method, congo red agar method and tube adherence method.

Results: Among 52 isolates, *S. epidermidis* (52%) was the most common species which was followed by *S. saprophyticus* (18%) and *S. haemolyticus* (14%). Antimicrobial susceptibility pattern of CoNS documented resistance of 80% to ampicillin. Resistance to cefoxitin and ceftriaxone was observed in 58% of the isolates. Biofilm formation was observed in 65.38% of the isolates. The accuracy of Congo red agar and tube adherence method for the detection of biofilm formation was 82% and 76% respectively.

Conclusion: CoNS isolates obtained from clinical samples should be processed routinely and antimicrobial susceptibility testing should be performed. Multidrug-resistant CoNS are prevalent. All the three methods i.e. tissue culture plate, Congo red agar and tube adherence method can be used in detecting biofilm formation.

Keywords: CoNS, Nosocomial infection, Biofilm

Background

Coagulase-negative staphylococci (CoNS) are the most abundant normal microbial flora of the human skin and mucous membranes. They were long regarded non-pathogenic as they are the commensals of human skin and mucosa. Due to the recent changes in the medical practice and changes in underlying host populations, they are being considered significant pathogens associated with a number of nosocomial infections [1, 2].

CoNS is now considered one of the most common causes of the device related infections in the recent two decades, especially in immunocompromised patients and the chronic debilitated patient who need the long-term central venous access [3]. They may adhere to medical devices and surfaces through slime layer which has a muco-polysaccharide structure, thus they may easily colonize and spread within the hospital environment. The slime factor also aids in pathogenicity by protecting them from phagocytosis, chemotaxis and also antimicrobial agents [4]. Studies suggest that selective advantage for CoNS in causing device associated infections is

* Correspondence: lok.shrestha@bpkihs.edu; drlok86@gmail.com
Microbiology & Infectious Diseases, B. P. Koirala Institute of Health Sciences (BPKIHS), Dharan, Nepal

achieved by its ability to adhere to plastic catheters more aggressively than any other organism [5].

CoNS isolated from nosocomial environments are usually resistant to multiple antimicrobial agents. About 80%–90% of CoNS isolates associated with hospital infections are methicillin resistant coagulase-negative staphylococci (MRCoNS) [4].

With the advancement of medical sciences, especially with the increasing use of medical devices, the infections caused by CoNS are ever increasing. The characterization of CoNS upto species level, their antimicrobial properties and biofilm production is very important for its diagnosis and treatment. The present study is therefore proposed to determine the species distribution, antimicrobial susceptibility and surface adherence property of CoNS isolated at BPKIHS hospital.

Methods

Isolates

The study was carried out in the Department of Microbiology, B.P. Koirala Institute of Health Sciences, Dharan, Nepal from July 2013 to June 2014. Consecutive sampling method was used i.e. all the clinically significant CoNS isolates obtained during the study period were enrolled. A total of 52 CoNS isolates were obtained from various clinical specimens (blood, pus, urine, CVC, tracheostomy tube, tissue) were included in the study.

Identification and characterization of CoNS

Bacterial isolates obtained were identified by colony morphology, gram staining and biochemical tests (catalase test, slide coagulase, tube coagulase and mannitol test). Once the identity of the isolate as CoNS was confirmed, several biochemical tests and antimicrobial discs were used for their characterization upto species level. All the tests were performed according to standard microbiological methodology [6, 7].

Antimicrobial susceptibility test: [8, 9]

Antimicrobial susceptibility testing of the isolates was performed on Mueller-Hinton Agar by.

Kirby-Bauer disk diffusion method recommended by clinical laboratory standard institution.

(CLSI) guidelines against following antimicrobial discs (HiMedia Laboratories): amikacin, ampicillin, ceftriaxone, ciprofloxacin, azithromycin, cotrimoxazole, vancomycin and linezolid.

Cefoxitin disc was used to detect methicillin resistance. *Staphylococcus aureus* ATCC 25923 and *Escherichia coli* ATCC 25922 were used as control strains and tested along with the test strains.

Determination of minimum inhibitory concentration (MIC) [10]

MIC of oxacillin and Vancomycin was determined by agar dilution technique as per CLSI guidelines. Oxacillin powder (815 μg/g) and Vancomycin powder (potency = 930 μg/g) was obtained from HiMedia laboratories India. The concentration at which complete inhibition of growth is achieved is considered the MIC. The results were interpreted according to the CLSI guidelines.

Study of biofilm formation

Biofilm production were investigated by the tube adherence test described by Christensen et al. (1982) and Congo red agar method as described by Freeman et al. (1989) and Tissue culture plate method as described by Christensen et al. (1985) [5, 11, 12]. Results were interpreted considering Tissue culture plate method as gold standard [13–15].

Tube adherence method [5]

A loopful of bacterial suspension from overnight culture were inoculated into the Trypticase.

Soy Broth with 1% glucose (TSBGlu, 10 mL) and incubated for 24 h at 37 °C. The tubes were gradually poured down and was washed with phosphate buffer solution (pH 7.3). After drying, the tubes were stained with 0.1% crystal violet. Excess stains were removed and tubes were washed away with water multiple times. Tubes were then kept in inverted position and finally observed for biofilm formation.

Congo red agar method [11]

Congo red agar was prepared by mixing 37 g Brain heart infusion broth (HiMedia), 50 g sucrose (HiMedia), 0.8 g congo red dye and 10 g agar in 1 l distilled water. The solution was then sterilized by autoclave (121 °C, 15 lbs. for 15 min) and dispensed onto 90 mm petri dishes. CoNS isolates were plated and were incubated at 37 °C for 24 h. Biofilm production was detected by culturing the CoNS isolates on congo red agar plates. The biofilm forming strains produced black colonies while non-forming strains developed red colonies.

Tissue culture plate (TCP) method [12]

Trypticase soy broth with 1% glucose (TSBglu) was used as culture media. Isolates from fresh agar plates were inoculated in TSBglu media and incubated for 18–24 h at 37 °C in aerobic condition. After incubation, 0.2 ml of culture was filled onto individual wells of 96 well flat-bottom tissue culture plates. For control to check sterility and non-specific binding of media, only broth without the bacteria was used. The tissue culture plates were incubated aerobically at 37 °C for 18–25 h. The plates were gently tapped for the removal of unbound content.

Table 1 Biochemical tests for the identification of CoNS isolates and their interpretation

Biochemicals															Identification
Urease	Acetoin production	Novobiocin	Polymyxin B	Slide coagulase	Tube coagulase	Alkaline phosphatase	Pyrrolidonyl aryiamidase	Ornithine Decaboxylase	Trehalose	Mannitol	Mannose	Xylose	Maltose	Sucrose	
+	+	S	R	–	–	+	–	–	–	–	+	–	+	+	*S. epidermidis* (*n* = 27)
+	+	R	S	–	–	–	–	–	+	–	–	–	+	+	*S. saprophyticus* (*n* = 10)
–	+	S	S	–	–	–	+	–	+	–	–	–	+	+	*S. haemolyticus*(*n* = 8)
+	–	S	S	–	–	–	–	–	–	–	–	–	+	+	*S. hominis* (*n* = 4)
–	–	S	S	–	–	–	–	–	–	+	+	–	–	+	*S. capitis* (*n* = 2)
+	+	S	S	–	–	–	–	–	+	–	–	–	+	+	*S. warneri* (*n* = 1)

[+ = Positive, – = negative, R = Resistant, S = Sensitive]

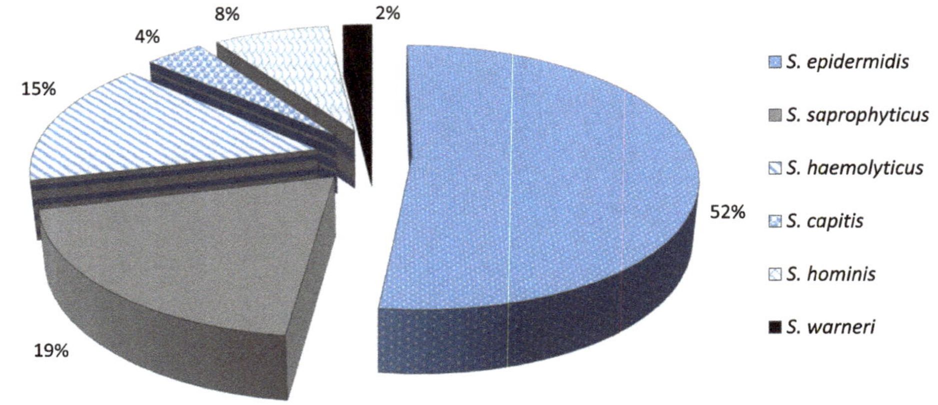

Fig. 1 Different species of coagulase-negative staphylococci (n = 52)

For the removal of free floating bacteria, the individual wells were cleaned four times with 0.2 ml of phosphate buffer saline (PBS pH 7.2). The biofilms formed by adherent organisms in tissue culture plate were fixed with sodium acetate (2%) and stained with 0.1% crystal violet. The plates were washed with water for excess stain and were left for drying. The isolates which formed biofilm were adherent on all side wells and stained uniformly with crystal violet.

Results

A total of 52 CoNS isolates were studied over the duration of 1 year (July 2013–june 2014). The species identification was done on the basis of standard guidelines [6, 7] using the biochemical tests which is interpreted in Table 1. Among them, *S. epidermidis* (52%) was the most common species, followed by *S. saprophyticus* (18%) and *S. haemolyticus* (14%). The overall species distribution is further elicitated on Fig. 1.

Antimicrobial susceptibility pattern of CoNS documented resistance of 80% of isolates to ampicillin. Resistance to ceftriaxone was observed in 58% of the isolates. Among 52 isolates,

Twenty two were susceptible to methicillin as indicated by cefoxitin disc diffusion (≤24 mm) and 30 were resistant. Methicillin resistance was confirmed by MIC of oxacillin against these isolates. All the isolates were susceptible to vancomycin and linezolid. Susceptibility to vancomycin was confirmed by calculating MIC of vancomycin against these isolates (Fig. 2).

The present study also showed that MRCoNS are comparatively more resistant to multiple antimicrobial agents. Isolates obtained from critical care units were more resistant strains as compared to isolates obtained from the outpatient department and wards.

Study of biofilm formation

Biofilm formation was studied in this study by three methods i.e. Tissue culture plate method,

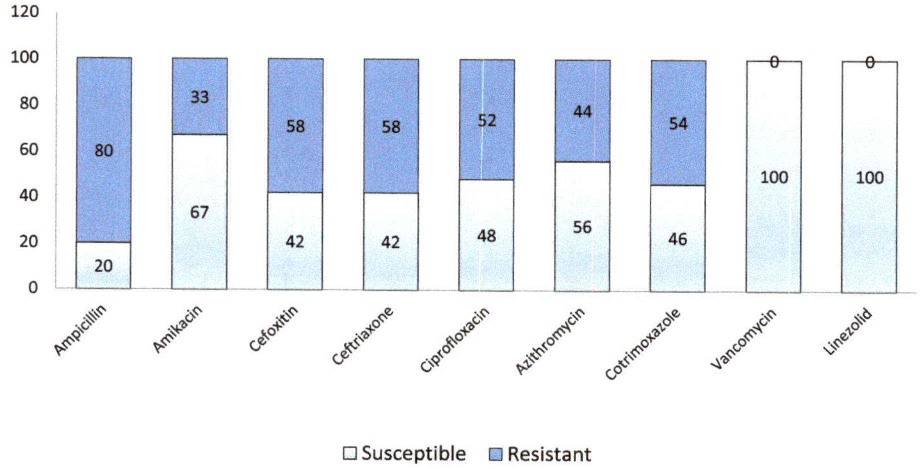

Fig. 2 Antimicrobial susceptibility pattern of different CoNS isolates against several antimicrobial agents (%)

Table 2 Biofilm formation by Congo red agar, tube adherence and tissue culture plate methods

		Tissue culture plate method	
		Positive	Negative
Congo red method	Positive	28	1
	Negative	6	17
Tube adherence method	Positive	26	1
	Negative	8	17

Congo red agar method and tube adherence method. Among 52 isolates, 34 isolates were biofilm formers; 34 of them were detected by tissue culture plate method, 29 by congo red agar method while 27 isolates were biofilm positive by tube adherence method.

The tissue culture plate method was used as the standard method to evaluate the congo red agar and tube adherence method [13–15]. Sensitivity, specificity, positive predictive value, negative predictive value, and accuracy were calculated by analysis of 2*2 table (Table 2). The sensitivity of congo red agar was 82.35% which is higher than tube adherence method 76.47%. The specificity of two tests was similar 94%. The accuracy of congo red agar method (86.5%) was also higher than tube adherence method (82.69%) (Table 3).

Biofilm formation was seen most commonly in *S. epidermidis* followed by *S. haemolyticus.*

The biofilm producers were resistant to multiple antibiotics in comparison to biofilm non- formers. Resistance to ampicillin and methicillin was seen in 100% and 86% of biofilm producers while only 42% and 30% resistance was seen in biofilm non-producers (Fig. 3).

The biofilm producer isolates were studied on the basis of the origin of the sample. All the isolates obtained from the intensive care unit (ICU) were biofilm former while no isolates obtained from outpatient department produced biofilm.

Discussion

General distribution and speciation

A total of 52 clinically significant isolates of coagulase-negative staphylococci obtained during the period of 1 year (July 2013–June 2014) were included in our study. Among the isolates, 6 different species of coagulase-negative staphylococci were encountered: *S. epidermidis* (27, 52%), *S. saprophyticus* (10, 19%), *S. haemolyticus* (8, 15%), *S. hominis* (4, 8%), S. capitis (2, 4%) and *S. warneri* (1, 2%). The findings of the present study are in agreement with the various studies which shows *S. epidermidis* as the most common coagulase-negative staphylococci [16, 17]. In contrast to the finding of our study, Jain A et al. isolated *S. haemolyticus* as (58%) as the most common isolate, followed by *S. epidermidis* (17%) [18]. *S. epidermidis* was isolated from various clinical specimens like blood, central venous catheter, pus and urine, while *S. saprophyticus* was predominantly obtained from urine samples (90%). The result correlates with the other studies which reported the pathogenic role of *S. epidermidis* in catheter related sepsis and that of *S. saprophyticus* in UTI [4, 5]. The higher incidence of *S. saprophyticus* in UTI is due to its colonization of the rectum or urogenital tracts of 5–10% of women [4].

Antimicrobial resistance

In our study, the antimicrobial susceptibility of isolates was tested against 9 antimicrobials in accordance with the CLSI guidelines [8]. AST pattern of the isolates showed 80% resistance to ampicillin, 55% to ceftriaxone. Fifty-eight percent of the isolates were characterized as methicillin-resistant CoNS. All the 52 isolates were susceptible to vancomycin and linezolid. The susceptibility of vancomycin was confirmed by MIC against the isolates. The result of our study is consistent with other research article [19]. However some studies have suggested that vancomycin resistance does exist and is in increasing trends. Natoli S et al. observed no resistance to vancomycin but 5.4% isolates had reduced susceptibility to vancomycin [20].

Isolates obtained from intensive care unit (ICU + NICU) were more resistant when compared to other wards and outpatient department. A similar pattern of drug resistance was documented by several other studies [19, 21]. The patients hospitalized in intensive care unit are managed with multiple indwelling medical devices for the medication, nutrition and respiration. They are more vulnerable to biofilm formation and subsequent infection [22].

Biofilm formation

Among the 52 isolates, 34 (65.38%) isolates were biofilm formers. Biofilm formation was detected by tissue culture plate method in 34 isolates, congo red agar in 29 isolates, while 27 isolates showed positive biofilm formation test by tube adherence method. Similar results were obtained in previous studies [23, 24].

Table 3 Statistical evaluation of Congo red agar and Tube adherence method for detection of biofilm lm formation in staphylococci using the tissue culture plate method as the standard method

	Sensitivity	Specificity	PPV	NPV	Accuracy
Congo red agar	82.35	94.5	96.5	43.47	86.5
Tube adherence method	76.47	94.44	96.29	68	82.69

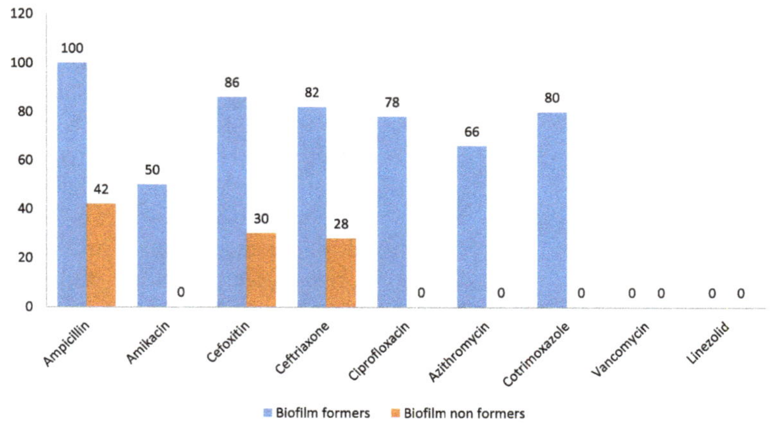

Fig. 3 Antimicrobial resistance pattern with relation to biofilm formation property

Congo red agar detected 85% (29/34) biofilm producer and tube adherence method detected 79% (27/34). Tissue culture plate is used as the standard method for detection of biofilm formation [13–15] and the results of our study supports the evidence. Similar results were documented in various studies [13, 17].

The sensitivity, specificity, accuracy of the two tests were calculated using tissue culture plate as the reference [13–15]. The sensitivity (82.35%) and accuracy (86.5%) of congo red agar were higher than tube adherence method (sensitivity = 76.47, accuracy = 82.69%), while no difference was observed in the specificity of these two methods. The positive predictive value of both congo red agar and tube adherence method is good (above 90), and they may therefore be used in clinical decision making. Similar results were documented by Saising et al. [24].

The present study also reveals that 100% of isolates obtained from intensive care units were biofilm formers while only 40% of isolates from surgery ward and none of the isolates obtained from the outpatient departments were biofilm formers. Similarly, the biofilm producers were more resistant to antimicrobial agents as compared to non-producers which agree with the study done in the past [5].

Conclusion

A total of 52 isolates of CoNS were studied, among which 6 species were identified. *S. epidermidis* (52%) was the most common species followed by *S saprophyticus* (19%), S. haemolyticus (15%) and *S. hominis* (8%). Antimicrobial susceptibility pattern of CoNS documented resistance of 80%, 58% and 58% resistance to ampicillin, ceftriaxone and cefoxitin respectively. All the isolates were susceptible to vancomycin and linezolid. Biofilm production was detected in 67% of the isolates. Tissue culture plate is the most effective method for the detection of biofilm formation while congo red agar and tube adherence method can also detect biofilm formation with an accuracy of 86% and 82% respectively.

Abbreviations

AMR: Antimicrobial resistance; ATCC: American type culture collection; CLSI: Clinical and laboratory standards institute; CoNS: Coagulase-negative Staphylococci; CVC: Central vascular catheter; FDA: Food and Drug Administration; HIV: Human immunodeficiency virus; ICU: Intensive Care Unit; MIC: Minimum Inhibitory Concentration; MRCoNS: Methicillin-resistant Coagulse-negative Staphylococci; MSCoNS: Methicillin-sensitive Coagulase-negative Staphylococci; NICU: Neonatal intensive care unit; UTI: Urinary tract infection

Acknowledgements

All members of the Department of Microbiology.

Funding

None.

Authors' contributions

Conceptualization: LBS, NRB, BK. Investigation: LBS. Methodology: LBS, NRB, BK. Resources: LBS, NRB, BK. Supervision: NRB, BK. Writing-original draft: LBS. Writing-review and editing: NRB, BK. All authors read and approved the final manuscript.

Consent for publication

Not applicable.

Competing interests

The authors declare that they have no competing interests.

References

1. Rupp ME, Archer GL. Coagulase-negative staphylococci: pathogens associated with medical progress. Clin Infect Dis. 1994;19(2):231–43. quiz 44-5. [PMID: 7986894]
2. Bannerman TL. Staphylococcus, micrococcus, and other catalasepositive cocci that grow aerobically. In: Murray PR, Baron EJ, Jorgensen JH, editors. Manual of medical microbiology. Washington, DC: American Society For Microbiology; 2003. p. 384–404.

3. Schulin T, Voss A. Coagulase-negative staphylococci as a cause of infections related to intravascular prosthetic devices: limitations of present therapy. Clin Microbiol Infect. 2001;7(Suppl 4):1–7. [PMID: 11688530]
4. Rupp ME, Fey PD. Staphylococcus Epidermidis and other Coagulase negative staphylococci. In: Mandell GL, Benett JE, Dolin R, editors. Mandell, Douglas and Bennett's principles and practice of infectious disease. 7th ed. Philadelphia: Churchill Livingstone Elsevier; 2010. p. 186.
5. Christensen GD, Simpson WA, Bisno AL, Beachey EH. Adherence of slime-producing strains of Staphylococcus Epidermidis to smooth surfaces. Infect Immun. 1982;37(1):318–26. [PMID: 6179880]
6. Kloos WE, Schleifer KH. Simplified scheme for routine identification of human staphylococcus species. J Clin Microbiol. 1975;1(1):82–8. PMID: 170303
7. Winn W, Allen S, Janda W. Koneman's color atlas and textbook of diagnostic microbiology. 6th ed. Philadelphia: Lippincott Williams and Wikins; 2006. p. 623–62.
8. Clinical and Laboratory Standard Institute. Performance standard for antimicrobial disk susceptibility tests, Document no M100-S23. 23rd ed. Wayne: Clinical and Laboratory Standard Institute; 2013.
9. Bauer AW, Kirby WMM, Sherris JC, Turck M. Antibiotic susceptibility testing by a standardized single disc method. Am J Clin Pathol. 1966;45:493.
10. Clinical and Laboratory Standards Institute. Methods for dilution antimicrobial susceptibility tests for bacteria that grow aerobically, CLSI document no M07-A9. 9th ed. Wayne: Clinical and Laboratory Standards Institute; 2012.
11. Freeman DJ, Falkiner FR, Keane CT. New method for detecting slime production by coagulase negative staphylococci. J Clin Pathol. 1989;42(8): 872–4. PMID: 2475530
12. Christensen GD, Simpson WA, Younger JJ, Baddour LM, Barrett FF, Melton DM, et al. Adherence of coagulase-negative staphylococci to plastic tissue culture plates: a quantitative model for the adherence of staphylococci to medical devices. J Clin Microbiol. 1985;22(6):996–1006. PMID: 3905855
13. Mathur T, Singhal S, Khan S, Upadhyay DJ, Fatma T, Rattan A. Detection of biofilm formation among the clinical isolates of staphylococci: an evaluation of three different screening methods. Indian J Med Microbiol. 2006;24(1):25–9. PMID: 16505551
14. Panda PS, Chaudhary U, Dube SK. Comparison of four different methods for detection of biofilm formation by uropathogens. Indian J Pathol Microbiol. 2016;59(2):177–9. PMID: 27166035
15. Hassan A, Usman J, Kaleem F, Omair M, Khalid A, Iqbal M. Evaluation of different detection methods of biofilm formation in the clinical isolates. Braz J Infect Dis. 2011;15(4):305–11.
16. Ferreira RB, Iorio NL, Malvar KL, Nunes AP, Fonseca LS, Bastos CC, et al. Coagulase-negative staphylococci: comparison of phenotypic and genotypic oxacillin susceptibility tests and evaluation of the agar screening test by using different concentrations of oxacillin. J Clin Microbiol. 2003; 41(8):3609–14. PMID: 12904363
17. Alcaraz LE, Satorres SE, Lucero RM, Centorbi OM. Species identification, slime production and oxacillin susceptibility in coagulase-negative staphylococci isolated from nosocomial specimens. Braz J Microbiol. 2003;34:45–1.
18. Jain A, Agarwal J, Bansal S. Prevalence of methicillin-resistant, coagulase-negative staphylococci in neonatal intensive care units: findings from a tertiary care hospital in India. J Med Microbiol. 2004; 53(Pt 9):941–4. PMID: 15314204
19. Jarlov JO. Phenotypic characteristics of coagulase-negative staphylococci: typing and antibiotic susceptibility. APMIS Suppl. 1999;91: 1–42. PMID: 10230367
20. Natoli S, Fontana C, Favaro M, Bergamini A, Testore GP, Minelli S, et al. Characterization of coagulase-negative staphylococcal isolates from blood with reduced susceptibility to glycopeptides and therapeutic options. BMC Infect Dis. 2009;9:83. PMID: 19497104
21. Zhao C, Sun H, Wang H, Liu Y, Hu B, Yu Y, et al. Antimicrobial resistance trends among 5608 clinical gram-positive isolates in China: results from the gram-positive Cocci resistance surveillance program (2005-2010). Diagn Microbiol Infect Dis. 2012;73(2):174–81.
22. Pfaller MA, Herwaldt LA. Laboratory, clinical, and epidemiological aspects of coagulase-negative staphylococci. Clin Microbiol Rev. 1988;1(3):281–99. PMID: 3058297
23. Karthik S, Bhattacharya S, Harish BN, Parija SC. Detection of slime production by coagulase-negative staphylococcus: an assessment of two methods. Indian J Pathol Microbiol. 2004;47(1):85–9. PMID: 15471145
24. Saising J, Singdam S, Ongsakul M, Voravuthikunchai SP. Lipase, protease, and biofilm as the major virulence factors in staphylococci isolated from acne lesions. Biosci Trends. 2012;6(4):160–4. PMID: 23006962

4

Phenotypic and genotypic characteristics of ESBL and AmpC producing organisms associated with bacteraemia in Ho Chi Minh City, Vietnam

Nguyen Phu Huong Lan[1,2†], Nguyen Huu Hien[1†], Tu Le Thi Phuong[2], Duy Pham Thanh[2], Nga Tran Vu Thieu[2], Dung Tran Thi Ngoc[2], Ha Thanh Tuyen[2], Phat Voong Vinh[2], Matthew J. Ellington[4], Guy E. Thwaites[2,3], Nguyen Van Vinh Chau[1], Stephen Baker[2,3,5] and Christine J. Boinett[1,2,3*]

Abstract

Background: Broad-spectrum antimicrobials are commonly used as empirical therapy for infections of presumed bacterial origin. Increasing resistance to these antimicrobial agents has prompted the need for alternative therapies and more effective surveillance. Better surveillance leads to more informed and improved delivery of therapeutic interventions, potentially leading to better treatment outcomes.

Methods: We screened 1017 Gram negative bacteria (excluding *Pseudomonas* spp. and *Acinetobacter* spp.) isolated between 2011 and 2013 from positive blood cultures for susceptibility against third generation cephalosporins, ESBL and/or AmpC production, and associated ESBL/AmpC genes, at the Hospital for Tropical Diseases in Ho Chi Minh City.

Results: Phenotypic screening found that 304/1017 (30%) organisms were resistance to third generation cephalosporins; 172/1017 (16.9%) of isolates exhibited ESBL activity, 6.2% (63/1017) had AmpC activity, and 0.5% (5/1017) had both ESBL and AmpC activity. *E. coli* and *Aeromonas* spp. were the most common organisms associated with ESBL and AmpC phenotypes, respectively. Nearly half of the AmpC producers harboured an ESBL gene. There was no significant difference ($p > 0.05$) between the antimicrobial resistance phenotypes of the organisms associated with community and hospital-acquired infections.

Conclusion: AmpC and ESBL producing organisms were commonly associated with bloodstream infections in this setting, with antimicrobial resistant organisms being equally distributed between infections originating from the community and healthcare settings. *Aeromonas* spp., which was associated with bloodstream infections in cirrhotic/hepatitis patients, were the most abundant AmpC producing organism. We conclude that empirical monotherapy with third generation cephalosporins may not be optimum in this setting.

Keywords: ESBL, AmpC, Bacteraemia, Antimicrobial resistance

* Correspondence: cboinett@oucru.org
[†]Equal contributors
[1]The Hospital for Tropical Diseases, 764 Vo Van Kiet, Quan 5, Ho Chi Minh City, Vietnam
[2]Oxford University Clinical Research Unit, The Hospital for Tropical Diseases, Wellcome Trust Major Overseas Programme, Ho Chi Minh City, Vietnam
Full list of author information is available at the end of the article

Background

Antimicrobial resistance (AMR) is an increasing problem in global health. Resistance against antimicrobials used for empirical therapy of invasive infections is increasing at an alarming rate and the provision of effective antimicrobials improves the likelihood of a better clinical outcome. To limit the possibility of poor outcomes, broad-spectrum antimicrobials, such as third generation cephalosporins, have become the most commonly used empirical drugs to treat non-specific febrile diseases but this has come at the cost of increased resistance to these drugs. The situation has been recognised internationally and the WHO have identified seven bacteria as the most important cause of AMR infections in hospitals and the community. This list includes *Escherichia coli* and *Klebsiella pneumoniae*, both commonly found to be resistant to third generation cephalosporins [1]. Resistance to third generation cephalosporins can be mediated by a class of serine hydrolases known commonly as the extended-spectrum β-lactamases (ESBLs), which act by cleaving the β-lactam ring, thereby rendering the drug inactive [2]. With the increasing threat of treatment failure, monitoring ESBL producing organisms in sentinel locations is imperative for surveillance and appropriate treatment strategies.

Routine susceptibility testing is usually capable of detecting the presence of ESBL activity, however false positives can occur. This lack of sensitivity is associated with plasmid-mediated ampicillinases known as AmpC. AmpC genes confer resistance to many β-lactams and β-lactam/β-lactamase inhibitor combinations, the latter of which render ESBL producing bacteria susceptible. AmpC genes are generally located chromosomally, however plasmid associated variants of the enzymes have become increasingly recognised. This observation is significant as these ampicillinases can be easily disseminated by horizontal gene transfer [3]. There are currently no standardised Clinical and Laboratory Standards Institute (CLSI) guidelines for AmpC detection, although several methods have been proposed to aid in the accurate detection of AmpC β-lactamases [4–6]. These phenotypic tests primarily use a cephalosporin with a β-lactamase inhibitor (e.g. clavulanate) or a non-β-lactamase inhibitor (e.g. boronic acid) and can be combined with molecular detection of the AmpC β-lactamases using multiplex PCR [7]. However, due to over-expression of AmpC genes, bacteria carrying an ESBL gene may test negative for ESBL production, resulting in misinterpretations of phenotypic AmpC methods [8–10], which can have significant consequences for patient care. The accurate testing and interpretation of AmpC and ESBL activity is vital for healthcare professionals to provide effective and appropriate treatment management. Here, we aimed to assess the distribution of AmpC and ESBL genes in organisms associated with bloodstream infections at the Hospital for Tropical Diseases (HTD) in Ho Chi Minh City (HCMC), Vietnam. Our data highlights the need for routine AmpC and ESBL gene surveillance in hospitals in low-middle income countries to ensure effective treatment and report on the incidence of drug resistant bacteraemia.

Methods

Ethics statement

Ethical approval for this study was provided by the ethical review board of HTD in Ho Chi Minh City (HCMC), Vietnam.

Study setting and patient population

HTD is a 550-bed infectious disease hospital that serves as a primary and secondary facility for the surrounding local population in HCMC and a tertiary referral centre for infectious diseases for the 17 southern provinces of the country. Neonates, patients without infectious diseases, including those with surgical requirements, tuberculosis, cancer, primary haematological disorders or immunosuppression (other than HIV) are referred to other hospitals in the city.

Blood cultures were performed for patients in whom an infection was suspected on the basis of a fever (> 38 °C) or who had evidence of sepsis on the basis of the presence of two or more of the following features: fever (> 38 °C) or low temperature (< 36 °C); tachycardia (exact level according to age); tachypnea (exact level according to age); an elevated white cell count (> 12,000 cells/mm^3) or depressed white cell count (< 4000 cells/mm^3). There was no systematic change in the application of these criteria during the time course of the study. All data originating from consecutive patients admitted to the hospital who had a blood culture performed for suspected bloodstream infection between January 1st 2011 and December 31st 2013 were included in this retrospective study. Routinely, a member of the hospital staff recorded the date of blood draw, the patient's age, sex, and suspected diagnosis, the number of blood culture bottles inoculated, the result of the culture (whether positive or negative) and the susceptibility of the isolate to commonly used antimicrobial agents. These are the source data for this study. For the purposes of these analyses blood samples taken for culture > 48 h after admission to HTD were classified as a Hospital Acquired Infection (HAI) and samples taken within 48 h of admission to HTD were classed as a Community Acquired Infection (CAI).

Blood culturing and bacterial identification

Venous blood cultures of 8–15 mL from adults and 2–5 mL of venous blood from infants and children were routinely obtained and inoculated into BACTEC*plus* aerobic bottles (Becton Dickenson, USA). Inoculated BACTEC bottles were incubated at 37 °C in a BACTEC 9050 automated analyser for up to 5 days and sub-cultured when the machine indicated a positive signal. All sub-cultures were plated onto fresh sheep blood agar (Oxoid Unipath, Basingstoke, United Kingdom). Plates were incubated at 37 °C in air for 5 days and organisms were subsequently identified by standard methods including API20E and API20NE identification kits (Bio-Mérieux, France). *Staphylococcus aureus* ATCC 29213 and *Pseudomonas aeruginosa* ATCC 27853 were used as controls.

Antimicrobial susceptibility testing

The susceptibility to relevant antimicrobial agents was determined by the modified Bauer-Kirby disc diffusion method. Enterobacteriaceae were tested with discs containing chloramphenicol (30 μg), ampicillin (10 μg), co-trimoxazole (trimethoprim 1.25 μg/sulfamethoxazole 23.75 μg), ceftriaxone (30 μg), ofloxacin (5 μg) and gentamicin (10 μg). The breakpoint zone sizes were interpreted according to CLSI guidelines [11].

The double disk diffusion method [12] was used to identify ESBL activity. This method was performed using a combination of cefepime (30 μg), ceftazidime (30 μg), ceftriaxone (30 μg), Amoxicillin (20 μg)/clavulanate (10 μg). ESBL producers were identified by reduced zone sizes to third-generation cephalosporins (ceftazidime and ceftriaxone), and expansion of these zones in the presence of an inhibitor (clavulanate). Confirmatory tests for ESBL producers were performed using oxyamino-cephalosporins/β-lactam inhibitor combinations, namely cefotaxime (30 μg)/clavulanate (10 μg) and ceftazidime (30 μg)/clavulanate (10 μg) (Additional file 1: Figure S1B). Zone sizes were measured and interpreted according to the CLSI guidelines [11].

Phenotypic AmpC activity was detected using two different tests. First, we measured zone sizes using a combination of cefoxitin and an alternative third- and fourth-generation cephalosporin, where an AmpC positive organism would be resistant to cefoxitin and exhibit reduced susceptibility to the alternative third generation cephalosporin (ceftriaxone 30 μg) and complete susceptibility to the fourth generation cephalosporin (cefepime). Secondly, we determined inducible AmpC phenotypes by assessing reduced zone sizes against a third generation cephalosporin (ceftriaxone 30 μg or ceftazidime 30 μg) in the presence of imipenem (30 μg) as an inducing substrate (Additional file 1: Figure S1A) [13, 14].

Genotypic screening of ESBL and AmpC genes

Blood isolates collected from the same patient at two different time-points with the same phenotypic AMR profile were denoted as duplicates and only one was subsequently selected for further PCR analysis. If the AMR profile of the two isolates selected differed, both were selected for PCR analysis. Multiplex PCR reactions were used to detect ESBL (*bla*$_{CTX-M}$ subtypes) [15] and AmpC [7] genes. Other β-lactamase genes, *bla*$_{TEM}$ [16], *bla*$_{OXA}$ [17], and *bla*$_{SHV}$ [16] were also detected by multiplex PCR using the following cycling conditions, initial denaturation step at 95 °C for 15 min, followed by 25 cycles of DNA denaturation at 94 °C for 30 s, primer annealing at 57 °C for 40 s, and primer extension at 72 ° C for 30 s. After the last cycle, a final extension step at 72 °C for 10 min was added. PCR amplicons were examined by agarose gel (BioRad) electrophoresis made up to a concentration of 1.5% (*w*/*v*). The primers used in this study are shown in Additional file 2: Table S1.

All positive ESBL (*bla*$_{CTX-M}$) and AmpC (*bla*$_{CIT}$) PCR amplicons were sequenced to further subtype these genes. DNA was extracted using the Agencourt AMPure XP PCR purification system (Beckman Coulter) and sequenced using the BigDye Terminator v3.1 cycle sequencing kit (Applied biosystems) on the 3130 genetic analyser (Applied biosystems). DNA sequences were compared against the National Centre of Biotechnology Information (NCBI) GenBank sequence database using the BLASTn algorithm and gene variants were subsequently deduced based on sequence similarity.

Statistical analysis

Statistical analysis was performed in R. Comparisons between HAI and CAI antimicrobial resistance instance rates was assessed using the Fisher's exact test (two-tailed). A *p*-value < 0.05 was considered statistically significant.

Results

Gram-negative organisms with reduced susceptibility against third generation cephalosporins isolated from bloodstream infections at the Hospital for Tropical Diseases

Between January 2011 and December 2013, 1690 non-contaminant bacteria were isolated from the blood of febrile patients attending HTD in HCMC. The overall isolation rate from blood during this period was 5.6% (1690/30,185); 1017 (60%) of these were Gram-negative (excluding *Pseudomonas* spp. and *Acinetobacter* spp.) (Table 1). In > 70% (783/1017) of cases, a member of the Enterobacteriaceae was found to be the causative agent, with *E. coli* accounting for 56% (445/783) of these infections. Nearly half of these isolates were resistant to at least three different antimicrobial classes, including third generation cephalosporins. *Aeromonas* spp. was the most abundant (59/234; 5.8%) non-Enterobacteriaceae Gram-negative genus isolated from the blood cultures, with 27/59 (46%) of the isolated *Aeromonas* spp. being resistant to a third generation cephalosporin.

Table 1 Summary of Gram-negative microorganisms isolated from blood cultures during the period of 2011–2013

				Resistance phenotype												
Species	CAI (*n* = 876)	HAI (*n* = 141)	Total (*n* = 1017)	amk	amc	caz	cip	cro	etp	fep	imp	mem	ofx	sxt	tcc	tzp
Enterobacteriaceae (*n* = 783)																
Edwardsiella spp.	2	0	2 (0.2%)	–	–	–	–	–	–	–	–	–	1	1	–	–
Enterobacter spp.	9	4	13 (1.3%)	–	8	8	1	10	–	1	–	–	1	4	5	1
E. coli	**392**	**53**	**445 (43.8%)**	2	80	201	196	203	5	179	1	1	200	298	262	24
***Klebsiella* spp.**	**127**	**27**	**154 (15.1%)**	1	15	23	19	24	3	18	2	3	19	51	30	8
Morganella morganii	2	1	3 (0.3%)	–	3	2	–	3	–	–	1	–	–	1	–	–
Proteus mirabilis	2	6	8 (0.8%)	–	–	1	3	1	–	1	–	–	3	5	1	–
Providencia spp.	1	1	2 (0.2%)	–	1	–	–	–	–	–	–	–	–	–	–	–
Non-typhoidal *Salmonella*	102	9	**111 (10.9%)**	–	–	1	3	1	–	1	–	–	3	29	28	–
Salmonella Typhi	40	4	44 (4.3%)	–	–	–	–	–	–	–	–	–	–	11	–	–
Serratia marcescens	0	1	1 (0.1%)	–	1	–	–	1	–	–	–	–	–	–	–	–
Non-Enterobacteriaceae (*n* = 234)																
***Aeromonas* spp.**	**51**	**8**	**59 (5.8%)**	–	24	23	–	27	–	–	–	–	1	9	20	–
Abiotrophia spp.	1	0	1 (0.1%)	–	–	–	–	–	–	–	–	–	–	1	–	–
Archromobacter xylosoxidans	1	1	2 (0.2%)	1	–	1	1	2	–	1	–	–	–	1	1	–
Alcaligenes spp.	8	3	11 (1.1%)	4	2	1	1	3	–	4	–	–	1	1	1	–
Brevundimonas vesicularis	2	0	2 (0.2%)	No information available												
Burkhoderia cepacia	**28**	**8**	**36 (3.5%)**	–	–	1	–	–	–	–	–	–		1	–	–
Burkhoderia pseudomallei	**51**	**0**	**51 (5.0%)**	–	–	–	–	–	–	–	–	–	–	–	–	–
Campylobacter spp.	13	0	13 (1.3%)	–	–	–	8	–	–	–	–	–	10	–	–	–
Chryseomonas spp.	2	2	4 (0.4%)	3	2	1	2	2	–	2	3	3	2	2	2	1
Comamonas spp.	1	1	2 (0.2%)	No information available												
Gemella spp.	1	0	1 (0.1%)	No information available												
Haemophilus spp.	9	2	11 (1.1%)	–	1	–	5	1	–	–	–	–	–	8	–	–
Moraxella spp.	1	1	2 (0.2%)	–	–	–	–	–	–	–	–	–	–	–	–	–
Neisseria meningitidis	5	0	5 (0.5%)	–	–	–	–	–	–	–	–	–	–	–	–	–
Pasteurella spp.	6	0	6 (0.6%)	1	–	–	–	1	–	1	–	–	–	–	–	–
Psychrobacter spp.	2	0	2 (0.2%)	No information available												
Ralstonia pickettii	4	2	6 (0.6%)	4	1	1	–	–	–	2	1	2	–	1	3	1
Roseomonas spp.	2	0	2 (0.2%)	1	–	–	–	–	–	–	–	–	–	–	–	–
Sphingomonas spp.	2	1	3 (0.3%)	–	1	2	–	–	–	2	–	–	–	–	–	1
Stenotrophomonas maltophilia	6	5	11 (1.1%)	–	–	7	–	–	–	–	–	–	–	2	6	–
Vibrio spp.	3	1	4 (0.4%)	–	–	–	–	–	–	–	–	–	–	1	–	–

Highlighted in bold are the top three Gram-negative microorganisms (Enterobacteriaceae and non-Enterobacteriaceae) isolated from blood cultures
Abbreviations: *amk* amikacin, *amc* amoxicillin-clavulanic acid, *caz* ceftazidime, *cip* ciprofloxacin, *cro* ceftriaxone, *etp* ertapenem, *fep* cefepime, *imp* imipenem, *mem* meropenem, *ofx* ofloxacin, *sxt* trimethoprim-sulfamethoxazole, *tcc* ticarcillin-clavulanic acid, *tzp* piperacillin-tazobactam

Ceftriaxone (or an alternative parenteral third generation cephalosporin) was (and remains) the empirical therapy for suspected bacteraemia/sepsis in this healthcare facility. Therefore, all Gram-negative organisms isolated from blood were routinely screened for susceptibility against various third generation cephalosporins. In total, nearly a third (304/1017; 30%) were found to exhibit reduced susceptibility against third generation cephalosporins, with > 90% (*n* = 280) of these exhibiting resistance to ceftriaxone and nearly 3% (*n* = 8) being intermediate according to current CLSI susceptibility breakpoints [11].

The 280 non-duplicate organisms exhibiting resistance to ceftriaxone were subjected to phenotypic screening using the double disk diffusion method to detect ESBL activity, and to identify a zone of reduced inhibition between the third generation cephalosporin and imipenem, indicative of AmpC activity (Additional file 1: Figure S1). In total 172/1017 (16.9%) isolates were phenotypically ESBL positive; 63/1017 (6.2%) were phenotypically AmpC positive and 5/1017 (0.5%) exhibited phenotypic evidence of both ESBL and AmpC activity. *E. coli* was the most common bacterial species exhibiting ESBL activity only, or both ESBL and AmpC activity, accounting for > 90% (162/177) of this group of ceftriaxone resistant organisms (Fig. 1). Approximately 40% (25/63) of the AmpC producing organisms were *Aeromonas* spp.; *E. coli* was the second most abundant species amongst the AmpC producers with 23/68 (> 30%) identified. The remaining organisms exhibiting AmpC activity belonged to a range of species, including *Enterobacter* spp. (9/68), *K. pneumoniae* (8/68), and *Morganella morganii* (2/68).

Molecular analysis of ESBL and AmpC genes conferring resistance to third generation cephalosporins

PCR amplification was performed on nucleic acid extracted from the 177 ESBL (172 ESBL and 5 producing both ESBL and AmpC) exhibiting phenotypic ESBL activity to identify the four most common ESBL gene groups (bla_{TEM}, bla_{SHV}, bla_{OXA}, and $bla_{CTX\text{-}M}$). These PCR amplifications demonstrated that $bla_{CTX\text{-}M}$ was the most prevalent ESBL gene family in these organisms, testing positive in 168/177 (95%) nucleic acid extractions; *E. coli* was the most frequently identified organism harbouring the $bla_{CTX\text{-}M}$ gene (Table 2). Sixty per cent (106/177) of these isolates had multiple ESBL genes, the most frequent combinations were $bla_{CTX\text{-}M}$ with bla_{TEM} (summarised in Additional file 3: Table S2). Subsequent sequencing of the $bla_{CTX\text{-}M}$ PCR amplicons revealed that $bla_{CTX\text{-}M\text{-}15}$ (n = 84) was the most common ESBL gene subtype. Other ESBL gene subtypes detected included $bla_{CTX\text{-}14}$ (n = 40), $bla_{CTX\text{-}24}$ (n = 6), $bla_{CTX\text{-}27}$ (n = 48), and $bla_{CTX\text{-}55}$ (n = 12) (Additional file 4: Table S3). Of the five isolates exhibiting both an ESBL and an AmpC phenotype, only two had genetic determinants that were associated with an AmpC phenotype, namely, bla_{CIT} (CMY-42), and bla_{EBC}. Two $bla_{CTX\text{-}M}$ variants ($bla_{CTX\text{-}M\text{-}15}$ and $bla_{CTX\text{-}M\text{-}27}$) were identified in these organisms as the genes most likely to confer resistance against third generation cephalosporins (Additional file 4: Table S3).

PCR amplification of nucleic acid extracted from the 68 organisms (63 AmpC and 5 isolates producing both ESBL and AmpC) with AmpC activity found that bla_{CIT} was the most common gene associated with this phenotype; this variant was detected in 19/68 (28%) of the isolates (Table 3). Sequencing of the AmpC amplicons determined that approximately half (11/19; 58%) of the isolates harboured the $bla_{CMY\text{-}2}$ subtype; the remainder (8/19; 42%) carried the $bla_{CMY\text{-}42}$ gene. Notably, more than half (37/68; 54%) of the organisms conferring an AmpC phenotype did not generate a PCR amplicon for any of the six AmpC genetic markers that were screened. The majority of the organisms exhibiting AmpC activity but not generating any detectable PCR products were *Aeromonas* spp. The remainder of the AmpC producing organisms harboured either bla_{DHA} (9/68; 13%) or bla_{EBC} (3/68; 4%) genes. Almost half (32/68; 47%) of the AmpC producing isolates also generated a PCR amplicon for an ESBL gene. The most commonly detected ESBL gene in these phenotypic AmpC organisms was the bla_{TEM} gene, found in 17/32 (53%) of these isolates (Table 4). Three *E. coli* isolates harboured three

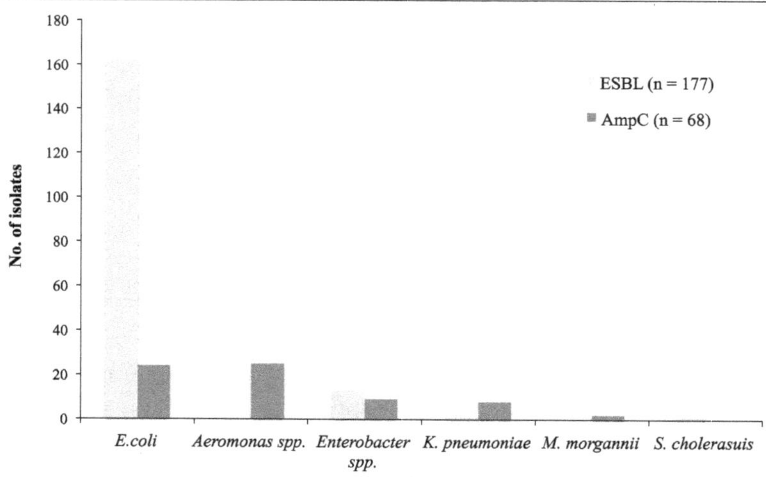

Fig. 1 The distribution of ESBL or AmpC producing bacteria isolated during the period of 2011–2013. Bar chart indicates the number and type of ESBL or AmpC producing bacteria isolated

Table 2 The distribution of β-lactamase genes from the 177 ESBLs producing bacteria identified

Gene	*E. coli*	*Klebsiella* spp.	*Enterobacter cloacae*	*Salmonella cholerasuis*	Total[a]
$bla_{CTX\text{-}M}$	157	9	1	1	168 (95%)
bla_{TEM}	70	7	1	1	79 (45%)
bla_{OXA}	33	2	1	–	36 (20%)
bla_{SHV}	1	4	–	–	5 (3%)
Not detected	3	1	–	–	4 (2%)

[a]The proportion of bacterial species harbouring a particular ESBL gene is expressed as a percentage of the total bacteria possessing an ESBL phenotype (n = 177)

different β-lactamase genes, $bla_{CTX\text{-}M}$, bla_{TEM}, and bla_{OXA}.

Hospital and community-acquired third-generation cephalosporin resistant infections

E.coli and *Aeromonas* spp. were the most common bacterial species identified as being ESBL or AmpC producing, respectively. Ninety-seven per cent (157/162) of the *E. coli* isolates with an ESBL phenotype harboured a $bla_{CTX\text{-}M}$ gene. Of the 162 phenotypically identified as ESBL producers, 140 were associated with a CAI and 22 were associated with a HAI. Hypothesising that organisms associated with HAI would have a broader AMR range, we compared the antimicrobial susceptibility profiles of organisms associated with CAIs and HAIs. However, after investigating susceptibility against a range of different antimicrobial classes in the ESBL producing organisms, we found no significant difference between the antimicrobial susceptibility profiles of organisms associated with CAI or HAI (p > 0.05; Fisher's exact test) (Additional file 5: Figure S2A). We additionally compared antimicrobial susceptibility phenotypes between *E. coli* associated with CAI and HAI for the isolates that were phenotypically AmpC positive. There was no significant difference in the antimicrobial susceptibility profiles between these groups (p > 0.05; Fisher's exact test)

Table 4 The distribution of the 68 AmpC producing bacteria harbouring an additional ESBL gene

Gene	*Aeromonas* spp.	*E. coli*	*Klebsiella* spp.	*Enterobacter* spp.	*M. morganii*	Total[a]
$bla_{CTX\text{-}M}$		3				3 (4%)
bla_{TEM}	–	15	–	1	1	17 (25%)
bla_{SHV}	–	–	4	1	–	5 (7%)
bla_{OXA}	–	2	–	–	–	2 (3%)
bla_{OXA} & bla_{TEM}	–	1	1	–	–	2 (3%)
bla_{OXA}, bla_{TEM} & $bla_{CTX\text{-}M}$	–	1	1	1	–	3 (4%)
Not detected[b]	25	2	2	6	1	36 (53%)

[a]The proportion of all bacterial species with AmpC phenotype (n = 68) gene is expressed as a percentage of the total bacteria possessing harbouring an additional ESBL gene
[b]These samples had an ESBLs phenotype but no detectable ESBL gene

(Additional file 5: Figure S2B). Lastly, we investigated the clinical source of the AmpC producing *Aeromonas* spp. in CAI and HAI. We found that 72% (18/25) of the AmpC expressing *Aeromonas* spp. were associated with patients with underlying liver cirrhosis or hepatitis (Fig. 2).

Discussion

With the ever-increasing reports of ESBL producing Gram-negative bacteria in clinical settings, identifying these organisms is imperative for disease monitoring and the provision of efficacious treatments. Although antimicrobial susceptibility profiling is still the most commonly used method, interpretation of AmpC production data can sometimes prove problematic and may lead to under-reporting or misdiagnosis as an ESBL phenotype [18]. This scenario could potentially lead to treatment failure due to the use of alternative fourth-generation cephalosporins or carbapenems. Here, we

Table 3 The distribution of β-lactamase genes from the AmpC producing bacteria identified

Gene	*Aeromonas* spp.	*E. coli*	*Klebsiella* spp.	*Enterobacter* spp.	*M. morganii*	Total[a]
bla_{CIT}	–	18	–	1	–	19 (28%)
Bla_{DHA}	–	1	6	–	2	9 (13%)
Bla_{EBC}	–	–	–	3	–	3 (4%)
Not detected	25	5	2	5	–	37 (54%)

[a]The proportion of bacterial species harbouring a particular AmpC gene is expressed as a percentage of the total bacteria possessing an AmpC phenotype (n = 68)

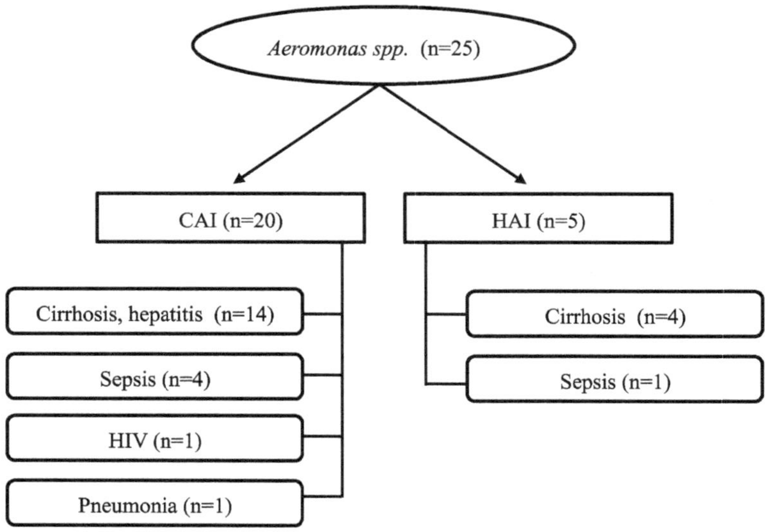

Fig. 2 The distribution of bacteremia infections where Aeromonas spp. was isolated from community (CAI) and hospital (HAI) patients. From 63 AmpC producing bacteria isolates, 25 were found to be *Aeromonas* spp. Indicated below the CAI/HAI designation, are the infections the patietns presented at the point of sample collection. We found cirrhosis/hepatitis to be significantly asosiated ($p < 0.001$) infection by *Aeromonas* spp.

aimed to investigate the prevalence and diversity of ESBL and AmpC producing isolates organisms isolated from bloodstream infections over a 3-year period at a major infectious disease hospital in Vietnam.

CTX-M type ESBLs are the most prevalent ESBL enzymes to be reported, with > 170 different subtypes assigned [19, 20]. Our study identified these enzymes to be largely associated with *E. coli* isolates originating from the community. This is not surprising, as a previous studies from the same region found that healthy individuals had a high carriage rate of ESBL producing *Enterobacteriaceae* in their gastrointestinal microbiota [21]. Furthermore, we found no statistical significance in overall AMR carriage between CAI and HAI in *E. coli* harbouring an ESBL or AmpC phenotype. This observation is important and suggests equilibrium between circulating AMR organisms with the potential to cause disease in the community and the clinical setting in this location. We identified an additional ESBL gene in approximately half of the AmpC producing organisms. The presence of a co-produced ESBL may affect the interpretation of a phenotypic AmpC detection test [8, 18, 22], therefore the treatment of infections associated with suspected AmpC producing organisms with cefepime requires additional microbiological assessment for production of an ESBL.

No plasmid associated resistance genes were detected for the most prevalent AmpC producing organism identified in this study, *Aeromonas* spp. We speculate that the AmpC phenotype in these organisms was mediated by a chromosomally located AmpC gene [4, 15]. Notably, when assessing the clinical presentations associated with the AmpC producing *Aeromonas* spp., these organisms were found to be associated with cirrhosis/hepatitis. *Aeromonas* spp. are commonly identified as the agent of spontaneous bacterial peritonitis with bacteraemia in patients with liver cirrhosis, and commonly has a higher mortality rate than infections caused by alternative pathogens [23, 24]. The high prevalence of *Aeromonas* spp. mediated cirrhotic infections suggests the spread of this bacterial organism within immunocompromised chronic liver patients in HCMC, a potential association that requires longitudinal surveillance.

Conclusions

We observed a high prevalence of AmpC and ESBL expressing organisms associated with CAI and HAI bloodstream infections hospitalised patients in HCMC. We additionally report that AmpC producing *Aeromonas* spp. are potentially associated with bacteraemia in patients with underlying cirrhosis/hepatitis. With febrile disease presentations, it is routine clinical practice in this location to prescribe a broad-spectrum antimicrobial, generally a third-generation cephalosporin, to increase the likelihood of a better clinical outcome [25, 26]. However, routine hospital data suggests that there has been in increase in the proportion of ESBL producing *E. coli* isolated from blood from 45 to > 60% between 2010 and 2014. Taken together we suggest that the use of third generation cephalosporins in monotherapy may not be an optimum approach and alternatives should be assessed carefully when there is a clinical suspicion of bacteraemia, irrespective of whether this is a suspected CAI or HAI.

Additional files

Additional file 1: Figure S1. Representative results of the double disk diffusion test (A) for ESBL production and the AmpC disk test (B). Abbreviations. AMC: amoxicillin, CTX: cefotaxime, CAZ: ceftazidime, CRO: ceftriaxone, CLA: clavulanate, FEP: cefepime, FOX: cefoxitin, IPM: imipenem.

Additional file 2: Table S1. The AmpC and ESBL primers used in this study.

Additional file 3: Table S2. Summary of ESBL genes identified in 177 ESBL producing isolates.

Additional file 4: Table S3. The genetic variants of the 177 ESBL producers. Key: * indicates the isolates that produce AmpC and ESBL phenotype: E063, E080, E081, E113 and E126 . #denotes ESBL encoding isolates that encoded an AmpC gene but did not have an AmpC phenotype. The bla_{EBC} variants includes (MIR-1 and ACT-1)

Additional file 5: Figure S2. Comparison of antimicrobial susceptibility profiles between CAI and HAI of the 177 ESBL (A) and 63 AmpC (B) producing *E. coli*. (A) The AMR phenotype of the ESBL producing *E. coli* (A) (n = 162) from CAI (n = 140) or HAI (n = 22) was scored for resistance to each drug and this was expressed as a percentage relative to the number of organisms in each group (CAI or HAI). (B) The AMR phenotype of the AmpC producing *E. coli* (n = 17) from CAI (n = 13) or HAI (n = 4) was scored for resistance to each drug and this was expressed as a percentage relative to the number of organisms in each group (CAI or HAI). No significant differences ($p > 0.05$) were found in antimicrobial resistance phenotype between CAI and HAI in either ESBL or AmpC producers.

Abbreviations
AmpC: Ampicillin-hydrolyzing cephalosporinase; AMR: Antimicrobial resistance; CAI: Community acquired infections; CSF: Cerebral spinal fluid; ESBLs: Extended-spectrum β-lactamases; HAI: Hospital acquired infections; HCMC: Ho Chi Minh City; HTD: Hospital of tropical diseases

Acknowledgements
The authors wish to thank all the staff at the Hospital for Tropical Diseases for assisting in sample and data collection and patient care.

Funding
SB is a Sir Henry Dale Fellow, jointly funded by the Wellcome Trust and the Royal Society (100,087/Z/12/Z). DPT is supported by an OAK foundation fellowship.

Authors' contributions
NPHL, NHH, MJE, SB were involved in study design. NHH, TLTP, DPT, NTVT, DTTN, HTT and PW performed the laboratory experiments. NPHL, NHH, TLTP and CJB performed the analysis. GET and NWC provided clinical input and supporting data for this work. NPHL, NHH, SB and CJB wrote the manuscript, all authors contributed to and approved the final version.

Consent for publication
Not applicable.

Competing interests
The authors declare that they have no competing interests.

Author details
[1]The Hospital for Tropical Diseases, 764 Vo Van Kiet, Quan 5, Ho Chi Minh City, Vietnam. [2]Oxford University Clinical Research Unit, The Hospital for Tropical Diseases, Wellcome Trust Major Overseas Programme, Ho Chi Minh City, Vietnam. [3]Centre for Tropical Medicine and Global Health, Nuffield Department of Clinical Medicine, Oxford University, Oxford, UK. [4]Antimicrobial Resistance and Healthcare Associated Infection Unit, National Infection Service, Public Health England, Public Health England, London, UK. [5]The Department of Medicine, Cambridge University, Cambridge, UK.

References
1. WHO. Antimicrobial Resistance: World Heal Organ; 2013. http://www.who.int/mediacentre/factsheets/fs194/en/
2. Bradford P. Extended spectrum beta-lactamase in the 21 century: characterization, epidemiology, and detection of this important resistant threat. Clin Microbiol Rev. 2001;14:933–51. https://doi.org/10.1128/CMR.14.4.933.
3. Doi Y, Paterson DL. Detection of plasmid-mediated class C β-lactamases. Int J Infect Dis. 2007;11:191–7.
4. Jacoby GA. AmpC β-Lactamases. Clin Microbiol Rev. 2009;22:161–82.
5. Gupta G, Tak V, Mathur P. Detection of AmpC β Lactamases in gram-negative bacteria. J Lab Physicians. 2014;6:1–6. https://doi.org/10.4103/0974-2727.129082.
6. Black JA, Moland ES, Thomson KS. AmpC disk test for detection of plasmid-mediated AmpC β-lactamases in Enterobacteriaceae lacking chromosomal AmpC beta-lactamases. J Clin Microbiol. 2005;43:3110–3.
7. Pérez-Pérez FJ, Hanson ND. Detection of plasmid-mediated AmpC beta-lactamase genes in clinical isolates by using multiplex PCR. J Clin Microbiol. 2002;40:2153–62. https://doi.org/10.1128/jcm.40.6.2153-2162.2002.
8. Song W, Moland ES, Hanson ND, Lewis JS, Jorgensen JH, Thomson KS. Failure of cefepime therapy in treatment of Klebsiella Pneumoniae bacteremia. J Clin Microbiol. 2005;43:4891–4. https://doi.org/10.1128/JCM.43.9.4891-4894.2005.
9. Steward CD, Rasheed JK, Hubert SK, Biddle JW, Raney PM, Anderson GJ, et al. Characterization of clinical isolates of Klebsiella Pneumoniae from 19 laboratories using the National Committee for clinical laboratory standards extended-spectrum beta-lactamase detection methods. J Clin Microbiol. 2001;39:2864–72. https://doi.org/10.1128/JCM.39.8.2864-2872.2001.
10. Thomson KS. Controversies about extended-spectrum and AmpC beta-lactamases. Emerg Infect Dis. 2001;7:333–6.
11. CLSI. Performance standards for antimicrobial susceptibility testing, M100-S20. Wayne: PA Clin Lab Stand Institute; 2010.
12. Jarlier V, Nicolas MH, Fournier G, Philippon A. Extended broad-spectrum beta-lactamases conferring transferable resistance to newer beta-lactam agents in Enterobacteriaceae: hospital prevalence and susceptibility patterns. Rev Infect Dis. 10:867–878. http://www.ncbi.nlm.nih.gov/pubmed/3263690. Accessed 21 Feb 2017
13. Ingram PR, Inglis TJJ, Vanzetti TR, Henderson BA, Harnett GB, Murray RJ. Comparison of methods for AmpC β-lactamase detection in enterobacteriaceae. J Med Microbiol. 2011;60:715–21.
14. Cantarelli W. Inamine E, Brodt TCZ, Secchi C, Cavalcante BC, Pereira F de S. Utility of the ceftazidime-imipenem antagonism test (CIAT) to detect and confirm the presence of inducible AmpC beta-lactamases among enterobacteriaceae. Braz J Infect Dis. 2007;11:237–9. https://doi.org/10.1590/S1413-86702007000200014.
15. Philippon A, Arlet G, Jacoby GA. Plasmid-determined AmpC-type beta-lactamases. Antimicrob Agents Chemother. 2002;46:1–11. https://doi.org/10.1128/aac.46.1.1-11.2002.
16. Xiong Z, Li T, Xu Y, Li J. Detection of CTX-M-14 extended-spectrum β-lactamase in Shigella sonnei isolates from China. J Inf Secur. 2007;55:7–10.
17. Lonchel Magou C, Melin P, Gangoue-Pieboji J, Okomo Assoumou M, Boreux R, De Mol P. Prevalence and spread of extended- spectrum b-lactamase-producing Enterobacteriaceae in Ngaoundere, Cameroon. Clin Microbiol Infect. 2013;19:E416–20.
18. Hanson ND. AmpC β-lactamases: what do we need to know for the future? J Antimicrob Chemother. 2003;52:2–4.
19. Pitout JDD, Laupland KB. Review extended-spectrum β-lactamase-producing Enterobacteriaceae: an emerging public-health concern. Lancet Infect Dis. 2008;8(3):159–66.
20. Lahey Clinic. ß-Lactamase classification and amino acid sequences for TEM, SHV and OXA extended-Spectrum and inhibitor resistant enzymes. 2016. https://www.lahey.org/studies/.
21. Le TMV, Baker S, Le TPT, Le TPT, Cao TT, Tran TTN, et al. High prevalence of plasmid-mediated quinolone resistance determinants in commensal members of the Enterobacteriaceae in ho chi Minh City, Vietnam. J Med Microbiol. 2009;58(Pt 12):1585–92. https://doi.org/10.1099/jmm.0.010033-0.

22. Thomson N, Baker S, Pickard D, Fookes M, Anjum M, Hamlin N, et al. The role of prophage-like elements in the diversity of salmonella enterica serovars. J Mol Biol. 2004;339:279–300.
23. Lau SM, Peng MY, Chang FY. Outcomes of Aeromonas bacteremia in patients with different types of underlying disease. J Microbiol Immunol Infect. 2000;33:241–7. http://www.ncbi.nlm.nih.gov/pubmed/11269369. Accessed 20 Feb 2017
24. Llopis F, Grau I, Tubau F, Cisnal M, Pallares R. Epidemiological and clinical characteristics of bacteraemia caused by Aeromonas spp. as compared with Escherichia Coli and Pseudomonas Aeruginosa. Scand J Infect Dis. 2004;36:335–41. http://www.ncbi.nlm.nih.gov/pubmed/15287377. Accessed 20 Feb 2017
25. Kollef MH. Broad-Spectrum antimicrobials and the treatment of serious bacterial infections: getting it right up front. Clin Infect Dis. 2008;47:S3–13. https://doi.org/10.1086/590061.
26. Kollef M. Appropriate empirical antibacterial therapy for nosocomial infections: getting it right the first time. Drugs. 2003;63:2157–68. http://www.ncbi.nlm.nih.gov/pubmed/14498753. Accessed 21 Feb 2017

5

Genotypic characterization of gentamicin and cephalosporin resistant *Escherichia coli* isolates from blood cultures in a Norwegian university hospital 2011–2015

Øyvind Andreas Fladberg[1,2], Silje Bakken Jørgensen[1] and Hege Vangstein Aamot[1,3*]

Abstract

Background: Cephalosporin resistance in clinical *E. coli* isolates is increasing internationally. The increase has been caused by virulent and often multidrug-resistant clones, especially the extended spectrum β-lactamase (ESBL) producing *E. coli* clone O25b-ST131.

Methods: In Norway, recommended empirical treatment of sepsis consists of gentamicin and penicillin combined, or a broad-spectrum cephalosporin. To investigate if increased gentamicin and cephalosporins resistance rates in our hospital could be caused by specific clones, we conducted a retrospective study on *E. coli* blood culture isolates from 2011 through 2015. All *E. coli* isolates non-susceptible to gentamicin and/or third-generation cephalosporins were genotyped using multiple-locus variable-number of tandem repeat analysis (MLVA) and compared with antibiotic susceptible isolates. The frequency of the most common genes causing ESBL production (bla_{CTX-M}, bla_{ampC}) was examined by Real-Time PCR.

Results: A total of 158 cephalosporin and/or gentamicin resistant and 97 control isolates were differentiated into 126 unique MLVA types. Of these, 31% of the isolates belonged to a major MLVA cluster consisting of 41% of the gentamicin resistant and 35% of the cephalosporin resistant isolates. The majority (65/80 isolates) of this MLVA cluster contained MLVA types associated with the *E. coli* O25b-ST131 clone. Genes encoding CTX-M enzyme phylogroups 1 and 9 occurred in 65% and 19% of cephalosporin resistant isolates, respectively, whereas $bla_{ampC-CIT}$ was identified in 3%.

Conclusion: No local *E. coli* bacteraemia clone was identified. Antibiotic resistance was dispersed over a variety of genotypes. However, association with the international *E. coli* O25b-ST131 clone was frequent and may be an important driver behind increased resistance rates. Monitoring and preventing dissemination of these resistant clones are important for continued optimal treatment.

Keywords: ESBL, CTX-M, AmpC, MLVA, Bacteraemia, *E. coli*, Antibiotic resistance, Genotyping, Surveillance

Background

Escherichia coli (E. coli) is the most common cause of bacteraemia [1–3]. In Norway, national recommendations for empirical treatment of sepsis are gentamicin and penicillin combined, or a broad-spectrum cephalosporin (https://helsedirektoratet.no/retningslinjer/antibiotika-i-sykehus, accessed 22. June 2017). According to the Norwegian surveillance programme for antimicrobial resistance in human pathogens (NORM), resistance to gentamicin in *E. coli* from blood cultures more than tripled the last decade from 2.0% in 2005 to 6.4% in 2015 [3, 4]. The prevalence of extended β-lactamases (ESBLs) increased from 0.5 to 6.5% in the same period. In 2015, approximately 40% of the gentamicin resistant isolates also produced ESBLs, but with large variations between different Norwegian hospitals [3].

* Correspondence: hege.vangstein.aamot@ahus.no
[1]Department of Microbiology and Infection Control, Akershus University Hospital, Lørenskog, Norway
[3]Department of Clinical Molecular Biology (EpiGen), Division of Medicine, Akershus University Hospital and University of Oslo, Lørenskog, Norway
Full list of author information is available at the end of the article

ESBLs are the leading cause of resistance to broad-spectrum cephalosporins in *E. coli*, together with AmpC-enzymes and enzymes also conferring resistance to carbapenems [5]. The most common ESBLs are the CTX-M enzyme family [2]. The family is divided into six phylogroups, where CTX-M phylogroup 1 is the most frequent. The dominance of CTX-M can be attributed to the successful *E. coli* clone O25b-ST131 carrying CTX-M-15, belonging to CTX-M-1 phylogroup, [6, 7] and the association with conjugative plasmids [8]. Among the plasmid-borne AmpC β-lactamases, there are six groups of AmpC genes of which the bla_{CMY-2} is the most common [2].

Use of molecular typing methods is essential in both surveillance and outbreak investigations as well as in tracking of evolutionary trends of microbes in both the community and healthcare settings. Pulsed field gel electrophoresis (PFGE), the previous "gold standard" typing method, has become outdated due to a time-consuming and labour-intensive protocol. Multilocus sequence typing (MLST) is widely used and has an advantage as the generated data can easily be shared between laboratories. However, this method does not give sufficient resolution for local outbreak investigations [9]. Whole genome sequencing is on the rise, but is still sub-optimal for small-scale surveillance and outbreak investigations in real-time. Multiple-locus variable-number of tandem repeat analysis (MLVA) has been performed to assess clonal relatedness between *E. coli* isolates. It has been reported as a rapid, accurate and cost-effective genotyping tool suitable as a "first-line-of-defense" method for epidemiological surveillance of multidrug-resistant *E. coli* [9–12]. In previous studies, *E. coli* O25b-ST131 has been shown to be associated with distinct MLVA types [9, 11–13].

Managing antibiotic resistance is a global issue and in order to limit dissemination effectively, monitoring genotypes and resistance mechanisms is vital [14]. To investigate if gentamicin resistance in *E. coli* bacteraemia was linked to one or several clones co-resistant to cephalosporins, we performed MLVA on all gentamicin and/or third-generation cephalosporin resistant *E. coli* from diagnostic blood cultures at our hospital from 2011 to 2015. MLVA analysis was chosen due to technological availability and low cost. In addition, the analysis is easy to perform and the data generated is simple to handle and interpret. We also wanted to investigate the prevalence of genes causing ESBL production.

Methods

Study design and setting

This retrospective cross-sectional study was performed at Akershus University Hospital (Ahus), Lørenskog, Norway. Ahus delivers public health services to ~ 500,000 people and is the largest acute care hospital in Norway.

Culturing and antibiotic susceptibility testing

All gentamicin non-susceptible ($N = 102$) and/or third-generation cephalosporin (ceftazidime and/or cefotaxime) non-susceptible ($N = 101$) *E. coli* from diagnostic blood cultures at Ahus from 2011 to 2015 were included (one isolate per patient per year). Co-resistance to gentamicin and cephalosporins were present in 45 isolates, hence a total of 158 non-susceptible isolates were included. Additionally, gentamicin sensitive and third-generation cephalosporin sensitive isolates ($n = 97$, ~ 20/year, one isolate per patient), were included as controls. A sample flow chart is presented in Fig. 1.

The samples were cultured in the BD BACTEC FX blood culture system (BD Diagnostics, Heidelberg, Germany) and identification was performed by conventional fermentation reactions or mass spectrometry (MALDI-TOF, Bruker Daltonics, Bremen, Germany). Phenotypic antibiotic susceptibility testing was determined using disk diffusion tests according to the Nordic committee on Antimicrobial Susceptibility Testing guidelines (www.NordicAST.org). ESBL phenotypes were detected by the disk approximation test [15], and AmpC phenotypes were detected by AmpC MIC strips (Etest, BioMérieux, Marcy l'Etolie, France and Mic Test Strip, Liofilchem, Roseto degli Abruzzi, Italy).

Intermediate and resistant (non-susceptible) phenotypes were combined in further analysis. Hence, in the following, all non-susceptible isolates, i.e. intermediate or resistant according to EUCAST (European Committee on Antimicrobial Susceptibility Testing) break points (www.eucast.org), are referred to as resistant.

Multiple-locus variable-number tandem repeat analysis (MLVA)

All isolates from blood cultures were stored at −80 °C. DNA was extracted by boil lysis before standardisation [10 ng/μL]. MLVA was performed according to published protocol by Linstedt and co-workers using seven alleles [16] with modification by Løbersli and co-workers [17]. Fragment analysis was performed by capillary electrophoresis on the 3130xl Genetic Analyzer (Applied Biosystems, Sint-Martens-Letem, Belgium). Determination of MLVA types and creation of minimum spanning trees were performed using BioNumerics software (Applied Biosystems 7.1). No PCR product was denoted as "-2", whereas no repeats was denoted as "0". Otherwise, the allele numbers reflect the number of repeats found in each locus. The MLVA types were numbered consecutively and designations are unique to this work (Additional file 1: Table S1). Dendrograms were constructed using categorical coefficients and the Ward algorithm and a standard minimum spanning tree was generated using categorical coefficients together with the single and double locus variance priority rules.

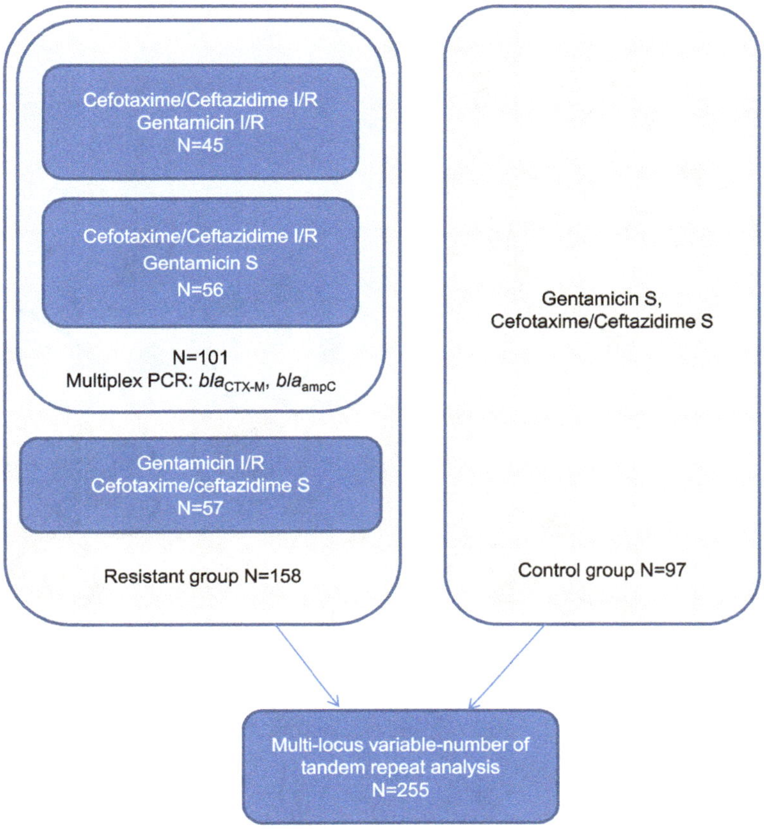

Fig. 1 Sample flow chart of the selected *E. coli* isolates from blood cultures. S = susceptible, I = intermediate, R = resistant

CTX-M Real-Time PCR

CTX-M Real-Time PCR was performed according to published protocol with minor modifications [18]. The original quadplex Real-Time PCR was divided into a duplex for CTX-M enzyme phylogroups 1 and 9, and a singleplex for CTX-M phylogroup 2. Due to low occurrence of CTX-M variants detected exclusively with the degenerate probe in the population, this probe was excluded. Analysis was performed on ABI PRISM 7900HT sequence detection system (Applied Biosystems, Foster City, CA, USA) with two detectors (FAM and VIC) in addition to ROX as passive reference.

AmpC Real-Time PCR

Detection of plasmid-borne AmpC was performed on phenotypically AmpC positive isolates according to published protocol with minor modifications [19]. The modified protocol was limited to detection of the most frequent genes previously described in Norway [20], bla_{DHA} and a combination of bla_{CIT} and bla_{CMY}.

Results

From 2011 to 2015, 1475 *E. coli* isolates were derived from blood cultures. Of these, 102 (6.9%) were resistant to gentamicin and 101 (6.8%) were resistant to third-generation cephalosporins. 45 (3.1%) of the isolates were co-resistant to both drugs. Of the 101 third-generation cephalosporins resistant isolates, 85 (84%) were phenotypically positive for ESBL and 13 (13%) positive for the AmpC phenotype test.

MLVA

Distribution of antibiotic resistance profiles by MLVA types (MTs) is presented in Fig. 2. The 158 antibiotic resistant isolates and 97 controls were differentiated into 126 unique MLVA types. A total of 65 (25%) of the isolates had MLVA types previously associated with O25b-ST131 (MT: 6, −2, −2, 14, 3, X, 5) [9, 11, 13] of which 7 (3%) were antibiotic susceptible controls. Of the gentamicin resistant isolates, 42/102 (41%) belonged to this cluster, as did 35/101 (35%) of the cephalosporin resistant isolates. For overview of all MLVA types see Additional file 1: Table S1. The occurrence of the ST131 associated MLVA types varied from seven to 17 per year (Fig 3) among the antibiotic resistant isolates and the number increased during the study period.

There was no exclusive association between MLVA type and phenotypic resistance, but resistance to third-

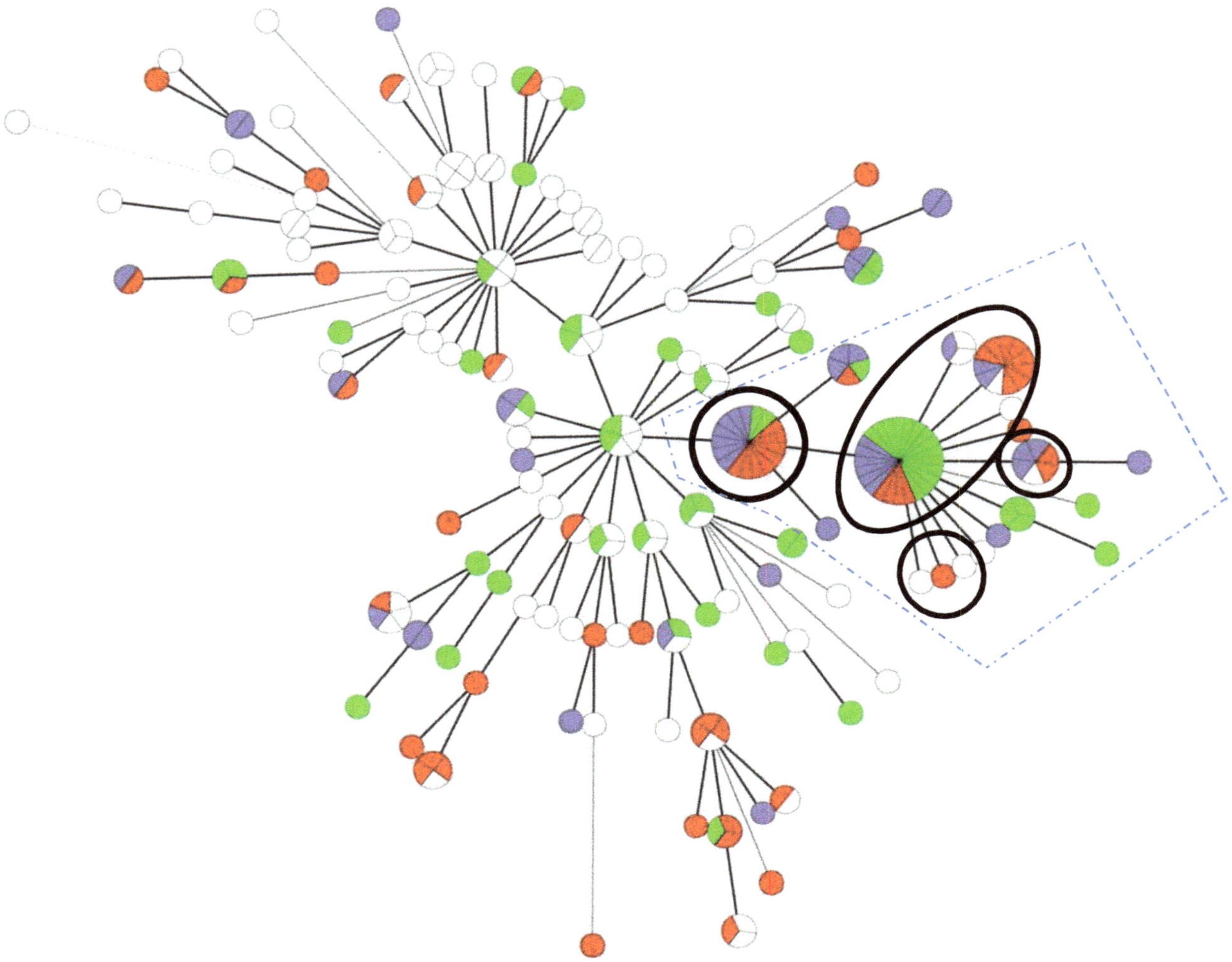

Fig. 2 Minimum spanning tree based on the 126 MLVA types (MTs) found in 256 *E. coli* bacteraemia isolates from 2011 to 2015. The isolates are coloured by phenotypic resistance. White: cephalosporin S and gentamicin S, *green* cephalosporin R and gentamicin S, *red*: cephalosporin S and gentamicin R, purple: cephalosporin R and gentamicin R. One disk represents one MT. Disk size indicates the number of isolates in the MT. The length of branches specifies how many Variable Number of Tandem Repeats (VNTR) loci are different, where the shortest branches indicate 1 VNTR loci separating MTs. This only applies to adjacent MLVA disks. Encircled MTs are associated with the international *E. coli* O25b-ST131 clone. *Dotted line* indicates the major MLVA cluster

generation cephalosporins dominated the largest MLVA type (MT 79, 20/24 isolates, Fig 2).

CTX-M and AmpC prevalence

A total of 85/101 (84%) of the isolates resistant to third-generation cephalosporin were positive for CTX-M genes corresponding to the 85 isolates positive for ESBL phenotype. CTX-M phylogroup 1 was most common with 66/101 isolates. CTX-M phylogroup 9 was identified in 18/101 isolates. In addition, one isolate was positive for both phylogroups 1 and 9. The remaining 16 isolates were negative for $bla_{\text{CTX-M}}$. None of the isolates were positive for CTX-M phylogroup 2.

Of the 13/101 third-generation cephalosporin resistant isolates that were phenotypically positive for the AmpC-test, three were positive for plasmid-borne AmpC genes, all of which were $bla_{\text{CIT/CMY2}}$. No isolate carried the combination of $bla_{\text{CTX-M}}$ and $bla_{\text{CIT/CMY2}}$ genes. However, two isolates that were phenotypically AmpC (presumptively identified as chromosomal-encoded AmpC) also contained genes from CTX-M phylogroup 1. With the combination of CTX-M Real-Time PCR and phenotypic AmpC, we identified the cause of resistance in 96/101 (95%) of the third-generation cephalosporin resistant isolates.

Discussion

The 7-locus MLVA identified several frequent clones in blood cultures at our hospital. They were found both in community-onset bacteremia and in hospital-acquired

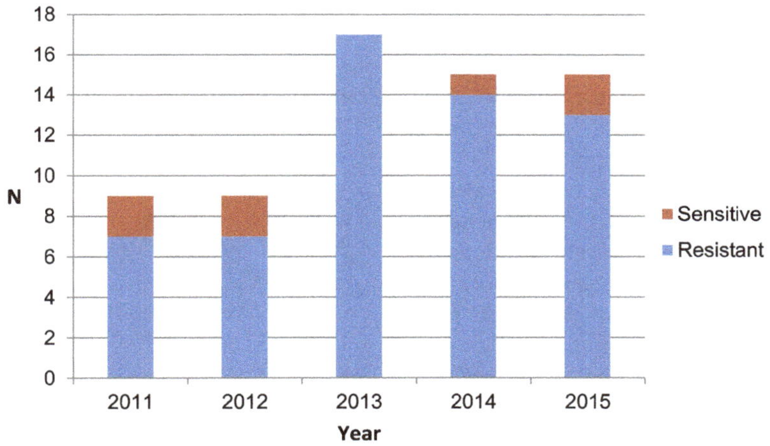

Fig. 3 Number of *E. coli* isolates with MLVA type associated with *E. coli* O25b-ST131 clone per year of inclusion

infections from different hospital wards and spread over a large time span. Hence, MLVA did not identify a hospital specific clone. However, MLVA did show that gentamicin and third-generation cephalosporin resistant isolates are more similar than antibiotic sensitive *E. coli*, i.e. they are more likely to belong to certain MLVA types. MLVA identified a large cluster that almost exclusively consisted of antibiotic resistant isolates. In this cluster, gentamicin resistance was more frequent than cephalosporin resistance or resistance to both drugs. An association between the O25b-ST131 clone and MTs (6, −2, −2, 14, 3, X, 5) has previously been described [6, 8, 11, 21] and the number of isolates with these MLVA types increased during the study period (Fig 3). Half (9/18) of the MLVA types in this cluster, containing 65/80 of the isolates, are associated with the pandemic O25b-ST131 clone, illustrating the considerable disease contribution from O25b-ST131 in an otherwise heterogenic population.

Gentamicin resistance was even more frequent than cephalosporin resistance in the O25b-ST131 associated MLVA types. Genes conferring aminoglycoside resistance and $bla_{\mathrm{CTX\text{-}M}}$ may occur on the same plasmids [22]. Gentamicin resistance can also be caused by adaptive mechanisms, such as membrane protein changes and regulation of genes involved in the anaerobic respiratory pathway.

Globally, the dominating cause of ESBL is the CTX-M enzyme family [2, 23]. The prevalence of the most common ESBL genes was as anticipated with CTX-M phylogroup 1 as the most frequent (65%) followed by CTX-M phylogroup 9 (19%) which is in accordance with previously published findings [3, 24]. CTX-M was highly prevalent (84%) among third-generation cephalosporin resistant isolates in this study. The absence of CTX-M phylogroup 2 was as expected. The Norwegian National Advisory Unit of Antimicrobial Resistance did not detect this CTX-M group in blood culture isolates from 2000 through 2014 [3] and a Swedish study reported that only 2 of 1003 (<0.002%) of urinary tract infection derived *E. coli* isolates were CTX-M phylogroup 2 [24]. With the combination of methods employed in this study we determined the cause of resistance in 95% of the isolates with third-generation cephalosporin resistance. The resistance mechanisms in the remaining isolates can possibly be explained by loss of porins resulting in lower permeability, loss of the resistance plasmid [25] or other CTX-M phylogroups.

Surveillance of plasmid-borne CTX-M and AmpC in combination with interventions to limit their dissemination can ensure longevity of the current recommendations for empirical sepsis treatment. Adequate, real-time surveillance should be employed in hospitals to identify outbreaks of antibiotic resistant and virulent strains in order to stop dissemination as early as possible. Parallel analysis of genotype and detection of resistance genes by Real-Time PCR is a pragmatic way of ensuring early outbreak detection. Using MLVA with only 3 VNTRs (CVN001, CVN004, CVN014) has been suggested to be adequate for epidemiological screening of ESBL-producing *E.coli* [9]. In our study, using the 3 VNTR MLVA would have given 84 MLVA types compared to the 126 MLVA types with all 7 VNTRs reducing the number of MLVA types with 33%. However, the differentiation of O25b-ST131 associated MLVA types was identical between 3 and 7 VNTR MLVA resulting in 9 MLVA types with both methods. As O25b-ST131 associated MLVA types comprised several major MLVA types in our study, complementary techniques may be necessary to differentiate among O25b-ST131 isolates in local outbreak investigations, as previously reported by Helldal and co-workers [9].

There are limitations to our study. Only a random selection of antibiotic sensitive *E. coli* bacteraemia isolates was included as controls for MLVA typing (~ 20 isolates per year of inclusion). Therefore, the specific MLVA types they represent may be biased. In general, however, they show more heterogeneity than the antibiotic resistant *E. coli* isolates. The Real-Time PCR for detection of CTX-M phylogroups was designed only to detect the three most common phylogroups (1, 2 and 9) leaving a possibility for false negatives. However, the prevalence of other phylogroups is low in Norway [3] and we detected the cause of resistance in 95% of the cephalosporin resistant isolates. The number of phenotypic AmpC positive *E. coli* to include in the study was scarce. Yet, over the 5 years included in the study, a total of 1475 *E. coli* was identified and they were all potential candidates for inclusion. The performed Real-Time PCR detected the two most common AmpC groups constituting 99% of previously reported cases [20]. Therefore, in the case of isolates negative for plasmid-borne AmpC, chromosome-encoded AmpC was presumptively identified. Extrapolation of data from this study should consider that isolates were extracted from individuals in a specific geographic region.

Conclusion

No local *E. coli* bacteraemia clone was identified. However, a large cluster of related MLVA types, comprising 25% of the isolates, was associated with the international *E. coli* O25b-ST131 clone suggesting that this clone is a major driver behind the increase in cephalosporin and gentamicin resistance in an otherwise heterogenic population. Resistance to third-generation cephalosporins was identified in 95% of the isolates with presence of genes coding for CTX-M phylogroup 1 as the most frequent cause of resistance. Monitoring and preventing dissemination of these resistant clones are important for continued optimal treatment.

Abbreviations

E. coli: *Escherichia coli*; ESBL: Extended spectrum β-lactamase; MLVA: Multiple-locus variable-number of tandem repeat analysis; MT: MLVA type; VNTR: Variable number of tandem repeat

Acknowledgements

The authors thank the Norwegian National Advisory Unit of Antimicrobial Resistance (K-res) for control isolates in connection with Real-Time PCR testing.

Funding

None

Authors contributions

Concept and design; SBJ, HVA. Laboratory analyses; ØAF, HVA. Data interpretation; ØF, SBJ, HVA. Writing and revising manuscript; ØF, SBJ, HVA. All authors read and approved the final manuscript.

Consent for publication

Not applicable

Competing interests

The authors declare that they have no competing interests.

Author details

[1]Department of Microbiology and Infection Control, Akershus University Hospital, Lørenskog, Norway. [2]Department of Medical Biochemistry and Microbiology, Uppsala University, Uppsala, Sweden. [3]Department of Clinical Molecular Biology (EpiGen), Division of Medicine, Akershus University Hospital and University of Oslo, Lørenskog, Norway.

References

1. Laupland KB, Gregson DB, Church DL, Ross T, Pitout JD. Incidence, risk factors and outcomes of *Escherichia coli* bloodstream infections in a large Canadian region. Clin Microbiol Infect. 2008; doi:10.1111/j.1469-0691.2008.02089.x.
2. European Center for Disease Prevention and Control. Antimicrobial resistance surveillance in Europe 2014. Annual report of the European antimicrobial resistance surveillance network (EARS-net). Stockholm: ECDC; 2015.
3. Norm/Norm-Vet 2015. Usage of antimicrobial agents and occurrence of antimicrobial resistance in Norway. Tromsø/Oslo; 2016. ISSN:1502-2307 (print) / 1890-9965 (electronic).
4. Norm/Norm-Vet 2005. Usage of antimicrobial agents and occurrence of antimicrobial Resistance in Norway. Tromsø/Oslo; 2006. ISSN:1502-2307.
5. Pitout JD. Infections with extended-spectrum beta-lactamase-producing enterobacteriaceae: changing epidemiology and drug treatment choices. Drugs 2010. doi:10.2165/11533040-000000000-00000.
6. Nicolas-Chanoine MH, Blanco J, Leflon-Guibout V, Demarty R, Alonso MP, Canica MM, Park YJ, Lavigne JP, Pitout J, Johnson JR. Intercontinental emergence of *Escherichia coli* clone O25:H4-ST131 producing CTX-M-15. J Antimicrob Chemother. 2008;61:273–81.
7. Coque TM, Novais A, Carattoli A, Poirel L, Pitout J, Peixe L, Baquero F, Canton R, Nordmann P. Dissemination of clonally related *Escherichia coli* strains expressing extended-spectrum beta-lactamase CTX-M-15. Emerg Infect Dis. 2008;14:195–200.
8. Rogers BA, Sidjabat HE, Paterson DL. *Escherichia coli* O25b-ST131: a pandemic, multiresistant, community-associated strain. J Antimicrob Chemother. 2011;66:1–14.
9. Helldal L, Karami N, Welinder-Olsson C, Moore ER, Ahren C. Evaluation of MLVA for epidemiological typing and outbreak detection of ESBL-producing *Escherichia coli* in Sweden. BMC Microbiol. 2017;17:8.
10. Christiansson M, Melin S, Matussek A, Lofgren S, Soderman J. MLVA is a valuable tool in epidemiological investigations of *Escherichia coli* and for disclosing multiple carriage. Scand J Infect Dis. 2011;43:579–86.
11. Naseer U, Olsson-Liljequist BE, Woodford N, Dhanji H, Canton R, Sundsfjord A, Lindstedt BA. Multi-locus variable number of tandem repeat analysis for rapid and accurate typing of virulent multidrug resistant *Escherichia coli* clones. PLoS One. 2012;7:e41232.
12. Karami N, Helldal L, Welinder-Olsson C, Ahren C, Moore ER. Sub-typing of extended-spectrum-beta-lactamase-producing isolates from a nosocomial outbreak: application of a 10-loci generic *Escherichia coli* multi-locus variable number tandem repeat analysis. PLoS One. 2013;8:e83030.
13. Jørgensen SB, Soraas A, Sundsfjord A, Liestol K, Leegaard TM, Jenum PA. Fecal carriage of extended spectrum beta-lactamase producing *Escherichia coli* and *Klebsiella pneumoniae* after urinary tract infection - a three year prospective cohort study. PLoS One. 2017;12:e0173510.
14. Mathers AJ, Peirano G, Pitout JD. The role of epidemic resistance plasmids and international high-risk clones in the spread of multidrug-resistant Enterobacteriaceae. Clin Microbiol Rev. 2015;28:565–91.
15. Jarlier V, Nicolas MH, Fournier G, Philippon A. Extended broad-spectrum beta-lactamases conferring transferable resistance to newer beta-lactam agents in Enterobacteriaceae: hospital prevalence and susceptibility patterns. Rev Infect Dis. 1988;10:867–78.
16. Lindstedt BA, Brandal LT, Aas L, Vardund T, Kapperud G. Study of polymorphic variable-number of tandem repeats loci in the ECOR collection and in a set of

pathogenic *Escherichia coli* and Shigella isolates for use in a genotyping assay. J Microbiol Method. 2007;69:197–205.
17. Løbersli I, Haugum K, Lindstedt BA. Rapid and high resolution genotyping of all *Escherichia coli* serotypes using 10 genomic repeat-containing loci. J Microbiol Methods. 2012;88:134–9.
18. Birkett CI, Ludlam HA, Woodford N, Brown DF, Brown NM, Roberts MT, Milner N, Curran MD. Real-time TaqMan PCR for rapid detection and typing of genes encoding CTX-M extended-spectrum beta-lactamases. J Med Microbiol. 2007;56:52–5.
19. Swayne R, Ellington MJ, Curran MD, Woodford N, Aliyu SH. Utility of a novel multiplex TaqMan PCR assay for metallo-beta-lactamase genes plus other TaqMan assays in detecting genes encoding serine carbapenemases and clinically significant extended-spectrum beta-lactamases. Int J Antimicrob Agents. 2013;42:352–6.
20. Norwegian National Advisory Unit of Antimicrobial Resistance. Summary and analysis of Enterobacteriaceae isolates with chromosomeal (cAmpC) or plasmid-mediated AmpC (ESBL M-C) sent to K-res in the period 2010–2012. 2013.
21. Johnson JR, Menard M, Johnston B, Kuskowski MA, Nichol K, Zhanel GG. Epidemic clonal groups of *Escherichia coli* as a cause of antimicrobial-resistant urinary tract infections in Canada, 2002 to 2004. Antimicrob Agents Chemother. 2009;53:2733–9.
22. Carattoli A. Resistance plasmid families in Enterobacteriaceae. Antimicrob Agents Chemother. 2009;53:2227–38.
23. Center for Disease Dynamics, Economics Policy. State of the World's Anitbiotics, 2015. Washington, D.C.: CDDEP; 2015.
24. Brolund A, Edquist PJ, Makitalo B, Olsson-Liljequist B, Soderblom T, Wisell KT, Giske CG. Epidemiology of extended-spectrum beta-lactamase-producing *Escherichia coli* in Sweden 2007-2011. Clin Microbiol Infect. 2014;20:O344–52.
25. Heesemann J. Mechanisms of resistance to beta-lactam antibiotics. Infection. 1993;21(Suppl 1):S4–9.

6

Prevalence of antimicrobial resistant pathogens from blood cultures: results from a laboratory based nationwide surveillance in Ghana

Japheth Awuletey Opintan* and Mercy Jemima Newman

Abstract

Background: Blood stream infections (BSI) are critical medical conditions with high morbidity and mortality. There is paucity of information on BSI from surveillance studies in Ghana.

Aim: This study sought to demonstrate how useful BSI data can be gleaned from population-based surveillance, especially from resource-limited settings.

Methods: Data from a nationwide surveillance of antimicrobial drug resistance (AMR) in Ghana were extracted and analyzed. Secondly, we revived archived *Staphylococcus aureus* isolates from blood cultures that were cefoxitin resistant (CRSA), and screened these for protein A (*spa*) and *mec* A genes.

Results: Overall blood culture positivity was 11.2% (714/6351). All together, participating laboratories submitted 100 multidrug resistant blood culture isolates (Gram-negative = 49 and Gram-positive = 51). Prevalence of some Gram-negative isolates was as follows; *Escherichia coli* (20.4%), *Pseudomonas aeruginosa* (16.3%), *Enterobacter* spp. (14.3%), *Salmonella* serotype Typhi (8.2%) and Non-typhoidal *Salmonella* [NTS] (8.2%). Gram-positive pathogens included *Staphylococcus aureus* (66.7%), coagulase negative *S. aureus* [CoNS] (17.6%) and *Streptococcus pneumoniae* (11.8%). No methicillin resistance was confirmed in our CRSA isolates. Most blood stream associated infections were from inpatients (75%) and cultured bacteria were resistant to common and cheaper antimicrobials.

Conclusion: *E. coli* and *S. aureus* are common pathogens associated with BSI in Ghana and they are resistant to several antimicrobials. Active and continuous AMR surveillance can serve multiple purposes, including data generation for BSI.

Keywords: Bloodstream infections, Antimicrobial drug resistance, Blood culture, Surveillance, Methicillin resistance

Background

Bloodstream infections (BSI) are important cause of morbidity and mortality, that require prompt and appropriate empiric therapy before blood culture results are ready. The management of BSI is further complicated in an era of increasing antimicrobial resistance (AMR) [1]. Empiric antimicrobial therapy when administered early in the course of BSI has the potential to save lives [2]. However, the epidemiology of the causative agents are not static, constantly changing over time [3]. Especially in resource limiting settings with inadequate laboratory support for culture and antimicrobial surveillance, BSI management is further complicated.

Several resource-rich countries have surveillance systems in place to monitor changing trends of infections including BSI. Examples include the Health Protection Agency (HPA) in England [3] and the Canadian Antimicrobial Resistance Alliance (CARA) [4]. These surveillance systems readily provide useful data on microorganisms of clinical significance, including those associated with BSI, providing clues on aetiological trends and AMR. Active surveillance systems are non-existent in most resource-limited countries including Ghana, in spite of the high disease in

* Correspondence: jaopintan@ug.edu.gh
Medical Microbiology Department, School of Biomedical and Allied Health Sciences, Korle-Bu, P. O. Box KB 4236, Accra, Ghana

these countries. Several local studies, especially in tertiary care facilities have been done in Ghana and elsewhere, but these are either disease condition or age specific [5–8]. In a previous study, we presented the overall results of a nationwide surveillance. In that study, only about 40% of participating hospitals provided data on blood culture results. In the present study, we focused on blood stream infections and analyzed the data on blood culture results that we did receive by those 40% of participating hospitals. We did this to emphasize the importance of more detailed information that can be obtained from more detailed reporting, and to encourage better participation in such nationwide surveillance.

Methods

Data on bloodstream infections (BSI), including patient information, bacterial isolates and their antibiogram were electronically extracted from our surveillance records [9]. The Department of Medical Microbiology, School of Biomedical and Allied Health Sciences (DM-SBAHS) coordinated this surveillance, June–November 2014. Participating laboratories used in-house standard operating procedures to culture and to identify bacteria from all specimens submitted for bacteriological analysis. Antimicrobial susceptibility testing was done by the disc diffusion test, in accordance with the Clinical and Laboratory Standards Institute [10] guidelines. Multiple drug resistant isolates, defined as resistance to more than two antimicrobial drug classes were submitted to DM-SBAHS. The location and description of participating laboratories are described elsewhere [9] and included Teaching, Regional, District and Faith-based hospitals in Ghana.

We analyzed data on all blood cultures submitted by participating laboratories to DM-SBAHS. To confirm methicillin resistant *Staphylococcus aureus* (MRSA), all stored cefoxitin-resistant *S. aureus* (CRSA) isolates were revived on blood agar plates. The identities of these CRSA were reconfirmed by Gram stain, catalase and tube coagulase tests. Genomic DNAs were extracted from pure CRSA isolates and were then screened by polymerase chain reaction for *Staphylococcus*-specific genes (*spa* and *mecA*), using previous protocols [11]. Data on BSI were stratified by age, isolate source and hospital facility and were summarized in tables or percentages.

Results

In total, 11 of 18 (61.1%) laboratories processed and submitted surveillance data on blood cultures. The overall culture positivity rate was 11.2% (714/6351) with great variabilities ranging between 4.7–27.3% (Table 1). Total number of non-duplicate multidrug resistant blood isolates received from participating laboratories was 100 (Gram-negative, n = 49; Gram-positive, n = 51). Blood culture Gram-negative (GN) isolates included *Escherichia coli* (20.4%), *Pseudomonas aeruginosa* (16.3%), *Enterobacter* spp. (14.3%), *Salmonella* Typhi (8.2%) and Non-Typhoidal Salmonella [NTS] (8.2%). *E. coli* was predominantly isolated from patients aged older than 10 years. Other GN rods like typhoidal and NTS were mostly recovered from children less than 10 years of age [Table 2]. Gram-positive (GP) isolates included *Staphylococcus aureus* (66.7%), coagulase negative *Staphylococcus* [CNS] (17.6%) and *Streptococcus pneumoniae* (11.8%). *Staphylococus* and *Streptococcus* were generally recovered from children less than 10 years. However many patients with staphylococcal associated BSI had missing data for age (Table 2). Multidrug resistant isolates were predominately recovered from inpatients (>70%). Tables 3 and 4 show the prevalence of antimicrobial drug resistance of epidemiologically important GN and GP bacterial isolates, respectively.

Table 1 Blood cultures processed and data submitted during surveillance

Laboratory code	Total blood cultures processed	Positives, rates (%)	Multi-drug resistant isolates submitted during surveillance
BaS	315	86 (27.3)	41
AcL	226	54 (23.9)	16
WsE	505	43 (8.5)	14
NoT	1376	102 (7.4)	13
AsK	3610	398 (11.0)	7
CeU	13	3 (23.1)	1
AsO	146	16 (10.9)	1
BaB	21	1 (4.7)	1
EaK	95	8 (8.4)	1
UeB	44	3 (6.8)	1
Total	6351	714	100

Teaching hospitals: Tamale (NoT) and Komfo Anokye (AsK). Regional hospitals: Sunyani (Bas), Eastern (EaK) and Upper East (UeB). District hospital: LEKMA (AcL), Faith base: St Patrick, Offinso (AsO), St Patrick Holy Family, Berekum (BaB). Quasi-government hospital: University, Cape Coast (CeU). Zonal public health reference laboratory: Sekondi (WsE)

In total, 4 of 6 CRSA were successfully revived and molecularly screened for MRSA (*mecA* and *spa* genes). None of these tested positive for MRSA, both negative for *mecA* and *spa* genes.

Discussion

To inform empiric antibiotic guidelines at institutional level, one requires regular review of pathogen spectrum and antibiogram. Critical medical information to manage BSI could be gleaned from population-based or nosocomial surveillance systems [6, 8, 12–16]. However, the current trend for investigating BSI is to use population-based approaches [15, 17]. Information from such systems becomes even more useful when they are designed

Table 2 Gram negative and positive multiple drug resistant isolates from surveillance records

Bloodstream isolates	n (%)	Isolate source			Age categories/years					
		In-patient	Out-patient	Not indicated[a]	< 1	1–10	11–30	31–50	> 50	Not indicated[a]
Gram negatives (n = 49)										
Escherichia coli	10	9	1	-	1	-	3	2	2	2
Salmonella Typhi	4	2	2	-	-	4	-	-	-	-
Non-Typhoidal Salmonella	4	4	-	-	2	2	-	-	-	-
Enterobacter spp	7	6	1	-	3	-	1	1	-	2
Serratia marcescens	4	4	-	-	-	2	-	-	1	1
Serratia spp	2	2	-	-	-	2	-	-	1	1
Klebsiella pneumoniae	2	2	-	-	-	2	-	-	-	-
Citrobacter korseri	1	-	1	-	1	-	-	-	-	-
Citrobacter spp	5	5	-	-	2	3	-	-	-	-
Acinetobacter	1	1	-	-	1	-	-	-	-	-
Pseudomonas aeruginosa	8	6	1	1	3	1	-	1	2	1
Proteus mirabilis	1	1	-	-	-	-	1	-	-	-
Gram positives (n = 51)										
Staphylococcus aureus	34	23	8	3	11	10	3	1	2	7
CNS	9	8	-	1	3	2	1	-	1	2
Streptococcus pneumoniae	6	5	1	-	2	3	-	-	-	1
Streptococcus pyogenes	1	1	-	-	1	-	-	-	-	-
Enterococcus spp	1	-	-	-	-	-	1	-	-	-
Totals	100	75	15	5	30	29	10	5	8	16

CNS, *Coagulase negative Staphylococcu*
-indicates not applicable
[a]unavailable date

to capture additional indicators. For example, illness severity as indicated by Pitt bacteraemia score, [18] receipt of adequate antimicrobial regimen, [19] primary source of infection, and the presence or absence of malignancies [20]. Previous studies on BSI in Ghana were limited to tertiary facilities and restricted to particular age category [8, 16, 21, 22]. The current study used population-based surveillance to investigate BSI.

Overall blood culture positivity rate was only about 11% with a wide variability range (between 4.7% to 27%)

Table 3 Antibiogram of epidemiologically important Gram negative blood culture isolates

Antimicrobial agent	*E. coli* (n = 10) n, (% resistant)	*S. Typhi* (n = 4) n, (% resistant)	NTS (n = 4) n, (% resistant)	*Pseudomonas* (n = 8) n, (% resistant)	*Enterobacter* (n = 7) n, (% resistant)
Ampicillin	10 (100)	4 (100)	3 (100)	8 (62.5)	7 (100)
Cefuroxime	8 (87.5)	3 (66.6)	3 (50)	6 (66.7)	7 (85.7)
Cefotaxime	9 (88.9)	4 (50)	3 (60)	8 (87.5)	7 (85.7)
Meropenem	8 (12.5)	3 (0)	4 (0)	5 (20)	5 (0)
Amikacin	8 (0)	2 (0)	2 (0)	8 (12.5)	3 (33.3)
Gentamicin	10 (30)	4 (25)	3 (50)	8 (25)	5 (80)
Ciprofloxacin	10 (60)	2 (100)	ND	8 (12.5)	4 (25)
Levofloxacin	7 (42.9)	2 (50)	ND	ND	ND
Trimethoprim/Sulfamethoxazole	10 (100)	4 (50)	3 (100)	8 (75)	7 (71.4)
Chloramphenicol	9 (100)	4 (50)	3 (100)	7 (71.4)	7 (57.2)
Tetracycline	10 (100)	4 (50)	3 (50)	8 (62.5)	5 (80)

NTS Non-typhoidal Salmonella, *ND* indicates not done

Table 4 Antibiogram of epidemiologically Gram positive blood culture isolates

Antimicrobial agent	*Staph aureus* (*n* = 34)	CNS (*n* = 9)	*S. pneumoniae* (*n* = 6)
	n, % resistance	n, % resistance	n, % resistance
Penicillin	26 (23.1)	6 (0)	6 (0)
Ampicillin	30 (100)	8 (100)	6 (0)
Cloxacillin	14 (100)	4 (0)	ND
Flucloxacillin	17 (14.3)	1 (0)	ND
Augmentin	12 (75)	ND	ND
Cefuroxime	26 (53.8)	6 (16.7)	ND
Cefotaxime	14 (71.4)	8 (62.5)	ND
Gentamicin	30 (30)	8 (25)	6 (16.7)
Ciprofloxacin	29 (34.5)	8 (62.5)	6 (50)
Trimethoprim/Sulfamethoxazole	30 (70)	8 (100)	6 (0)
Erythromycin	5 (64)	8 (83.3	6 (66.7)
Tetracycline	31 (77.5)	8 (100)	6 (83.3)
Vancomycin	15 (0)	ND	2 (0)

CNS Coagulase negative Staphylococcus, *ND* indicates not done

across the 10 surveillance sites in Ghana. These rates have serious implications on patient care and also reflect blood culture capabilities in the respective hospitals. A combination of the following reasons may apply; some patients already on antibiotics prior to specimen collection, misdiagnosis from clinicians or laboratories using inadequate culture methods. It is worth noting that most of the regional hospitals in this study use the BACTEC blood cultures systems, but are usually short of one supply or the other. Alizadeh and colleagues however showed that both BACTEC and conventional blood culture methods have high validity [23]. We propose that the BACTEC and conventional blood culture methods should be used complementarily, especially in resource-limited countries, where consumables for the BACTEC are often in short supply. Infrastructure for blood culture services, whether BACTEC or conventional should be available for BSI diagnosis and management. Several studies in Ghana [8, 22] had blood culture positivity rates greater than 20% and in a large Indian study with over 135,000 cultures, a 14% rate was observed [24]. In a meta-analysis review, Reddy and colleagues identified bloodstream infections in 13.5% and 8.2% adults and children, respectively, with overall in-hospital case fatality rate of about 18% [25]. Our analysis did not follow up on patient outcomes but poor laboratory infrastructure and inadequate diagnostics, often results in poor treatment outcomes, sometimes confusing malaria bloodstream infections with other pathogens [25].

We found slightly more Gram-positive bacteria (GPB) in association with BSI in the current study, contrary to the Gram-negative bacteria (GNB) observed in several studies in Ghana [8, 22] and elsewhere [26]. Among the GNB, *E coli* was responsible for about a fifth of the BSI in the current study. Elsewhere, patient specific studies have generally associated *E. coli* to BSI [6, 8, 22]. On the contrary, in Europe, though *E coli* was previously topping the list of organisms associated with BSI, this has currently given way to MRSA [3, 14]. *E coli* associated BSI in most cases is secondary to focal infections such as urinary tract, abdominal, hepato-biliary sepsis, or surgical site infections [3]. An association with central vascular lines has also been reported [13]. Besides *E. coli*, *S. Typhi* and NTS were other GNB with higher prevalence, especially among children with ages less than 10 years. Compared to resource-rich countries where *Salmonella* (whether typhoidal or nontyphoidal) is almost never implicated in BSI [3, 4, 14], persistently, this organism is a common cause of GN sepsis in resource limiting countries [7, 8, 22, 24, 27]. It is generally difficult to distinguish between community and hospital acquired BSI. However, *Pseudomonas* is often associated with hospital-acquired BSI, often related to indwelling devices. In the current study *Pseudomonas* was responsible for more than 16% of all GN BSI.

Among the GPB, *Staphylococcus* and CNS were the predominant organisms, together accounting for greater than 80% of all GP sepsis. *Staphylococcus* was found more in patients less than 30 years of age, whilst CNS was found in children less than 10 years. Higher frequencies of GPB have been implicated in some earlier BSI studies from the USA and Canada [14]. GPB dominates in places where more prosthetic devices, mainly intravenous catheters, invasive procedures and specific procedures are done [28]. We did not confirmed MRSA in the current study. Meanwhile, studies from the largest tertiary hospital in Ghana have reported MRSA, primarily based on cefoxitin resistance [8, 22]. This tertiary hospital did not submit data for the current surveillance. MRSA associated BSI has been reported elsewhere. In England, mandatory and voluntary surveillance systems helped in reducing high MRSA bacteraemia [29]. *Streptococcus pneumoniae*, the next frequent GPB were predominantly found in children less than 5 years of age, comparable to other observations [8].

The high prevalence of antimicrobial drug resistance (AMR) observed in the GNB associated with BSI is alarming. Among the GNB, it appears meropenem and amikacin are the last resort antimicrobials. The hospitals in our surveillance reported and submitted data only on multi-drug resistant isolates, and we did not have information on the isolates susceptible. However, management of BSI in these patients with these high resistant bacteria will be difficult and may have bad outcomes. Extended spectrum beta-lactamase (ESBLs) and carbapenemase producing enterobacteriaceae (CRE) isolates in the current analysis is a worrying concern. These hydrolyzing enzymes render these antimicrobials ineffective, but are sparingly screened for in Ghana, especially, in bloodstream infections [8, 30]. Elsewhere, relatively high levels of these enzymes have been found in bloodstream isolates [31]. Scaling up of laboratory capacity in resource-limited countries like Ghana is urgently needed. In the absence of molecular assays for these enzymes, phenotypic assays would be helpful for patient management. GPB like *Staphylococcus* and CNS were also resistant to older antibiotics. We did not observe any MRSA (by molecular assay) and vancomycin resistant *Staphylococcus* in the current study, contrarily to other investigations in Ghana [8]. However, it is important to highlight that all *Staphylococcus aureus* isolates submitted by participating laboratories were resistant to cloxacillin (Table 4). Since cefoxitin is a better inducer for *mecA* (MRSA), it is currently preferred to oxacillin. A polymerase chain reaction (PCR), targeting the *mecA* gene remains the gold standard for MRSA confirmation [32]. However, PCR is seldom used in routine clinical laboratories because of logistics and inability to standardized laboratory protocols. The current study is not without limitations, which includes incomplete data sets and detailed clinical information. No clinical information was available about the patients from the participating laboratories. It is therefore difficult to differentiate between community acquired and hospital acquired BSIs [15, 17]. Complete clinical information, if available will help in ruling out some possible skin contaminants, which many include some CNS. Information on blood culture contaminants has implication on cost and practice. Finally, the relatively fewer numbers of bacterial isolates tested in any particular species limits the power of our study.

Conclusion

E. coli and *Salmonella* (typhoidal and NTS), *Staphylococcus aureus*, CNS and *Streptococcus pneumoniae* are often associated with BSI in Ghana. Most of these organisms are resistant to common antibiotics. Active and continuous surveillance systems will play a dual role in monitoring BSI and AMR.

Acknowledgement

We acknowledge all the laboratories that participated in this study. Reuben Arhin Essel, Amos Akanwena, Mary Osei and Abena Lawson are appreciated for providing technical assistance. Beverly Egyir performed MRSA screening test and we are grateful to her.

Funding

None to declare.

Authors' contributions

JAO and MJN designed the study. JAO analyzed data and drafted manuscript. Both authors read and approved the final manuscript.

Competing interests

The authors declare that they have no competing interests.

Consent for publication

Not applicable.

References

1. Fabbro-Peray P, Sotto A, Defez C, Cazaban M, Molinari L, Pinède M, et al. Mortality attributable to nosocomial infection: a cohort of patients with and without nosocomial infection in a French university hospital. Infect Control Hosp Epidemiol. 2007;28:265–72.
2. Munson EL, Diekema DJ, Beekmann SE, Chapin KC, Doern GV. Detection and treatment of bloodstream infection: laboratory reporting and antimicrobial management. J Clin Microbiol. 2003;41:495–7.
3. Wilson J, Elgohari S, Livermore DM, Cookson B, Johnson A, Lamagni T, et al. Trends among pathogens reported as causing bacteraemia in England, 2004-2008. Clin Microbiol Infect. 2011;17:451–8.
4. Adam HJ, DeCorby M, Rennie R, Karlowsky JA, Hoban DJ, Zhanel GG, et al. Prevalence of antimicrobial resistant pathogens from blood cultures from Canadian hospitals: results of the CANWARD 2007-2009 study. Diagn Microbiol Infect Dis. 2011;69:307–13.
5. Hamer DH, Darmstadt GL, Carlin JB, Zaidi AK, Yeboah-Antwi K, Saha SK, et al. Etiology of bacteremia in young infants in six countries. Pediatr Infect Dis J. 2015;34:e1–8.
6. Krakash KP, Vinod A, Geethanjali PP. Bloodstream bacterial pathogens and their antibiotic resistance pattern in Dhahira Region, Oman. Oman Med J. 2011;26:240–79.
7. Nielsen MV, Sarpong N, Krumkamp R, Dekker D, Loag W, Amemasor S, et al. Incidence and characteristics of bacteremia among children in rural Ghana. PLoS One. 2012;7:e44063.
8. Obeng-Nkrumah N, Labi AK, Addison NO, Labi JE, Awuah-Mensah G. Trends in paediatric and adult bloodstream infections at a Ghanaian referral hospital: a retrospective study. Ann Clin Microbiol Antimicrob. 2016;15:49.
9. Opintan JA, Newman MJ, Arhin RE, Donkor ES, Gyansa-Lutterodt M, Mills-Pappoe W. Laboratory-based nationwide surveillance of antimicrobial resistance in Ghana. Infect Drug Resist. 2015;8:379–89.
10. CLSI. Clinical Laboratory Standards Institute: Performance standards for antimicrobial susceptibility testing: twenty-second informational supplement;[. provides updated tables for. M02-A11 and M07 .... (2012).
11. Egyir B, Guardabassi L, Sørum M, Nielsen SS, Kolekang A, Frimpong E, et al. Molecular epidemiology and antimicrobial susceptibility of clinical Staphylococcus aureus from healthcare institutions in Ghana. PLoS One. 2014;9:e89716.
12. Al-Hasan MN, Lahr BD, Eckel-Passow JE, Baddour LM. Seasonal variation in Escherichia coli bloodstream infection: a population-based study. Clin Microbiol Infect. 2009;15:947–50.

13. Albrecht SJ, Fishman NO, Kitchen J, Nachamkin I, Bilker WB, Hoegg C, et al. Reemergence of gram-negative health care-associated bloodstream infections. Arch Intern Med. 2006;166:1289–94.
14. Biedenbach DJ, Moet GJ, Jones RN. Occurrence and antimicrobial resistance pattern comparisons among bloodstream infection isolates from the SENTRY Antimicrobial Surveillance Program (1997-2002). Diagn Microbiol Infect Dis. 2004;50:59–69.
15. Goto M, Al-Hasan MN. Overall burden of bloodstream infection and nosocomial bloodstream infection in North America and Europe. Clin Microbiol Infect. 2013;19:501–9.
16. Gross U, Amuzu SK, de Ciman R, Kassimova I, Gross L, Rabsch W, et al. Bacteremia and antimicrobial drug resistance over time, Ghana. Emerg Infect Dis. 2011;17:1879–82.
17. Laupland KB, Church DL. Population-based epidemiology and microbiology of community-onset bloodstream infections. Clin Microbiol Rev. 2014;27:647–64.
18. Paterson DL, Ko WC, Von Gottberg A, Mohapatra S, Casellas JM, Goossens H, et al. International prospective study of Klebsiella pneumoniae bacteremia: implications of extended-spectrum beta-lactamase production in nosocomial Infections. Ann Intern Med. 2004;140:26–32.
19. Kang CI, Kim SH, Park WB, Lee KD, Kim HB, Kim EC, et al. Bloodstream infections caused by antibiotic-resistant gram-negative bacilli: risk factors for mortality and impact of inappropriate initial antimicrobial therapy on outcome. Antimicrob Agents Chemother. 2005;49:760–6.
20. Al-Hasan MN, Lahr BD, Eckel-Passow JE, Baddour LM. Predictive scoring model of mortality in Gram-negative bloodstream infection. Clin Microbiol Infect. 2013;19:948–54.
21. Acquah SE, Quaye L, Sagoe K, Ziem JB, Bromberger PI, Amponsem AA. Susceptibility of bacterial etiological agents to commonly-used antimicrobial agents in children with sepsis at the Tamale Teaching Hospital. BMC Infect Dis. 2013;13:89.
22. Labi AK, Obeng-Nkrumah N, Bjerrum S, Enweronu-Laryea C, Newman MJ. Neonatal bloodstream infections in a Ghanaian Tertiary Hospital: are the current antibiotic recommendations adequate. BMC Infect Dis. 2016;16:598.
23. Alizadeh AM, Kabiri Movahed R, Mohammadnia M. Comparative evaluation of conventional and BACTEC methods for detection of bacterial infection. Tanaffos. 2016;15:112–6.
24. Gandra S, Mojica N, Klein EY, Ashok A, Nerurkar V, Kumari M, et al. Trends in antibiotic resistance among major bacterial pathogens isolated from blood cultures tested at a large private laboratory network in India, 2008-2014. Int J Infect Dis. 2016;50:75–82.
25. Reddy EA, Shaw AV, Crump JA. Community-acquired bloodstream infections in Africa: a systematic review and meta-analysis. Lancet Infect Dis. 2010;10:417–32.
26. Luzzaro F, Ortisi G, Larosa M, Drago M, Brigante G, Gesu G. Prevalence and epidemiology of microbial pathogens causing bloodstream infections: results of the OASIS multicenter study. Diagn Microbiol Infect Dis. 2011;69:363–9.
27. Negussie A, Mulugeta G, Bedru A, All I, Shimeles D, et al. Bacteriological Profile and Antimicrobial Susceptibility Pattern of Blood Culture Isolates among Septicemia Suspected Children in Selected Hospitals Addis Ababa, Ethiopia. Int J Biol Med Res. 2015;6:4709–17.
28. Muñoz P, Cruz AF, Rodríguez-Créixems M, Bouza E. Gram-negative bloodstream infections. Int J Antimicrob Agents. 2008;32(Suppl 1):S10–4.
29. Pearson A, Chronias A, Murray M. Voluntary and mandatory surveillance for methicillin-resistant Staphylococcus aureus (MRSA) and methicillin-susceptible S. aureus (MSSA) bacteraemia in England. J Antimicrob Chemother. 2009;64(Suppl 1):i11–7.
30. Obeng-Nkrumah N, Twum-Danso K, Krogfelt KA, Newman MJ. High levels of extended-spectrum beta-lactamases in a major teaching hospital in Ghana: the need for regular monitoring and evaluation of antibiotic resistance. Am J Trop Med Hyg. 2013;89:960–4.
31. Myat TO, Hannaway RF, Zin KN, Htike WW, Win KK, et al. ESBL- and carbapenemase-producing enterobacteriaceae in patients with bacteremia, Yangon, Myanmar, 2014. Emerg Infect Dis. 2017;23:857–9.
32. Chomvarin C, Siripornmongcolchai T, Chaicumpar K, Limpaiboon T, Wongkham C, et al. Evaluation of polymerase chain reaction, conventional and MRSA screen latex agglutination methods for detection of methicillin-resistant, –borderline and -susceptible Staphylococcus aureus. Southeast Asian J Trop Med Public Health. 2004;35:879–85.

7

Pet owner and vet interactions: exploring the drivers of AMR

Matt Smith[1*], Caroline King[1], Mark Davis[2], Adele Dickson[1], Jeni Park[1], Fraser Smith[1], Kay Currie[1] and Paul Flowers[1]

Abstract

Background: Antimicrobial resistance (AMR) is a growing public health problem across the world. As the negative consequences of AMR become apparent at local, national and international levels, more attention is being focussed on the variety of mechanisms by which AMR is potentiated. We explore how interactions between pet owners and veterinarians represent a key arena in which AMR-related behaviours can be shaped.

Methods: In depth semi-structured interviews were carried out with pet owners ($n = 23$) and vets ($n = 16$) across the UK in 2017. A thematic analysis approach was taken, with inductively gathered data analysed deductively using a behavioural framework to identified key behaviours emerging from participant accounts which were amenable to change.

Results: Interactions between vets and pet owners were characterised by misunderstandings and misconceptions around antibiotics by pet owners, and a lack of clarity about the positions and intentions of the other party. Vets and pet owners had differing perceptions of where pressure to prescribe antibiotics inappropriately originated. Vets perceived it was mostly pet owners who pushed for inappropriate antibiotics, whereas pet owners reported they felt it was vets that overprescribed. Low levels of understanding of AMR in general were apparent amongst pet owners and understandings with regard to AMR in pets specifically were almost non-existent in the sample.

Conclusions: Improved use of antibiotics could be assisted by educating the pet owning public and by guideline development for companion animal vets, concurrent development of mandatory legislation, increased consultation time to facilitate better communication, development of vet training on antimicrobial therapy and stewardship led interactions with pet owners, and increased levels of knowledge of pet-related AMR amongst pet owners.

Keywords: Antibiotic resistance, Pets, Vets, Behaviour, AMR

Background

Interdisciplinary consensus identifies AMR as an increasingly severe global concern [1, 2]. Antibiotics have facilitated revolutionary improvements in medical practice in many areas (from routine to critical care) by protecting patients from the threat of bacterial infection [1]. However, due to various biological mechanisms (dependent on the infective organism and class of antimicrobial agent), there are now an increasing variety of microbes that display resistance to antimicrobial drugs [3–5]. The process that drives this resistance is selective pressure (causing differential mortality and growth stasis of non-resistant organisms which then causes genetic change in the overall population) of antimicrobial use, resulting in successive generational increases in resistance to mortality in bacteria [6]. Antimicrobial resistance (AMR) threatens to undo decades of medical progress, resulting in substantial increases of dangerous infections in the course of previously routine treatment [7, 8]. Resistant organisms are linked to increased disease severity due to lessened treatment efficacy, longer hospitalisation and increased costs in treatment and post disease care [7].

Animal health care is implicated in the problem of AMR. Animals have been shown to have potential to act as reservoirs for resistant organisms, especially when infections are not comprehensively and successfully treated. Moreover, veterinary science acknowledges that a unique and critical aspect of AMR in pets is their close physical contact with humans [9, 10]. This can lead to an increased potential for transmission of resistant microorganisms between humans and their pets [11], especially those that

* Correspondence: matt.smith@gcu.ac.uk; Matt.smith@gcu.ac.uk
[1]Institute for Applied Health Research, Glasgow Caledonian University, Glasgow, Scotland G4 0BA, UK
Full list of author information is available at the end of the article

reside on the skin or in saliva [12]. In addition, pet numbers have substantially increased in the modern age, and more efforts are devoted to pet welfare, meaning higher levels of treatment for sick animals, and more frequent use of antibiotics for pets [9]. This is of particular concern for antibiotics also used in human medicine, especially those known as "last resort" treatments for potentially fatal infections [10]. Growing resistance to these antibiotics in particular is likely to result in increased human mortality [10]. Interspecies transmission can result in an increase of AMR through a feedback loop of resistance reservoirs and evolving generations of increasingly resistant bacteria [13–15].

To combat these drivers of AMR, the effective use of antibiotics in animal health depends on pet-owners and their collaborations with prescribing vets. Pet owners mediate the treatment of their animals; they control antibiotic usage and other actions that can directly determine potential for AMR in their animals [14]. In the absence of more effective antimicrobials as a solution to AMR, understanding the behaviours of pet owners in collaboration with vets could become an important part of the global effort to reduce AMR. Responsible use of antibiotics, or "Antimicrobial Stewardship" [16] will be referred to in this paper. Fishman [16] defines it as directly related to prescribing practices that ensure that antibiotics will continue to be effective for future generations. Here we conceive of it more broadly, as also taking into account responsible use by patients and pet owners to the same ends. In what follows, we investigate how pet-owners and vets talk about animal health care, antibiotics and antimicrobial resistance to advance understanding of AMR-related behaviour and opportunities for change.

Study aims

This paper addresses the pet-owner – vet prescribing interaction through qualitative interviews focussed on experiences and knowledge of antibiotics and AMR, to i) shed light on pet-owners and vets experiences, beliefs and intentions with regard to their interactions on antibiotic prescription, and ii) to identify approaches for behaviour change interventions targeting pet owner-vet interactions as a primary site for mutual understanding between parties to develop more responsible antibiotic use in pets.

Research questions

1) What do vets believe are the most important aspects of interaction between pet owners and themselves that can lead to increases in AMR?
2) What do the pet owning public believe are the most important aspects of interactions between themselves and vets that can lead to increases in AMR?
3) How do these aspects help or hinder the development and maintenance of antimicrobial stewardship?

Methods

We took a qualitative approach, using semi-structured interviews with two types of study group: pet owners ($n = 22$) and small animal vets ($n = 16$) across the UK in 2017.

Ethical approval and recruitment

Ethical approval for the study was granted from the ethics committee for Nursing and Community Health at Glasgow Caledonian University (Reference number: HLS/NCH/16/001).

Pet owners were recruited through: adverts on social media (Facebook and Twitter); convenience sampling at a veterinary practice; snowballing via recruited participants; and through personal contacts from the research team. Inclusion criteria for pet owners were: having a dog, cat or rabbit; having received antibiotics for their pet in the last year; and not having recently bereaved of a pet. Vets were recruited through: nationwide veterinary practices, networks and connections from Health Protection Scotland (HPS) and the wider Control of Antimicrobial Resistance Scotland (CARS) programme Animal Health and AMR group. The vet inclusion criterion was that they had to be in small animal practice.

Data collection

Topic guides for interviews were developed with expert advice from the study advisory group. Both topic guides were used to balance participant led data with our focus upon understandings and perceptions of AMR and the drivers of AMR.

Twenty one pet owner participants were interviewed of which 14 were female and seven were male. For pet owners, eight face to face interviews and 13 phone interviews were carried out. The duration of the interviews ranged from 28 min to one hour and 30 min. Pet owners ranged in age from 32 to 77 years old.

Sixteen vets took part in interviews. Nine of the participants were male and seven were female. Eleven of the vets were based in Scotland, four in England and one in Northern Ireland. Recruited participants were identified as holding various positions within the industry including: front-line ($n = 10$), Second opinion ($n = 2$), vet hospital ($n = 1$), emergency out of hours ($n = 1$) and vet school ($n = 1$). These interviews lasted between 25 min and 40 min.

Data analysis

Data were analysed thematically, as defined by Braun & Clarke [17], in two main stages. Initially three researchers independently coded a selection of transcripts looking for an agreed range of broad inductively developed descriptive themes, generating a list of codes. These broad codes were applied to all the remaining data using NVivo qualitative analysis software [18]. Coding was quality checked as an ongoing process by multiple researchers within the team.

Subsequently, within the second stage of analysis, the broad inductively derived data were analysed deductively using a behavioural analytic approach. Data relating to specific behavioural domains were identified amongst both samples. For vets, these included the following behavioural domains: prescribing; use of diagnostic testing; and interactions with pet owners. For pet owners, these included: appropriate use of antibiotics; AMR transmission related behaviours (between owner and pet); and interacting with vets. This paper examines the behavioural domain of interactions from the perspectives of both groups of participants. A continuous process of cross checking was carried out between researchers to ensure analytical rigour.

Results

The following sections consider important AMR-related aspects of the broad behavioural domain of interactions between vets and pet owners, firstly from the perspective of vets, then from the perspective of pet owners.

Vet perspectives on AMR-related interactions with pet owners

Vets gave their perspectives on their interactions with pet owners, and identified the behaviours, and barriers and facilitators they thought contributed to inappropriate antibiotic decision-making. These relate primarily to perceived pressures from pet owners and possible discussions around antimicrobial resistance.

Perceived pressures from pet owners that influence antibiotic decision making

Vets reported that their interactions with pet owners were complex when it came to their decision making concerning antibiotics. There was a common tension between an awareness of the need for AMR stewardship and the perceived satisfaction of the pet owner. The satisfaction of the pet owner, from a vet perspective, was dependent on a myriad of factors which extended beyond the appropriate use of an antibiotic relating to clinical need, including: payment for consultation and the expectation of active treatment; ease of administering the treatment; previous experiences with receiving antibiotics for their pets; and pet owners' emotional connections with their animals. Vets commonly reported prescribing 'just in case' in response to their perceptions of client anxiety about pet health and welfare. From the vet's point of view, clients appeared to expect the provision of a clearly defined treatment (i.e. an antibiotic prescription), as the following example indicates:

> There's a pressure when an owner comes in and pays 35 or 40 pounds , for a consultation, because their animal is unwell, that they want to go home with a medication that in inverted commas "fixes" their animal, and even though the bill will be higher with that medication, so you sort of have that feeling that if you have an unwell animal and if you send it home with nothing then you'll get a raised eyebrow, or for example they will say to you, "Well, so and so , the senior partner gave my older dog antibiotics just last week for similar symptoms" so, you know whatever, but there is a sort of general expectation I think of owners, that you will treat their animal when they pay for a consultation. (Vet 10)

As this extract suggests, expectations from clients to prescribe antibiotics were often inferred rather than explicitly stated. Vets saw that pet owners appeared to perceive prescription as a binary of presence or absence of treatment and therefore action versus inaction. Prescription appeared to be received as a measurable, visible action taken for the health of the pet, whereas a lack of prescription meant nothing was being done to help the animal.

Tacit pressure was also framed by vets in terms of pet owners' expectations for transaction, that is, payment exchanged for a tangible outcome in the form of medicine for the pet. This expectation was exacerbated by the fact that veterinarian practices are profit making enterprises, and seeking to keep customers loyal, sometimes against appropriate clinical action. This pressure was felt by vets because customers are able to go to other practices where they may get what they want:

> Yeah, I mean these people are our customers and they are, what keeps the business going, so if we annoy them and there is another vet practice they can go to where they may just be handed out antibiotics, and [the vet] might take the opinion "well, here's a client, if I give him a course of antibiotics, he'll just take his dog to me from now on and I've gained a client" (Vet 1)

These market pressures can therefore be construed as potential drivers of inappropriate antibiotic prescribing among other mechanisms. Other vet accounts show that the AMR related consequences of over-prescription are not high on their agenda when acquiescing to pet owner pressure to provide treatment. Vets cited professional tendencies to prescribing, i.e., giving animals antibiotics as a quick and easy way to deal with an infection, even if that was not necessarily the best course of action:

> So for example, if you've got a cat with cystitis and a lot of [vets] will give them antibiotics when actually a lot of them don't need antibiotics. So I think a lot of is through fear as well. You want to make the animal better, therefore you think oh sod it, I'll just give them a jag. (Vet 13)

As this quotation indicates, the risks involved in inappropriate use of an antibiotic were outweighed by the risk losing a client. Potential, ambiguous and non-present consequences of AMR for vets were not as salient as the present lived experiences of pressure from pet owners, and business pressures around client satisfaction.

Discussion of AMR with pet owners that influence antibiotic decision making

Vets were asked to what extent they felt they could use the concept of AMR to negotiate with pet owners in the interactions described above, to improve overall antimicrobial stewardship. Vets identified that pet owner understanding and willingness to discuss antibiotics and AMR were important determinants of their eventual prescribing decisions. The majority of vets reported that their clients tended to have some knowledge of the importance of correct antibiotic use; particularly that partial use of a course of antibiotics, or using them unnecessarily, had some kind of negative effects concerning future treatment outcomes. However vets reported a general lack of knowledge of the wider and longer term, inter specifies effects of over- or mis-use of antibiotics, and an almost total lack of knowledge of about the phenomena of AMR. This was also borne out in data from pet owners. Vet accounts also reported that clients were often unaware of disease processes. The limits of pet owners' knowledge about appropriate antibiotic use could lead them to believe that an antibiotic would be appropriate treatment when it would not be suitable, for example, for a viral infection:

> They'll be a little bit annoyed that I haven't really given them anything, even though there's nothing that I could really give them that would improve their cat's position. And a lot of the time, they will sort of be like, well, what about some antibiotics, what about this, what about that, and I'll have to be, like, well, no, your cat doesn't need it and it's not going to help. But they sort of feel like I'm not really listening to their issue or that I'm not trying to help their cat because I'm not giving them this medicine that they perceive will be helpful to them, basically. (Vet 3)

Most vets in the sample perceived that whilst this lack of knowledge was an issue, awareness was improving, making it easier to carry out AMR negotiations without jeopardising pet owner satisfaction. However, some vets reported that there were still those who would not engage in discussion about appropriate use of antibiotics:

> You can tell very quickly if someone's going to be receptive to that [appropriateness of antibiotics] conversation or not, and if they're not, then obviously sometimes you just have to accept that that's what the client wants, and if we don't do that then the animal is going to suffer anyway, so we just say, well, there's no point even discussing this. (Vet 15)

This extract shows that vets are required to make judgements which balance outcomes for clients and pets, revealing prescribing decisions to be complexly embedded in management of the pet's illness, the owner's expectations and the reality of a competitive business environment. Antimicrobial stewardship does not easily factor into these complex deliberations.

Vets also reported that their professional experience played an important role in empowering them to be able to assert a more appropriate course of action, skills which took time to develop:

> I think a lot of it boils down to communication, and it does get easier as you get older. As a younger vet - I'm kind of middle aged now, somewhere in the middle - as a younger vet, it's difficult, you often feel pressured from clients, you feel pressured to conform to what the older vets would do, if they would do something in a certain way. But now that I'm an established vet in my own right with my own ideas and opinions, as long as I get the time to actually communicate that with the client and talk effectively, I can usually talk them round to my point of view and they will see that's reasonable enough, yeah. And I think it depends where you work. If you're in a very busy practice or if you're a younger vet feeling pressure from clients or from senior staff, then it is going to be difficult, you're just going to grab the antibiotics, that's the easy option. (Vet 2)

This account reflects the social norms and dynamics which influence prescribing decisions and underlines that the development of communication skills was an important factor in being able to negate pressures from misinformed pet owners and, it seemed, other vets. Identifying and sharing these skills could be a useful tactic for the advancement of stewardship.

Pet owner's perspectives on AMR-related interactions with vets

Pet owners also gave their perspectives on their interactions with vets, and identified the behaviours, and barriers and facilitators they thought contributed to antibiotic decision-making and antibiotic use for their pets. These relate primarily to pet owner expectations around antibiotic prescribing and discussions related to antimicrobial resistance.

Pet owners' expectations of antibiotic use

In contrast to vet perspectives that pet owner satisfaction was the main source of inappropriate prescribing, pet owners, on the whole, denied that they would be dissatisfied if their pets were not prescribed antibiotics. The majority of our respondents indicated that they would follow the vet's instructions because they perceived vets to have expertise in an area where they had little to no knowledge.

> I would say ultimately it's my decision but the vet is the expert… I mean if they tell me it's needed, I'll not, I'm not going to, I might try and ask sensible questions… but I'm not going to dispute that. (Laura, dog owner).

However, some participants reported that they thought it was vets who promoted antibiotics unnecessarily:

> But I have been to the vet before and got antibiotics and questioned it and asked why they were taking them, when, where… they said right we'll put them on antibiotics and I said I'm not really sure that they need them and do we really need to go ahead with them and they said to me, yes we really, really, need to go ahead, then I would go ahead with it. But there has been instances where I've said, I don't, I'm not sure that we need them, are you absolutely sure? And they said OK, no. We'll wait a while. (Andrea, dog owner).

Andrea's account of questioning the prescription was rare in our interviews as most reported that they had not had any disagreements with vets over their expectations that antibiotics would be prescribed. Some pet owners reported assuming that antibiotics were required and had those assumptions negated by the expertise of the vet. However, in contrast to vet perceived risks of not keeping the client satisfied, there were no cases where pet owners had major disagreements which resulted in moving to other vets. These accounts indicate that pet owners may differ markedly from vets regarding their experiences of interactions and that there was a shared tendency among pet-owners and vets to externalise the drivers of inappropriate prescribing. This understandable self-protecting bias among both vets and owners is an important consideration for the development of effective stewardship, as we discuss below.

Pet owners' understanding of AMR

As with vets, being able to understand and discuss AMR was seen by pet owners as an important factor for their own enactment of stewardship principles.

The majority of pet owners reported that they did not know about AMR, particularly in relation to their pets, confirming the reports of vets described above. While most pet owners did not know about AMR, the majority of participants did have an awareness of "superbugs", which they described as being primarily hospital-based resistant infections such as MRSA. This awareness was mainly credited to news media. Only a few spoke in specific terms about AMR, for example, the mechanisms through which it might develop and what impact improper use of antibiotics might have on its development. It was usually discussed in more general terms:

> "I think we're just reaping the [consequences] of maybe people having antibiotics unnecessarily." (*Maura, dog and cat owner*).

Even fewer pet owners had an understanding that AMR was an issue for animals and a very small minority knew about interspecies transmission. When participants were prompted about AMR specifically in animals, the large majority referred to antibiotic use in farming:

> I'm sure there was something on the BBC news about pigs, I'm sure there was pig farming because I was just tuning in and out of it. I wondered why they had pigs and then they had people in a hospital bed and I was getting them confused. I know it was something about pigs being prescribed antibiotics and that is somehow having a knock on effect for us [laughter] but the steps on that chain I'm not sure about. (*Rosemary, Dog owner*)

This lack of awareness of AMR in pets, let alone interspecies transmission risks, implied that it was highly unlikely that pet owners would be able to broach the topic with vets, take AMR into account in the treatment of their pets, and participate in decision making concerning antibiotics. These perspectives indicate that AMR literacy and scaffolding of antibiotic decision making may be important for pet owners.

Another challenge for pet-owners was the long term and collective nature of AMR which was not easily related to their own immediate predicament with their pet in the present:

> I suppose with any of these future problems, problems are easily described as being something that'll affect us in the distant future, there's an issue

> with knowing how serious a risk is this, how much needs to be done *now* (*Dave, Dog Owner*)

As in this example, for most pet owners, AMR was perceived as distant, future problem, with many ambiguous and unknown dimensions. Some participants contrasted the seemingly distant threat of AMR with the immediacy of their pets' health, which was more directly experienced as part of their everyday lives, and therefore of a bigger influence on decision-making processes about antibiotics. AMR was of such negligible concern, due to its abstract, complex and temporally distant nature, that it did not influence decisions about the immediate concern of pet health and wellbeing. In contrast, the suffering of the animal that many considered to be "part of the family" was a visceral, potently experienced phenomenon that pushed individuals to make financial and other sacrifices to ensure their pet got better.

Figure 1 summarises results influences on pet owner and vet behaviours.

Discussion

This paper is the first of its kind to examine *how* vets and pet-owners experience antibiotic decision-making, and identifying their subjective views on the factors which influence effective stewardship. This novel and inductive approach makes a valuable contribution by identifying the antecedents which underpin antibiotic prescribing behaviour (in vets) and usage (in pet owners). As such, it identifies several key ingredients for future intervention development.

First, it is important to acknowledge the interaction between pet owners and vets in relation to behaviours which might drive AMR. Vets appeared focussed upon the prescribing of antibiotics. They attributed over-prescribing to the complexity of the following drivers; perceived client satisfaction, commercial pressures to retain clients, the symbolic value of giving treatment, the influence of senior vets within practice, under-developed communication and persuasion skills, pet owners partial knowledge of appropriate antibiotic use and their very poor knowledge of antimicrobial resistance and interspecies transmission. Second, we must consider the nature of the interaction between pet owners and vets which may in itself facilitate AMR. For example, in the current study, pet owners had very poor knowledge and understanding of AMR and inter-species transmission but were aware of the negative consequences of inappropriate antibiotic use. They considered vets as being fundamentally responsible for prescribing decisions (attributing responsibility to their professional expertise). Pet owners did not report having high expectations of receiving antibiotic prescription.

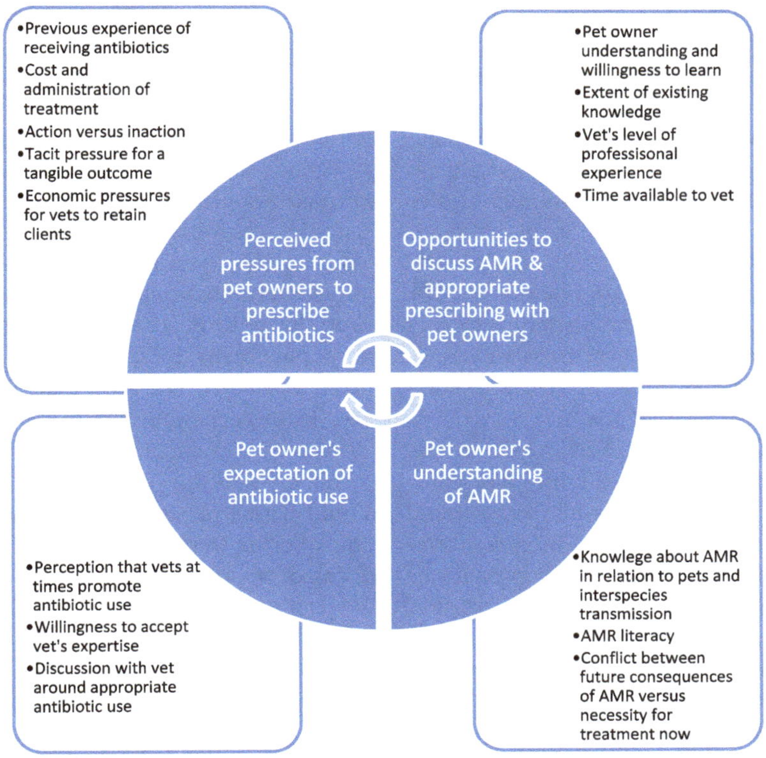

Fig. 1 Factors shaping vet and pet owner interactions in relation to antibiotic prescribing and use

Finally, several key points are illuminated in terms of antimicrobial stewardship. Dissonance between the pet owner and vet appears to exist between their perceptions of where responsibility should rest in relation to the decision to prescribe antibiotics. Low levels of knowledge and understanding of AMR and its drivers amongst pet owners are important to note in this regard as they have the potential to constrain antimicrobial stewardship.

The apparent dissonance in perceptions of responsibility for antibiotic decision making for pets should be factored into effective stewardship interventions. Alternatively, vets and pet-owners only notice differing prescribing decisions which conflict with their a priori expectations (i.e. vets notice pressure to prescribe from pet-owners; pet-owners notice what they see as over-prescription). This possible explanation for dissonance implies that future work should focus on sensitising vets and owners to these situations. Dissonance may also result from a breakdown in communication, that is, misinterpretation of behavioural cues, mistaken inferences and so on, undertaken in the challenging context of time limited consultations with a pet-owner and their pet. The facilitation of more effective discussions between pet owner and vets around antibiotics might therefore be useful. Interventions should include professional development for vets, particularly those new to practice, to specifically facilitate more effective discussion around antibiotics. This may enable a more accurate identification and mitigation of pet owner pressures to prescribe. Potentially, standardised guidelines, vignettes and protocols could help pet owners and vets manage their interactions more effectively. Concurrent to the development of guidelines, there is potential to develop mandatory legislation, however this is contingent on political will and identifying suitable bodies to legislate and enforce. Specific training and guidelines with step-by-step protocols for engaging in conversations about antibiotic prescription have the potential to assist professionals and their clients ensure better decisions on antibiotics [19, 20]. As our research highlights, however, any attempt to shift the behaviours of vets will need support from clients, so interventions for vets should be run in parallel with complementary ones for owners.

Raising awareness and knowledge of AMR in pet owners themselves could be key to facilitating more productive interactions and discussions with vets around appropriate antibiotic use for their pets. Increased emphasis on appropriate, responsible stewardship could be especially effective in countering potential vet pressures to overprescribe, as pet owners might be more likely to resist with better knowledge resources. If negative consequences of over prescription were framed in terms of side effects for the animal (lessened future efficacy of antibiotics) it might be particularly effective. In this regard, increasing the self-efficacy of pet owners by teaching skills to participate in consultations might be useful. For example, vets claimed pet owners were unsatisfied if they did not receive antibiotics as they did not get "their money's worth". If pet owners' awareness of the vets' diagnostic processes was improved and therefore understanding of the informed decisions vets make was increased, potentially they would be more likely to perceive vet's expertise as a reasonable outcome for the money they have spent.

There are some possible barriers to enhancing antibiotic decision-making, however. Research in other areas has shown that awareness alone is not sufficient to change individual behaviours [21], particularly for issues, like AMR, that are highly complex and seen to be a distant ambiguous risk. It is likely, therefore, that enhanced regulation of antibiotic prescribing in animal health will also be of value. In addition, standardisation and regulation of prescribing could be met with resistance by vets due to perceived to impositions on their autonomy and business models [22]. In addition, the governance of veterinary practice in the UK is fragmented into many different bodies, so cross practice guidelines would be challenging to develop and enact.

It is important to consider the key strengths and limitations of the current study. First, this paper presents a novel piece of work, original in its inductive, qualitative approach and innovative in its dual-focus (considering both the vet and pet-owners perspectives). This study contributes a rich, insightful understanding of AMR enabling behaviours from the perspectives of the participants themselves. It promotes increased awareness of the key drivers for antibiotic use/prescription, including underlying cognitive processes such as decision making and dissonance.

Various limitations have been identified for this study, primarily sources of bias within samples. The pet-owner sample were predominantly from middle-class, well-educated backgrounds (due to relatively poor success of other recruitment approaches). Vets who were recruited were likely to be already interested in AMR, and therefore potentially biased towards stewardship. Vets may have also been reserved in their disclosure due to a desire to project professionalism. The sample size reflects accepted standards for exploratory, theory-building qualitative health research. However, a larger sample could have alleviated some of the issues. The next step in exploring this topic would be a quantitative design informed by this research exploring behaviours of pet owners and vets regarding antibiotics use.

Conclusions

This paper provides original evidence of the power of interactions between vets and pet owners to influence appropriate antibiotic prescribing and use in companion animals. In the absence of open communication, both vets and pet owners are inclined to misinterpret the intentions of the other, potentially leading to unnecessary prescription and inappropriate use of antibiotics.

Targeted multi-modal strategies which increase knowledge and awareness of antimicrobial resistance and appropriate antibiotic use in the pet owning public are important. These would provide a strong foundation on which effective interactions between vets and pet owners can be built, thus enhancing antibiotic stewardship behaviours. In addition, adequate time within consultations is required to enable vets to provide relevant information and to educate per owners around alternatives to antibiotic use.

By tackling the barriers of potential misunderstandings, lack of awareness of AMR, and lack of opportunity or capacity to discuss AMR during consultations, whilst enhancing the enablers of skilled communication which focuses on best clinical judgement as a precursor to client satisfaction, more effective antimicrobial stewardship can be achieved.

Abbreviations

AMR: Antimicrobial Resistance; CARS: Control of Antimicrobial Resistance in Scotland; CVMP: Committee for Medicinal Products for Veterinary Use; HPS: Health Protection Scotland

Acknowledgements

The authors are particularly grateful to all our participants for volunteering to give up their time to be interviewed and to share their story & their enthusiasm for their pets, with us.
We would also like to express our appreciation to the members of the Control of Antimicrobial Resistance in Scotland (CARS) team at Health Protection Scotland for their support and advice.

Funding

Research funded by a grant from the Control of Antimicrobial Resistance in Scotland (CARS) group at Health Protection Scotland (Reference CARS_2016-06-08/RIE 15-127).
The opinions expressed in this publication are those of Glasgow Caledonian University and are not necessarily those of Health Protection Scotland. Through iterative discussions with the research team the funding body shaped the broad research focus -to develop insights into potential areas for behaviour change interventions. Regular discussions between the funding body and the team provided a forum to discuss data collection and analysis. The interpretation of the data was amongst the research team only.

Authors' contributions

Matt Smith (MS), Caroline King (CK), Mark Davis (MD), Adele Dickson (AD), Fraser Smith (FS), Jeni Park (JP), Kay Currie (KC), Paul Flowers (PF). MS carried out data collection, led on data analysis and interpreted data, and was primary author. CK made a major contribution to data analysis and data interpretation; she was a major contributor to the manuscript. MD contributed to data analysis and drafting the manuscript. AD analysed and interpreted data and contributed to the manuscript. FS carried out data collection and contributed to the manuscript. JP organised recruitment, data preparation and mace a major contribution to the manuscript. KC contributed to data analysis and drafting the manuscript. PF was the principle investigator and was awarded the funding. He led the overall design and development of the project, managed the whole study, was involved in data collection, data analysis and made a major contribution to the manuscript. All authors read and approved the final manuscript.

Consent for publication

All data has been anonymised, participants all provided written consent for content of their interviews to be used in analysis, report and paper writing.

Competing interests

The authors declare that they have no competing interests.

Author details

[1]Institute for Applied Health Research, Glasgow Caledonian University, Glasgow, Scotland G4 0BA, UK. [2]School of Social Sciences, Monash University, Melbourne 3800, Australia.

References

1. Marston HD, Dixon DM, Knisely JM, Palmore TN, Fauci AS. Antimicrobial resistance. JAMA. 2016;316(11):1193–204.
2. Jasovsky D, Littmann J, Zorzet A, Cars O. Antimicrobial resistance-a threat to the world's sustainable development. Upsala J Med Sci. 2016;121(3):159–64.
3. Holmes AH, Moore LS, Sundsfjord A, Steinbakk M, Regmi S, Karkey A, Guerin PJ, Piddock LJ. Understanding the mechanisms and drivers of antimicrobial resistance. Lancet. 2016;387(10014):176–87.
4. Beever L, Bond R, Graham PA, Jackson B, Lloyd DH, Loeffler A. Increasing antimicrobial resistance in clinical isolates of Staphylococcus intermedius group bacteria and emergence of MRSP in the UK. Vet Rec. 2015;176(7):172.
5. Roca I, Akova M, Baquero F, Carlet J, Cavaleri M, Coenen S, Cohen J, Findlay D, Gyssens I, Heuer OE, et al. The global threat of antimicrobial resistance: science for intervention. New Microbes New Infect. 2015;6:22–9.
6. Hawkey PM. The growing burden of antimicrobial resistance. J Antimicrob Chemother. 2008;62(suppl_1):i1–9.
7. Umber JK, Bender JB. Pets and antimicrobial resistance. Vet Clin North Am. 2009;39(2):279–92.
8. Laxminarayan R, Matsoso P, Pant S, Brower C, Rottingen JA, Klugman K, Davies S. Access to effective antimicrobials: a worldwide challenge. Lancet. 2016;387(10014):168–75.
9. Guardabassi L, Schwarz S, Lloyd DH. Pet animals as reservoirs of antimicrobial-resistant bacteria. J Antimicrob Chemother. 2004;54(2):321–32.
10. Commitee for Medicinal Products for Veterinary Use (CVMP): Reflection paper on the risk of antimicrobial resistance transfer from companion animals. London: European Medicines Agency; 2013.
11. Wieler LH, Ewers C, Guenther S, Walther B, Lubke-Becker A. Methicillin-resistant staphylococci (MRS) and extended-spectrum beta-lactamases (ESBL)-producing Enterobacteriaceae in companion animals: nosocomial infections as one reason for the rising prevalence of these potential zoonotic pathogens in clinical samples. Int J Med Microbiol. 2011;301(8):635–41.
12. Walther B, Hermes J, Cuny C, Wieler LH, Vincze S, Abou Elnaga Y, Stamm I, Kopp PA, Kohn B, Witte W, et al. Sharing more than friendship–nasal colonization with coagulase-positive staphylococci (CPS) and co-habitation aspects of dogs and their owners. PLoS One. 2012;7(4):e35197.
13. Van Duijkeren E, Wolfhagen MJHM, Box ATA, Heck MEOC, Wannet WJB, Fluit AC. Human-to-dog transmission of methicillin-resistant Staphylococcus aureus. Emerg Infect Dis. 2004;10(12):2235–7.
14. Lloyd DH. Reservoirs of antimicrobial resistance in pet animals. Clin Infect Dis. 2007;45(Supplement_2):S148–52.
15. Van Balen J, Landers T, Nutt E, Dent A, Hoet A. Molecular epidemiological analysis to assess the influence of pet-ownership in the biodiversity of Staphylococcus aureus and MRSA in dog- and non-dog-owning healthy households. Epidemiol Infect. 2017;145(06):1135–47.
16. Fishman N. Antimicrobial stewardship. Am J Infect Control. 2006;34(5):S55–63.
17. Braun V, Clarke V. Using thematic analysis in psychology. Qual Res Psychol. 2006;3(2):77–101.
18. Welsh E. Dealing with Data: Using NVivo in the qualitative data analysis process [12 paragraphs]. Forum Qualitative Sozialforschung / Forum. Qual Soc Res. 2012;3(2):26. http://nbn-resolving.de/urn:nbn:de:0114-fqs0202260.
19. Hughes LA, Williams N, Clegg P, Callaby R, Nuttall T, Coyne K, Pinchbeck G, Dawson S. Cross-sectional survey of antimicrobial prescribing patterns in UK small animal veterinary practice. Prev Vet Med. 2012;104(3–4):309–16.
20. Chipangura JK, Eagar H, Kgoete M, Abernethy D, Naidoo V. An investigation of antimicrobial usage patterns by small animal veterinarians in South Africa. Prev Vet Med. 2017;136(Supplement C):29–38.

8

Inappropriate use of antibiotics among communities of Gondar town, Ethiopia: a threat to the development of antimicrobial resistance

Daniel Asfaw Erku[1,3*], Abebe Basazn Mekuria[2] and Sewunet Admasu Belachew[1]

Abstract

Background: The emergence of antimicrobial resistance, the main cause of morbidity and mortality from otherwise treatable infections, is largely attributed to the inappropriate use of antimicrobials. However, data on the extent of inappropriate use of antibiotics in the community is scarce in Ethiopia. The aim of present study is to document the extent of inappropriate use of antibiotics and its associated factors among the communities of Gondar, Northwest Ethiopia.

Methods: A community based cross-sectional survey was conducted on a total of 650 participants in Gondar town, northwest Ethiopia from December 1, 2016 to January 30, 2017. Descriptive statistics, univariate and multivariate logistic regression analysis were also performed to express different variables and to examine factors associated with inappropriate use of antibiotics.

Results: According to the finding of our study, 315 (48.5%) of the participants took antibiotics in the past 1 year, of which 115 (35.9%) of them used inappropriately. Amoxicillin (72%) was the most commonly utilized antibiotics and respiratory tract infection (40.9%) was the most common disease condition to which antibiotics had been sought. About 36.8% of the respondents got antibiotics from community drug retail outlets without a prescription and 67.9% of respondents had discontinued the use of antibiotics once their symptoms subside. Low educational status (AOR = 5.01, 95% CI = 2.62–9.34), being employed (AOR = 2.12, 95% CI = 1.81–7.29) and unsatisfied with health care services provided (AOR = 5.41, 95% CI = 2.71-14.21) were found to be strong predictors of inappropriate use of antibiotics use among the community.

Conclusion: Inappropriate use of antibiotics was found to be considerably high in the communities of Gondar, northwest Ethiopia. Taking into consideration the heightened importance of comprehensive knowledge in the rational use of antibiotics, different stakeholders working in the public health sectors should provide a comprehensive and customized education to the public so as to improve their knowledge about antibiotics. It is also essential to adopt a strong and explicit line of actions towards the accessibility of antibiotics without a valid prescription in community medicine retail outlets.

Keywords: Inappropriate use, Antimicrobials, Drug resistance, Community, Ethiopia

* Correspondence: daniel.asfaw05@gmail.com
[1]Department of Clinical Pharmacy, School of Pharmacy, University of Gondar Chechela Street, Lideta Sub city Kebele, 16 Gondar, Ethiopia
[3]Department of clinical pharmacy, School of Pharmacy, College of Medicine and Health Sciences, University of Gondar, P.O. Box: 196, Gondar, Ethiopia
Full list of author information is available at the end of the article

Background

The emergence of antimicrobial resistance (AMR), the main cause of morbidity and mortality from otherwise treatable infections, is largely attributed to the use, over use or misuse of antimicrobials [1]. The development of AMR coupled with the downturn in the development of new antimicrobials in the pharmaceutical industry creates unexpected challenges in the effective management of infections [2]. Annually, multi-drug resistant (MDR) bacteria is estimated to claim the lives of more than 20,000 patients in North America, 25,000 patients in Europe and more than 90,000 patients in Southern Asia [3, 4].

A number of researchers underlined the relationship between the inappropriate use of antimicrobials in the community and the emergence of antimicrobial resistance [5]. According to WHO (World Health Organization), more than two third of all antibiotics are used in the community, of which about 30% is used inappropriately [2]. Due to this, interventions focusing on the in the community such as improving access to medical services, reducing unnecessary use of antibiotics, taking a full course of treatment, and not sharing medications with other people are recommended [6]. Many previous studies documented factors associated with inappropriate use of antibiotics including culture [7], educational status [8], residency [9], marital status [8], age [10], health insurance [8] and level of satisfaction with the health care services [11, 12], and storing antibiotics at home [13].

In Ethiopia, there are signs of irrational use of antibiotics by the community, patients as well as by health care providers. According to the baseline survey conducted by Food, Medicine and Healthcare Administration and Control Authority of Ethiopia (FMHACA), about two third of patients (70%) patients who visited outpatient clinics have had one or more antibiotics prescribed with a percentage of irrational prescribing close to 40% [14]. A number of studies underlined the role of the general public in the emergence and spread of antibiotic resistance [15–18]. According to WHO, improving public access to medical facilities, reducing unnecessary and irrational use of antimicrobials, taking prescribed antimicrobials to their full course of therapy and not sharing medication with other people are some of the key issues of the general public in the fight against antimicrobial resistance [19]. However, the extent of inappropriate use of antibiotics in the urban and rural community settings has not yet been fully explored in Ethiopia. The present study aimed to document inappropriate use of antibiotics and its associated factors among the communities of Gondar, Northwest Ethiopia.

Methods

Study design and setting

A community based cross-sectional survey was conducted from December 1, 2016 to January 30, 2017 to determine inappropriate use of antibiotic among the communities Gondar town, northwest Ethiopia. We collected data between December 2016 and January 2017 as this season is associated with higher cases of infectious disorders and other common parasitic infections in Ethiopia. This study was approved by the ethical committee of School of Pharmacy, University of Gondar with an approval number of UoG-SoP-123/2016. Written informed consent from the participants was also obtained before conducting this study. Participants' information obtained was kept confidential.

Population and sampling

Gondar town, the study area, is found in Amhara regional state and is located 750 km Northwest of Addis Ababa (the capital city of Ethiopia). According the recent population and housing census report, Gondar town has a total of 207, 000 population [20]. The town has a total of 12 administrative zones (areas),1 referral hospital, and 1 defense hospital and 5 health centers. Single population proportion formula was used with the assumption of 95% confidence interval, 5% margin of error, the prevalence (p) of inappropriate use of antibiotics (30.9%) [21] and 5% for possible non-response to determine a final sample size of 720. Multistage stratified random sampling technique was used to select households in administrative areas (kebeles). Five administrative areas were selected randomly to get a representative sample. The number of households to be interviewed in each administrative area was determined in proportion with the total number of households found in each kebeles. A systematic random sampling method was then used to select the study participants. Lottery method was used to select a respondent whenever more than one eligible respondent found in the selected household.

Survey instrument

Data collection was performed by five well trained final year pharmacy students through interviewer-administered questionnaire. The tool was created by modifying items in a previously used instrument regarding knowledge and use of antibiotics in the community [21], and items were thoroughly reviewed for relevance by a team of experts including experienced clinical pharmacists and public health experts. The survey instrument was further pre-tested on 45 households who were not included in the final analysis and relevant modifications were instituted before the commencement of actual data collection. The questionnaire asks respondents about the socio-demographic characteristics and knowledge as well as the use of antibiotics. Investigators took different antibiotics (in all dosage forms) with them to show participants whether they know and/or use the antibiotics in the last 1 year. In our study, inappropriate use of antibiotics is defined as the non-prescription use of antibiotics for themselves and/or their family members, or the use of leftover antibiotics or the use of prescribed antibiotics for a reason other than its intended for [22].

Statistical analysis

All the statistical analyses were done using Social Sciences (SPSS) software version 21.0 for Windows (SPSS Inc., Chicago, IL). Frequencies and percentages were used to express different variables. Uivariate and multivariable logistic regressions were used to come up with predictors of inappropriate use of antibiotics. Associations with significance level of less than 0.20 ($p < 0.20$) in the univariate analysis were included in the multivariate logistic regression analysis. The results were adjusted for patients' demographic and disease characteristics. OR with 95% CI were also computed along with corresponding p-value ($p < 0.05$) as cut off points for determining statistical significance.

Results

Out of 720 households approached, 650 of them give consent and included in the study giving a response rate of 90.3%. The mean age of participants was 33.19 years with a standard deviation of ± 10.82. The majority of respondents were females (74.9%) and the mean family size was 4.2 with a standard deviation of ± 2.32. Details of socio-demographic characteristics of study participants are shown in Table 1.

According to the finding of our study, nearly half (48.5%) of the participants took antibiotics in the past 1 year, of which 200 (63.5%) used for themselves and 115 (36.6%) used for family members. Amoxicillin (72%) was the most commonly utilized antibiotics followed by Amoxicillin-clavulanate combination (26%) and Doxycycline (19%). Commonly utilized antibiotics are depicted in Fig. 1. Respiratory tract infection (40.9%), mechanical injury/wound (27%) and acute diarrhea (19.1%) were the three most common disease conditions to which antibiotics had been taken. More than half of the respondents (53%) got antibiotics from community drug retail outlets without a prescription (36.8%) or shared from family member or neighbor (19.1%) (Table 2).

Among participants who took antibiotics, 115 (35.9%) of them used inappropriately. Majority of participants answered incorrectly on the use of amoxicillin (80.8%) tetracycline (60.9%) and ciprofloxacin (76%). Nearly two-third of respondents (67.9%) responded that they had discontinued the use of antibiotics once their symptoms gone.

Predictors of inappropriate antibiotics use

Logistic regression analysis was employed to assess possible associations between different sociodemographic variables and respondent' inappropriate use of antibiotics (Table 1). According to the results from bivariate logistic regression, factors that were associated with inappropriate use of antibiotics included age, educational status, employment status and satisfaction with health care services. Variables that were significantly associated with inappropriate use of antibiotics in the bivariate analysis (those with p-value < 0.20) were further examined in multivariate logistic regression. Having other variables controlled, educational status, employment status and satisfaction with health care services remained to be significant in the multivariate logistic model. The odds for inappropriate antibiotics use among respondents who were unable to read and write were 4.01 times higher than respondents with tertiary education. Similarly, the odds for inappropriate antibiotics use among respondents who are employed were 2.12 times higher than respondents who are unemployed. Furthermore, those who are unsatisfied with the health care services provided were 4.41 times more likely to practice inappropriate use of antibiotics than those who are satisfied with the health care services provided.

Discussion

Inappropriate use of antibiotics, the key driver of antimicrobial resistance, is mounting at an alarming rate and the condition is conceivably worse in many developing countries including Ethiopia [23]. According to the finding of our study, 315 (48.5%) of respondents took antibiotics in the past 1 year, of which 200 (30.8%) used for themselves and 115 (17.7%) used for family members. The prevalence of self-medication reported in this study is comparable to the study done in three towns of northwest Ethiopia (27.5%) [24], but higher than studies conducted in Bahir Dar, Ethiopia (18%) [21], Portugal (19%) [25] and Euro-Mediterranean region (19.1%) [26]. Moreover, the prevalence of family medication in our study was slightly higher than the study done in Bahi Dar [21], but much lower than the study conducted in china (59.4%) [27]. Amoxicillin and Amoxicillin-clavulanate combination were the two most commonly utilized antibiotics and respiratory tract infection was the most common disease problem to which antibiotics had been sought. Similar findings were also reported in the study conducted in Uganda [28], Indonesia [29], Guatemala [30], and different parts of Ethiopia [31, 32], which reported that Amoxicillin was the most commonly used antibiotics. Similarly, in a study conducted in three selected towns of northwest Ethiopia, respiratory tract symptom was the most commonly reported complaint for self-medication [24].

It is widely believed that antimicrobial resistance can potentially arise from inadequate dosing and discontinuation of the full course of treatment [22, 33]. In our study, one third of respondents (32.1%) discontinued the

Table 1 Socio-demographic characteristics and factors associated with inappropriate antibiotic among study participants, Gondar, Ethiopia 2017 ($N = 650$)

Variables	Total ($n = 650$)	Inappropriate use		AOR (95%CI)
		No ($n = 200$)	Yes ($n = 115$)	
Gender				
Male	163(25.9%)	127	36	–
Female	487 (74.9%)	408	79	–
Age				
< 29	132 (20.3%)	108	24	1.02 (0.38–1.92)
30–39	247 (38%))	212	35	1.13 (0.46–2.02)
40–49	123 (18.9)	98	25	1.01 (0.30–1.41)
50-59	89 (13.7%)	70	19	0.98 (0.27–1.71)
> 60	59 (9.1%)	47	12	1
Number of family size				
1–2	156 (24%)	121	35	–
3–5	383 (58.9%)	339	44	–
> 5	111 (17.1)	75	36	–
Family monthly income (in USD)				
< 100	331 (50.9%)	282	49	–
101–150	201 (30.9%)	170	31	–
> 150	118 (18.2%)	83	35	–
Education status				
Unable to read and write	182 (28%)	125	57	5.01 (2.62–9.34)
Primary education	201 (30.9%)	180	21	2.81 (1.32–6.146)
Secondary education	179 (27.5%)	159	20	1.96 (0.91–4.51)
Tertiary (college) education	88 (13.5%)	71	17	1
Employment status				
Unemployed	253 (38.9%)	209	44	1
Employed	397 (61.1%)	326	71	2.12 (1.81–7.29)
Marital status				
Ever married	513 (78.9%)	444	69	–
Unmarried	137 (21.1%)	91	46	–
Frequency of visiting health care institution (in a year)				
Never	240 (36.9%)	201	39	–
Once	130 (20%)	96	34	–
Twice	119 (18.3%)	106	13	–
Three times	96 (14.8%)	80	10	–
More than three times	65 (10%)	46	19	–
Level of healthcare service satisfaction				
Satisfied	234 (36%)	121	22	1
Averagely satisfied	114 (17.5%)	78	36	3.01 (2.17–7.25)
Not satisfied	302 (46.5%)	245	57	5.41 (2.71-14.21)

use of antibiotics once their symptoms were gone. This finding is higher compared with the study done in in Kuwait (24%) [34]. But, it is lower than other studies conducted in Malaysia and Greece [35, 36]. This antibiotic misuse may put the patient at risk of relapse with drug resistant bacteria.

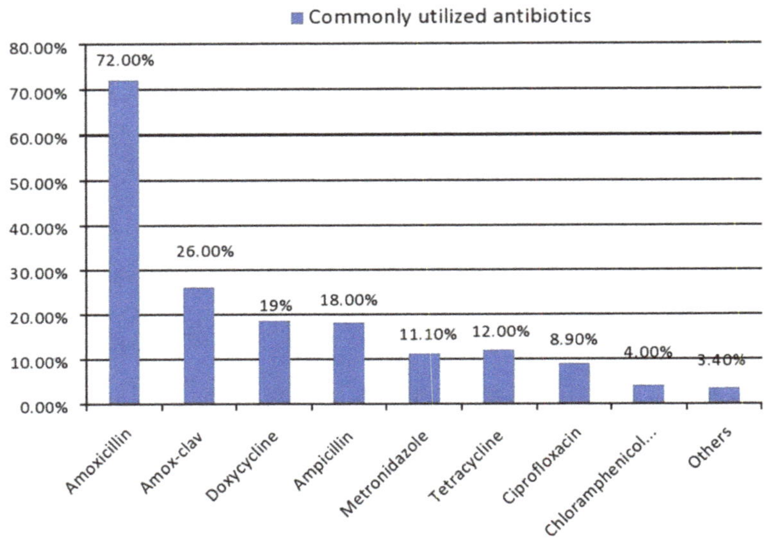

Fig. 1 Commonly utilized antibiotics among participants

Several studies conducted in different parts of the globe reported that antimicrobials are purchased without a valid prescription and could be simply possessed regardless of policies prohibiting such practice [37–39]. In our study, over half of the respondents got antibiotics from community drug retail outlets without a valid prescription or shared from family member or neighbor. In a simulated study conducted in Addis Ababa, Ethiopia to assess the non-prescription sale of medications, antibiotics were obtained without any valid prescription from 75.9% of community pharmacies [40]. Similar findings were also reported in studies conducted elsewhere [41–43]. The high prevalence of non-prescription sale and access of antibiotics in our study could be due, in part, to the lack of appropriate national regulations and explicit line of actions in the sales of antimicrobials in community drug retail outlets. Furthermore, patients may prefer to go directly to pharmacies rather than visiting a hospital due to a number of reasons including ease of accessibility, shorter waiting time and accommodate patients' ability to pay [44, 45].

According to the finding of our study, 115 (35.9%) of respondents used antibiotics inappropriately. Having other variables controlled, low educational status, being employed and unsatisfied with health care services provided are found to be strong predictors of inappropriate use of antibiotics use in the multivariate logistic model. Several other studies have also reported that lower educational status [46, 47], engagement with regular job [48, 49] and being unsatisfied with health care services [11, 12] were associated with inappropriate use of antibiotics. The low educational status of participants, which may render them to have insufficient knowledge on use of antibiotics, could have a weighty impact on the rational use of antimicrobials and development of antimicrobial resistance in the community. Hence, a customized educational campaign regarding the rational use of antibiotics and its impact on the development of antimicrobial resistance should be provided to the community. Furthermore, the relative lack of time to visit health care facilities during working hours, along with having pocket money in respondents with a regular job may render them to purchase antibiotics directly from community drug retail outlets without visiting health care facilities, ultimately increasing the potential for inappropriate use of these medications. Moreover, lack of satisfaction with health care services provided may discourage people to seek medical care from hospitals, encouraging them to look for other options for the management of their medical condition [50].

Limitation of the study

Even though this survey highlights an area of research where there is lack of literature in Ethiopia, caution should be exercised when generalizing to other regions in Ethiopia as the study was a cross-sectional and conducted only in Gondar, northwest Ethiopia. Nevertheless, this survey has significant implications for promoting the rational use of antibiotics and contain the development of antimicrobial resistance in the community.

Table 2 Extent of inappropriate use of antibiotic among study participants, Gondar, Ethiopia 2017 ($N = 650$)

Variables	Frequency (%)
Use of antibiotics in the last 1 year	
No	335 (51.5%)
Yes	315 (48.5%)
Mode of antibiotics use	
Self-medication	200 (63.5%)
Family member medication	115 (36.6%)
Purpose of antibiotics use	
Respiratory tract symptoms	129 (40.9%)
Acute diarrhea	60 (19.1%)
Mechanical injury/wound	85 (27%)
Urinary tract symptoms	34 (10.8%)
Colic	5 (1.6%)
Headache	9 (2.9%)
I could not remember	41 (13%)
Source of antibiotics	
Prescribed by health care professional	139 (44.1%)
Bought from pharmacy without prescription	116 (36.8%)
Shared from family member or neighbor	60 (19.1%)
Discontinue treatment after symptoms subside ($N = 315$)	
No	214 (67.9%)
Yes	101 (32.1%)
Amoxicillin cure common cold	
No	125 (19.2%)
Yes	525 (80.8%)
Tetracycline cure all diseases	
No	254 (39.1%)
Yes	396 (60.9%)
Ciprofloxacin cure all types of diarrhea	
No	156 (24%)
Yes	494 (76%)

Conclusion

The results of the present study revealed that inappropriate use of antibiotics is high and associated with low educational status, engagement in regular job and being unsatisfied with health care services. Our findings emphasize the need to form and deliver a comprehensive and multifaceted interventions including providing a customized education to the public so as to improve their knowledge about antibiotics and change their attitude to limit self-medication. Moreover, it is essential to adopt a strong and explicit line of actions towards the accessibility of antibiotics without a valid prescription. A larger national scale and multi centered survey that includes more diverse participants is warranted to validate our findings and to provide more accurate findings. In addition, we do recommend upcoming studies to focus on identification of areas to antibiotic treatment failure and referral to healthcare facilities due to infectious diseases like tuberculosis.

Abbreviations

AMR: Antimicrobial resistance; AOR: Adjusted odds ratio; CI: Confidence interval; FMHACA: Food, medicine and healthcare administration and control Authority of Ethiopia; MDR: Multi-drug resistant; OR: Odds ratio; SPSS: Statistical package for the social sciences; USD: United States Dollar; WHO: World Health Organization

Acknowledgements

The authors are thankful to all the participants of the survey. The authors also acknowledge the support of School of pharmacy, University of Gondar in facilitating the data collection process.

Funding

No financial support was gained to conduct the study.

Authors' contributions

All the authors involved in the conceptualization of the study, data collection supervision and write up of the first draft of the manuscript as well as submission of the manuscript. All authors read and approved the final manuscript.

Consent for publication

Not applicable

Competing interests

The authors declare that they have no competing interests.

Author details

[1]Department of Clinical Pharmacy, School of Pharmacy, University of Gondar Chechela Street, Lideta Sub city Kebele, 16 Gondar, Ethiopia. [2]Department of Pharmacology, School of Pharmacy, University of Gondar Chechela Street, Lideta Sub city Kebele, 16 Gondar, Ethiopia. [3]Department of clinical pharmacy, School of Pharmacy, College of Medicine and Health Sciences, University of Gondar, P.O. Box: 196, Gondar, Ethiopia.

References

1. Centers for Disease Control and Prevention. Antibiotic resistance threats in the United States, 2013.
2. WHO. The world health report 2007. A safer future: global public health security in the 21st century, vol. 2007: World Health Organization (WHO). Available http://www.who.int/whr/2007/en/. Accessed Jan 2017.
3. Leung E, Weil DE, Raviglione M, Nakatani H. The WHO policy package to combat antimicrobial resistance. Bull World Health Organ. 2011;89:390–2.
4. Zaidi AK, Awasthi S, de Silva HJ. Burden of infectious diseases in South Asia. BMJ. 2004;328:811–5.
5. Goldstein EJ. Beyond the target pathogen: ecological effects of the hospital formulary. Curr Opin Infect Dis. 2011;24:S21–31.
6. WHO. WHO. World Health Organization report on infectious diseases overcoming antimicrobial resistance: World Health Organization; 2000. Available http://apps.who.int/iris/handle/10665/66672. Accessed Jan 2017.
7. Cizman M. The use and resistance to antibiotics in the community. Int J Antimicrob Agents. 2003;21(4):297–307. PMID: 12672574
8. Jafari F, Khatony A, Rahmani E. Prevalence of self-medication among the elderly in Kermanshah-Iran. Global J. Health Sci. 2015;7(2):360–5.
9. Yu M, Zhao G, Stalsby Lundborg C, Zhu Y, Zhao Q, Xu B. Knowledge, attitudes, and practices of parents in rural China on the use of antibiotics in children: a

cross-sectional study. BMC Infect Dis. 2014;14:112. Epub 2014/03/01. doi: 10.1186/1471-2334-14-112.
10. Grosso G, Marventano S, Ferranti R, Mistretta A. Pattern of antibiotic use in the community: nonadherence and self-prescription rates in an Italian urban population. Mol Med Rep. 2012;5(5):1305–10. doi:10.3892/mmr.2012.818. Epub 2012/03/08. PMID: 22395156
11. Fernandes M, Leite A, Basto M, Nobre MA, Vieira N, Fernandes R, et al. Non-adherence to antibiotic therapy in patients visiting community pharmacies. Int J Clin Pharm. 2014;36(1):86–91. doi: 10.1007/s11096-013-9850-4. Epub 2013/10/09. PMID: 24101031
12. Pechere JC. Patients' interviews and misuse of antibiotics. Clinical infectious diseases. 2001; 33 Suppl 3:S170–S173. doi: 10.1086/321844 Epub 2001/08/29. PMID: 11524715.
13. Togoobaatar G, Ikeda N, Ali M, Sonomjamts M, Dashdemberel S, Mori R, et al. Survey of non-prescribed use of antibiotics for children in an urban community in Mongolia. Bull World Health Organ. 2010;88(12):930–6. doi: 10.2471/blt.10.079004. Epub 2010/12/03. PMID: 21124718; PubMed Central PMCID: PMCPmc2995192
14. DACA. Antimicrobials use, resistance and containment baseline survey synthes of findings. Addis Ababa: DACA (Drug Administration and Control Authority) in collaboration with Management Science for Health, Stregthening Pharmacutical Systems (MSH/SPH); 2009.
15. You JH, Yau B, Choi KC, Chau CT, Huang QR, et al. Public knowledge, attitudes and behavior on antibiotic use: a telephone survey in Hong Kong. Infection. 2008;36:153–7.
16. Davey P, Pagliari C, Hayes A. The patient's role in the spread control of bacterial resistance to antibiotics. Clin Microbiol Infect. 2002;8:43–68.
17. Hawkings NJ, Butler CC, Wood F. Antibiotics in the community: a typology of user behaviours. Patient Educ Couns. 2008;73:146–52.
18. McNulty CA, Boyle P, Nichols T, Clappison P, Davey P. Don't wear me out—the public's knowledge of and attitudes to antibiotic use. J Antimicrob Chemother. 2007;59:727–38.
19. World Health Organization (2001) WHO global strategy for containment of antimicrobial resistance. WHO/CDS/CSR/DRS/2001.2. Available: http://www.who.int/drugresistance/WHO_Global_Strategy_English.pdf. Accessed Jan 2017.
20. Federal Democratic Republic of Ethiopia. Population census commission: summary and statistical report of the 2007 population and housing census. Addis Ababa: UNFPA; 2008. p. 9–10.
21. Gebeyehu E, Bantie L, Azage M. Inappropriate use of antibiotics and its associated factors among urban and rural communities of Bahir Dar City Administration, Northwest Ethiopia. PLoS One. 2015;10(9):e0138179. doi: 10.1371/journal. pone.0138179.
22. Ayukekbong JA, Michel Ntemgwa M, Atabe AN. The threat of antimicrobial resistance in developing countries: causes and control strategies. Antimicrobial Resistance and Infection Control. 2017;6:47. DOI 10.1186/s13756-017-0208.
23. Byarugaba DK. A view on antimicrobial resistance in developing countries and responsible risk factors. Int J Antimicrob Agents. 2004;24:105–10.
24. Abula T, Worku A. Self-medication in three towns of north West Ethiopia. Ethiop J Heal Dev. 2001;1(15):25–30.
25. Ramalhinho I, Cordeiro C, Cavaco A, Cabrita J. Assessing determinants of self-medication with antibiotics among Portuguese people in the Algarve region. Int J Clin Pharm. 2014;36(5):1039–1047. Epub 2014/08/26. doi: 10.1007/s11096-014-9992-z.
26. Scicluna EA, Borg MA, Gur D, Rasslan O, Taher I, Redjeb SB, et al. Self-medication with antibiotics in the ambulatory care setting within the euro-Mediterranean region; results from the ARMed project. Journal of infection and public health. 2009;2(4):189–197. Epub 2009/01/01. doi: 10.1016/j.jiph.2009.09.004.
27. Bi P, Tong S, Parton KA. Family self-medication and antibiotics abuse for children and juveniles in a Chinese city. Soc. Sci. Med. (1982). 2000;50(10): 1445–50. Epub 2000/03/31
28. Ocan M, Bwanga F, Bbosa GS, Bagenda D, Waako P, Ogwal-Okeng J, et al. Patterns and predictors of self-medication in northern Uganda. PLoS One. 2014;9(3):e92323. Epub 2014/03/25. doi: 10.1371/ journal.pone.0092323.
29. Widayati A, Suryawati S, de Crespigny C, Hiller JE. Self medication with antibiotics in Yogyakarta City Indonesia: a cross sectional population-based survey. BMC. Res. Notes. 2011;4:491. Epub 2011/ 11/15. doi: 10.1186/1756-0500-4-49.
30. Ramay BM, Lambour P, Ceron A. Comparing antibiotic self-medication in two socio-economic groups in Guatemala City: a descriptive cross-sectional study. BMC Pharmacol. Toxicol. 2015;16(1):11. Epub 2015/05/01. doi: 10.1186/s40360-015-0011-3.
31. Desalegn AA. Assessment of drug use pattern using WHO prescribing indicators at Hawassa university teaching and referral hospital, south Ethiopia: a cross-sectional study. BMC Health Serv Res. 2013;13:170. Epub 2013/05/08. doi: 10.1186/1472-6963-13-170.
32. Fenta A, Belay M, Mekonnen E. Assessment of antibacterial drug exposure patterns of patient encounters seen by different categories of prescribers at health institutions in Bahir Dar, Ethiopia. Ethiop Med J. 2013;51(1):33–9. Epub 2013/08/13
33. Kardas P, Devine S, Golembesky A, Roberts C. A systematic review and meta-analysis of misuse of antibiotic therapies in the community. Int J Antimicrob Agents. 2005;26(2):106–113. Epub 2005/07/13. doi: 10.1016/j.ijantimicag.2005.04.017.
34. Awad AI, Aboud EA. Knowledge, attitude and practice towards antibiotic use among the public in Kuwait. PLoS One. 2015;10(2):e0117910. doi: 10.1371/journal.pone.0117910.
35. Fatokun O. Exploring antibiotic use and practices in a Malaysian community. Int J Clin Pharm. 2014;36(3):564–569. Epub 2014/04/05. doi: 10.1007/s11096-014-9937-6.
36. Mitsi G, Jelastopulu E, Basiaris H, Skoutelis A, Gogos C. Patterns of antibiotic use among adults and parents in the community: a questionnaire-based survey in a Greek urban population. Int J Antimicrob Agents. 2005;25(5): 439–443. Epub 2005/04/26. doi: 10.1016/j.ijantimicag.2005.02.009.
37. Contopoulos-Ioannidis DG, Koliofoti ID, Koutroumpa IC, Giannakakis IA, Ioannidis JP. Pathways for inappropriate dispensing of antibiotics for rhinosinusitis: a randomized trial. Clin Infect Dis. 2001;33(1):76–82.
38. Lansang MA, Lucas-Aquino R, Tupasi TE, Mina VS, Salazar LS, Juban N, Limjoco TT, Nisperos LE, Kunin CM. Purchase of antibiotics without prescription in Manalia, the Philippines. Inappropriate choices and doses. J Clin Epidemiol. 1990;43:61–7.
39. Morgan DJ, Okeke IN, Laxminarayan R, Perencevich EN, Weisenberg S. Non-prescription antimicrobial use worldwide: a systematic review. Lancet Infect Dis. 2011;11:692–701.
40. Erku DA, Mekuria AB, Surur AS, Gebresillassie BM. Extent of dispensing prescription-only medications without a prescription in community drug retail outlets in Addis Ababa, Ethiopia: a simulated-patient study. Drug, Health care and Patient Safety. 2016;8:65–70.
41. Kagashe GAB, Minzi O, Matowe L. An assessment of dispensing practices in private pharmacies in Dar-es-salaam, Tanzania. Int J Pharm Pract. 2011;19:30–5.
42. Volpato DE, de Souza BV, Dalla Rosa LG, Melo LH, Daudt CA, Deboni L. Use of antibiotics without medical prescription. Braz J Infect Dis. 2005;9(4):288–91.
43. Llor C, Cots JM. The sale of antibiotics without prescription in pharmacies in Catalonia, Spain. Clin Infect Dis. 2009;48(10):1345–9.
44. Goel P, Ross-Degnan D, Berman P, Soumerai S. Retail pharmacies in developing countries: a behavior and intervention framework. Soc Sci Med. 1996;42:1155–61.
45. Kwena Z, Sharma A, Wamae N, Muga C, Bukusi E. Provider characteristics among staff providing care to sexually transmitted infection self-medicating patients in retail pharmacies in Kibera slum, Nairobi. Kenya Sex Transm Dis. 2008;35:480–3.
46. Panagakou SG, Papaevangelou V, Chadjipanayis A, Syrogiannopoulos GA, Theodoridou M, Hadjichristodoulou CS. Risk factors of antibiotic misuse for upper respiratory tract infections in children: results from a cross-sectional knowledge-attitude-practice study in Greece. ISRN Pediatrics. 2012;2012: 685302. Epub 2012/12/05. doi: 10.5402/2012/685302.
47. Barah F, Goncalves V. Antibiotic use and knowledge in the community in Kalamoon, Syrian Arab Republic: a cross-sectional study. East Mediterr Health J. 2010;16(5):516–21. Epub 2010/08/ 31
48. Berzanskyte A, Valinteliene R, Haaijer-Ruskamp FM, Gurevicius R, Grigoryan L. Self-medication with antibiotics in Lithuania. Int J Occup Med Environ Health. 2006;19(4):246–53. Epub 2007/04/04
49. Jose J, Jimmy B, Alsabahi AG, Al Sabei GA. A study assessing public knowledge, belief and behavior of antibiotic use in an omani population. Oman Med J. 2013;28(5):324–330. Epub 2013/09/18. doi: 10.5001/omj.2013.95.
50. Lyu H, Wick EC, Housman M, Freischlag JA, Makary MA. Patient satisfaction as a possible indicator of quality surgical care. JAMA Surgery. 2013;148(4): 362–367. Epub 2013/05/30. doi: 10.1001/2013.jamasurg.270.

9

Prevalence, identification of virulence factors, O-serogroups and antibiotic resistance properties of Shiga-toxin producing *Escherichia coli* strains isolated from raw milk and traditional dairy products

Reza Ranjbar[1], Farhad Safarpoor Dehkordi[2], Mohammad Hossein Sakhaei Shahreza[3*] and Ebrahim Rahimi[4,5]

Abstract

Background: Shiga-toxigenic *Escherichia coli* strains are one of the most important foodborne bacteria with an emergence of antibiotic resistance. Foodborne STEC strains are mainly associated with presence of certain virulence factors and O-seogroups. The present investigation was done to study the distribution of virulence factors, O-serogroups and antibiotic resistance properties of Shiga-toxigenic *Escherichia coli* isolated from milk and dairy products.

Methods: Six-hundred samples were randomly collected and immediately transferred to laboratory. All samples were cultured and *E. coli* strains were isolated. STEC strains were identified based on the presence of putative virulence factors and subtypes. STEC isolates were subjected to multiplex PCR and disk diffusion methods.

Results: One-hundred and eighty-one out of 600 samples (30.16%) harbored *E. coli*. Prevalence of STEC strains was 10.66%. O157 (43.75%) and O26 (37.50%) were the most frequently identified serogroups. *Aac(3)-IV* (100%), *CITM* (96.87%) and *tetA* (76.56%) were the most commonly detected antibiotic resistance genes. STEC strains had the highest prevalence of resistance against ampicillin (100%), gentamicin (100%) and tetracycline (96.87%).

Conclusions: Kashk and dougn were negative for presence of *E. coli* strains. High prevalence of resistant-O157 strains and simultaneous presence of multiple virulence factors pose an important public health problem regarding the consumption of raw milk and dairy products.

Keywords: Shiga toxin producing *Escherichia coli*, Molecular characterization, Antibiotic resistance

Background

Billions of people consuming milk and dairy products every day. Milk and dairy products are full from valuable nutritional factors such as proteins, lipids, minerals, and vitamins. Researches showed that consumption of milk and dairy products is useful for human [1, 2]. There are several types of dairy products such as cheese, cream, butter, yoghurt, and ice cream, with high beneficial effects for human health [3, 4]. Kashk and dough are two important traditional dairy products in Iran and some other sites of the world. Kashk comes in liquid or dried forms and is traditionally made with the milk left over from cheese-making. Dough is a popular salty yogurt-based beverage amongst the Iranian people [3, 4]. Based on the high consumption rate of milk and dairy products, it is important to ensure from the microbial quality of these types of food samples [5].

Escherichia coli (*E. coli*) strains are one of the most important cause of foodborne diseases al-around the world

* Correspondence: Dr.mh_sakhaieshahreza@yahoo.com
[3]Doctor Veterinary Medicine, Faculty of Veterinary Medicine, Shahrekord Branch, Islamic Azad University, Shahrekord, Iran
Full list of author information is available at the end of the article

[5–7]. Milk and dairy products are one of the main sources of transmission of the *E. coli* strains into the human [5–7]. *E. coli* is a Gram-negative, non-sporulating, flagellated, rod-shaped and facultative anaerobic bacterium which belongs to Enterobacteriaceae family. Enterohemorrhagic *E. coli* (EHEC) strains are a subtype of the Vero (Shiga) toxin (Vtx or Stx)-producing *E. coli* (VTEC or STEC) [5, 6, 8]. EHEC bacteria are causative agents of severe syndromes including Hemolytic Uremic Syndrome (HUS), Thrombotic Thrombocytopenic Purpura (TTP), Hemorrhagic Colitis (HC) and bloody and non-bloody diarrhea [5, 6, 9].

E. coli strains isolated from milk and dairy products harbored the high prevalence of intimin (*eaeA*), Vero or Shiga toxins (*vtx1* and *vtx2* or *stx1* and *stx2*) and hemolysin (*hlyA*). These factors can cause bacterial adhesion and invasion into the intestinal epithelial cells which cause severe attaching-effacing (A/E) lesions [9–11]. Attaching and effacing lesions are mainly caused by certain types of the STEC bacteria called Attaching-Effacing *E. coli* (AEEC) [9–11]. Expression of the *eae* gene is the main factor for occurrence of A/E lesions [9–11].

Occurrence of foodborne diseases caused by this bacterium are mainly occurred due to the activity of certain O-serogroups including non-O157 (O103, O26, O113, O91, O145, O111, O121, O128 and O45) and also O157 [5, 6, 12].

STEC strains are mainly resistant against several types of antibiotics. Documented data revealed that STEC strains isolated from milk and dairy products and also other types of food samples harbored the high prevalence of resistance against different types of antibiotics including aminoglycosides, fluoroquinolone, tetracyclines, trimethoprim, ampicillin, cephalothin, sulfonamides, gentamicin and chloramphenicol [5–13]. Molecular epidemiological researches showed that presence of certain antibiotic resistance genes including the genes that encode resistance against fluoroquinolone (*qnr*), trimethoprim (*dfrA1*), cephalothin (*blaSHV*), tetracycline (*tetA* and *tetB*), ampicillin (*CITM*), gentamicin (*aac(3)-IV*), sulfonamide (*sul1*), chloramphenicol (*cat1* and *cmlA*), aminoglycosides (*aadA1*), and erythromycin (*ereA*) is the most important reason for occurrence of antibiotic resistance in STEC strains [5–13].

According to an uncertain role of STEC strains in milk and dairy products and deficiency of similar microbiological and epidemiological surveys in Iran, the current examination was done to molecular characterization of O-serogroups, virulence genes and antibiotic resistance properties of STEC bacteria recovered raw milk and traditional dairy products.

Methods

Samples and *Escherichia coli* identification

From March 2015 to March 2016, a total of 600 different types of raw milk and traditional dairy product samples including raw bovine ($n = 70$), raw ovine ($n = 60$), raw caprine (n = 60), raw buffalo ($n = 40$) and raw camel ($n = 30$) milk samples and traditional cheese ($n = 50$), yoghurt ($n = 60$), kashk ($n = 50$), dough ($n = 50$), butter ($n = 40$), cream ($n = 40$) and ice-cream ($n = 50$) samples were randomly collected from Isfahan province, Iran. Samples collection was done according to the instruction introduced by International Dairy Federation [14]. Samples (100 mL) were transferred to laboratory at 4 °C. All food samples showed normal physical characters including odor, color and consolidation.

Twenty-five milliliters of raw milk samples and 25 mg of homogenized dairy products were added to sterilized tubes containing 225 ml of Buffered Peptone Water (BPW, Merck, Germany) and hatched aerobically at 37 °C for 24 h. Then, samples were cultured on 5% sheep blood and MacConkey agar (Merck, Germany) media and incubated at 37 °C for 24 h. Colonies with the typical color and appearance of *E. coli* were picked and streaked again on blood agar plates and re-streaked on EMB agar (Merck, Germany). All plates were further incubated for 24 h at 37 °C. The green metallic sheen colonies were considered as *E. coli*. The presumptive colonies were biochemically tested for growth on triple sugar iron agar (TSI) and lysine iron agar (LIA), oxidative/fermentative degradation of glucose, citrate utilization, urease production, indol fermentation, tryptophan degradation, glucose degradation (methyl red test) and motility.

PCR confirmation of *E. coli* isolates

Colonies were further confirmed using the *16S rRNA*-based Polymerase Chain Reaction (PCR) according to the method described previously [15]. Bacterial strains were sub-cultured overnight in Luria-Bertani broth (Merck, Germany) and further incubated for 48 h at 37 °C. Genomic DNA was extracted from bacterial colonies using the DNA extraction kit (Thermo Fisher Scientific, St. Leon-Rot, Germany) according to manufacturer's instruction. DNA quality and concentration were examined using the spectrophotometer [16]. The 10 ml bacterial DNA extract and controls were amplified with 0.5 mM primers (Forward: 5'-AGTTTGATCCTGGCTCAG-3′ and Reverse: 5'-AGGCCCGGGAACGTATTCAC-3′) (1343 bp) [15], 200 mM of each dNTP (Thermo Fisher Scientific, St. Leon-Rot, Germany), 2 mM MgCl2, 10 mM KCl PCR buffer and 1.0 U Taq polymerase (Thermo Fisher Scientific, St. Leon-Rot, Germany). The DNA was amplified in a programmable thermal cycler (Eppendorf, Mastercycler® 5330, Eppendorf-Netheler-Hinz GmbH, Hamburg, Germany) PCR device using the following protocol: 94 °C for 5 min, 40 cycles of 94 °C for 1 min, 55 °C for 1 min, 72 °C for 2 min, and final 72 °C for 5 min.

Detection of virulence factors, O-serogroups and antibiotic resistance genes

Table 1 indicates list of primers and PCR conditions used for detection of O-serogroups, virulence genes and antimicrobial resistant genes [17, 18]. Fifteen microliters of amplified PCR products were subjected to electrophoresis in a 1.5% agarose gel in 1X TBE buffer at 80 V for 30 min, stained with SYBR Green (Thermo Fisher Scientific, St. Leon-Rot, Germany) [17, 18]. All runs included a negative DNA control consisting of PCR grade water and strains of *E. coli* O157:K88 ac:H19, CAPM 5933 and *E. coli* O159:H20, CAPM 6006 were used as positive controls.

Disk diffusion test

Antibiotic resistance pattern of *E. coli* isolates was determined by simple disk diffusion method. The Mueller–Hinton agar (Merck, Germany) media were used for antibiotic susceptibility test. Principles of the Clinical and Laboratory Standards Institute (CLSI) were used for this purpose [19]. Susceptibility of *E. coli* isolates were tested against tetracycline (30 u/disk), ampicillin (10 u/disk), cefotaxime (30 μg/disk), gentamicin (10 μg/disk), ciprofloxacin (5 μg/disk), amikacin (30 u/disk), ceftazidime (30 μg/disk), imipenem (30 u/disk), cotrimoxazole (30 μg/disk), enrofloxacin (5 μg/disk), sulfamethoxazole (25 μg/disk), trimethoprim (5 μg/disk), streptomycin (10 μg/disk) and chloramphenicol (30 μg/disk) antibiotic agents (Oxoid, UK). All of the inoculated plates were aerobically incubated at 37 °C for 18-24 h. Results were interpreted based on the instruction provided by CLSI [19]. *E. coli* ATCC 25922 was used as positive control.

Statistical analysis

Data obtained from all tests were transferred to the Microsoft Excel spreadsheet (Microsoft Corp., Redmond, WA) for analysis. At first, all data were subjected to Kolmogorov-Smirnov test to study their distribution. Then, the statistical analysis was performed using SPSS/20.0 software (SPSS Inc., Chicago, IL). *P*-values were calculated using Chi-square and Fisher's exact tests. Statistical analysis was used to find any significant relationship for prevalence of *E. coli* and also STEC strains between different samples, seasonal distribution of bacteria, distribution of O-serogroups, virulence factors and antibiotic resistance. The *P*-value less than 0.05 was considered statistically significant.

Results

Table 2 represents the prevalence of *E. coli* strains in different types of milk samples and dairy products. One-hundred and eighty-one out of 600 samples (30.16%) were positive for *E. coli* strains. Cheese (80%) and raw buffalo milk (50%) samples had the highest prevalence of *E. coli*, while raw camel milk (6.66%) had the lowest. There were no positive results for Kashk and dough samples. Statistical significant difference was seen between types of samples and prevalence of *E. coli* ($P < 0.05$).

Figure 1 revealed the seasonal prevalence of *E. coli* strains. Raw milk and traditional dairy product samples which were collected through the summer season had the highest prevalence of *E. coli* (62.50%). Statistical significant difference was seen for the prevalence of *E. coli* strains between hot and cold seasons ($P = 0.018$).

Table 3 represents the prevalence of EHEC and AEEC subtypes in the *E. coli* strains isolated from raw milk and traditional dairy product samples. Prevalence of EHEC subtype in raw bovine, ovine, caprine and buffalo milk and traditional cheese, yoghurt, butter, cream and ice-cream samples was 25%, 22.22%, 27.27%, 35.71%, 32%, 33.33%, 16.66%, 25% and 22.22%, respectively. Prevalence of AEEC subtype in raw bovine, ovine, caprine and buffalo milk and traditional cheese, yoghurt, butter, cream and ice-cream samples was 31.25%, 33.33%, 36.36%, 35.71%, 36%, 33.33%, 50%, 50% and 55.55%, respectively. *E. coli* strains of the EHEC subtype were positive for all *stx1*, *eae* and *ehly* virulence genes. Statistical significant difference was seen between the prevalence of EHEC and AEEC subtypes ($P < 0.01$). Sixty-four out of 181 *E. coli* isolates (35.35%) were positive for AEEC and EHEC subtypes. These isolates were determined as STEC strains. There were no STEC strains in the raw camel milk samples. *E. coli* strains of the EHEC subtype were recognized as O157 serogroup.

Table 4 represents the prevalence of O157 and non-O157 serogroups in the STEC strains isolated from raw milk and traditional dairy product samples. O157 (43.75%) and O26 (37.50%) were the most commonly detected O-serogroups. Prevalence of O111, O45, O113 and O121 serogroups were 9.37%, 1.50%, 1.50% and 6.25%, respectively. There were no positive results for O145, O91 and O128 serogroups. Statistical significant difference was seen between types of samples and prevalence of O-serogroups ($P < 0.05$).

Table 5 shows the distribution of antibiotic resistance genes amongst the STEC strains isolated from raw milk and traditional dairy product samples. *Aac(3)-IV* (100%), *CITM* (96.87%) and *tetA* (76.56%) were the most commonly detected antibiotic resistance genes. Prevalence of *cmlA* (1.50%), *cat1* (18.75%) and *tetB* (20.31%) antibiotic resistance genes were low. Statistical significant difference was seen between the types of samples and distribution of antibiotic resistance genes ($P < 0.05$).

Table 6 indicates the prevalence of antibiotic resistance in the STEC strains isolated from raw milk and traditional dairy product samples. STEC strains harbored the highest prevalence of resistance against ampicillin (100%), gentamicin (100%) and tetracycline (96.87%) antibiotics. Statistical significant difference was seen between

Table 1 Primers and PCR conditions used for characterization of virulence genes, O-serogroups and antibiotic resistance genes in the STEC strains isolated from raw milk and traditional dairy product samples

Target gene	Primer sequence (5′-3′)	PCR product (bp)	PCR programs	PCR Volume (50 µL)
O157	F: CGGACATCCATGTGATATGG R: TTGCCTATGTACAGCTAATCC	259	1 cycle: 95 °C ———— 3 min. 30 cycle: 95 °C ———— 20 s 58 °C ———— 40 s 72 °C ———— 30 s 1 cycle: 72 °C ———— 8 min	5 µL PCR buffer 10X 2 mM $Mgcl_2$ 150 µM dNTP (Fermentas) 0.75 µM of each primers F & R 1.5 U Taq DNA polymerase (Fermentas) 3 µL DNA template
O145	F: CCATCAACAGATTTAGGAGTG R: TTTCTACCGCGAATCTATC	609		
O103	F: TTGGAGCGTTAACTGGACCT R: GCTCCCGAGCACGTATAAG	321		
O26	F: CAGAATGGTTATGCTACTGT R: CTTACATTTGTTTTCGGCATC	423		
O111	F: TAGAGAAATTATCAAGTTAGTTCC R: ATAGTTATGAACATCTTGTTTAGC	406		
O91	F: GCTGACCTTCATGATCTGTTGA R: TAATTTAACCCGTAGAATCGCTGC	291	1 cycle: 94 °C ———— 6 min. 34 cycle: 95 °C ———— 50 s 58 °C ———— 70 s 72 °C ———— 55 s 1 cycle: 72 °C ———— 10 min	5 µL PCR buffer 10X 2 mM $Mgcl_2$ 150 µM dNTP (Fermentas) 0.75 µM of each primers F & R 1.5 U Taq DNA polymerase (Fermentas) 3 µL DNA template
O128	F: GCTTTCTGCCGATATTTGGC R: CCGACGGACTGATGCCGGTGATT	289		
O121	F: TGGCTAGTGGCATTCTGATG R: TGATACTTTAGCCGCCCTTG	322		
O113	F: GGGTTAGATGGAGCGCTATTGAGA R: AGGTCACCCTCTGAATTATGGCAG	771		
O45	F: CCGGGTTTCGATTTGTGAAGGTTG R: CACAACAGCCACTACTAGGCAGAA	527		
stx1	F: AAATCGCCATTCGTTGACTACTTCT R: TGCCATTCTGGCAACTCGCGATGCA	366	1 cycle: 95 °C ———— 3 min. 34 cycle: 94 °C ———— 60 s 56 °C ———— 45 s 72 °C ———— 60 s 1 cycle: 72 °C ———— 10 min	5 µL PCR buffer 10X 2 mM $Mgcl_2$ 150 µM dNTP (Fermentas) 0.75 µM of each primers F & R 1.5 U Taq DNA polymerase (Fermentas) 3 µL DNA template
stx2	F: CGATCGTCACTCACTGGTTTCATCA R: GGATATTCTCCCCACTCTGACACC	282		
eaeA	F: TGCGGCACAACAGGCGGCGA R: CGGTCGCCGCACCAGGATTC	629		
ehly	F: CAATGCAGATGCAGATACCG R: CAGAGATGTCGTTGCAGCAG	432		
aadA1	F: TATCCAGCTAAGCGCGAACT R: ATTTGCCGACTACCTTGGTC	447	1 cycle: 94 °C ———— 8 min. 32 cycle: 95 °C ———— 60 s 55 °C ———— 70 s 72 °C ———— 2 min 1 cycle: 72 °C ———— 8 min	5 µL PCR buffer 10X 2 mM $Mgcl_2$ 150 µM dNTP (Fermentas) 0.75 µM of each primers F & R 1.5 U Taq DNA polymerase (Fermentas) 3 µL DNA template
tetA	F: GGTTCACTCGAACGACGTCA R: CTGTCCGACAAGTTGCATGA	577		
tetB	F: CCTCAGCTTCTCAACGCGTG R: GCACCTTGCTGATGACTCTT	634		
dfrA1	F: GGAGTGCCAAAGGTGAACAGC R: GAGGCGAAGTCTTGGGTAAAAAC	367		
qnr	F: GGGTATGGATATTATTGATAAAG R: CTAATCCGGCAGCACTATTTA	670		
aac(3)-IV	F: CTTCAGGATGGCAAGTTGGT R: TCATCTCGTTCTCCGCTCAT	286		
sul1	F: TTCGGCATTCTGAATCTCAC R: ATGATCTAACCCTCGGTCTC	822		
blaSHV	F: TCGCCTGTGTATTATCTCCC R: CGCAGATAAATCACCACAATG	768		
CITM	F: TGGCCAGAACTGACAGGCAAA R: TTTCTCCTGAACGTGGCTGGC	462		
cat1	F: AGTTGCTCAATGTACCTATAACC R: TTGTAATTCATTAAGCATTCTGCC	547		
cmlA	F: CCGCCACGGTGTTGTTGTTATC R: CACCTTGCCTGCCCATCATTAG	698		

Table 2 Prevalence of *Escherichia coli* strains isolated from raw milk and traditional dairy product samples

Types of samples	No. samples collected	No positive strains (%)
Raw bovine milk	70	30 (42.85)
Raw ovine milk	60	21 (35)
Raw caprine milk	60	23 (38.33)
Raw buffalo milk	40	20 (50)
Raw camel milk	30	2 (6.66)
Cheese	50	40 (80)
Yoghurt	60	5 (8.33)
Kashk	50	–
Dough	50	–
Butter	40	10 (25)
Cream	40	15 (37.50)
Ice-cream	50	15 (30)
Total	600	181 (30.16)

the types of samples and prevalence of antibiotic resistance ($P < 0.05$).

Figure 2 shows the prevalence of multi-drug resistant STEC strains isolated from raw milk and traditional dairy product samples. All of the STEC strains were resistant to at least an antibiotic, while prevalence of resistance against more than 7 antibiotics was 43.75%.

Discussion

As far as we know, the current research is the most comprehensive report of the molecular characterization and study the phenotypic and genotypic properties of antibiotic resistance of the STEC strains isolated from raw milk and traditional dairy product samples. We found that 30.16% of raw milk and traditional dairy product samples were contaminated with *E. coli* strains. We also found that the prevalence of STEC strains were 35.35% (64/181). Ombarak et al. (2016) [20] reported that the prevalence of *E. coli* strains in various types of dairy products had a range of 21 to 77%. Elhadidy and Mohammed (2012) [21] revealed that 11.29% of cheese samples were contaminated with the STEC strains which was lower than our findings (34%). Total prevalence of *E. coli* strains in raw milk and traditional dairy product samples of studies conducted on Switzerland [22], Iran [23], Italy [24], Egypt [25], Turkey [26], China [27], and Spain [28] had range between 1% to 27% which were lower than our reported prevalence rate.

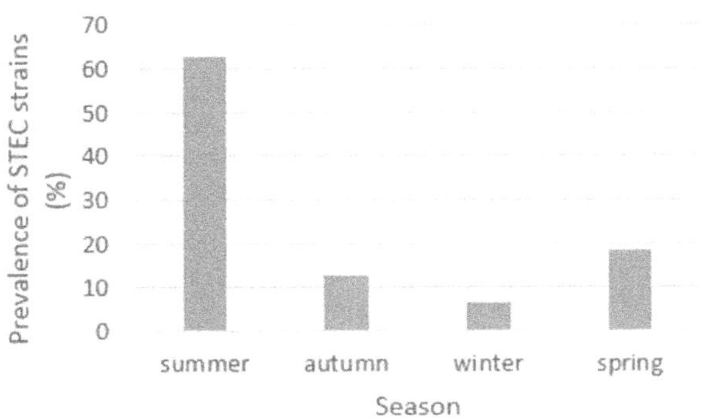

Fig. 1 Seasonal prevalence of *Escherichia coli* strains in raw milk and traditional dairy product samples

There were some probable explanations for the high prevalence of *E. coli* and also STEC strains in raw milk and traditional dairy product samples of our study [5, 7, 29]. At first. Iranian ranchers used from their hand and also traditional equipment for milking procedure which increase the risk of transmission of bacteria into the milk and dairy products [5, 7, 29]. At second, lack of maintenance of raw milk samples at temperatures below than 4 °C which facilitates survival and proliferation of bacteria [5, 7, 29]. At third, using from unpasteurized milk for production of dairy products which facilitates the survival of bacteria in dairy products. [5, 7, 29]. Transmission of pathogenic agents from the infected staffs of the milking halls and also factories is another important risk factor. There were no positive results for kashk and dough samples. Production of these two dairy products need high thermal processing which caused to destruction of pathogenic agents.

We found marked seasonality in the distribution of *E. coli* strains in raw milk and traditional dairy product samples. High prevalence of *E. coli* strains in summer season (64.10%) could be related to the low levels of individual hygiene in this season. The higher prevalence of STEC strains may be due to the higher activity of bacteria in hot seasons. Of studies which have been conducted in this field [29–31], all have shown a seasonal distribution for *E. coli* strains with a higher prevalence of bacteria in warmer seasons [32–34].

Results of the current research revealed that raw milk and traditional dairy product samples harbored the high prevalence of virulent STEC strains. We found that STEC strains harbored the high prevalence of *stx1, stx2, eaeA* and *ehlyA* virulence factors. Some isolates were positive for multiple virulence genes which represented their high pathogenicity. Momtaz et al. [5] revealed that *stx1, papA, cnf1, traT, cnf2, eaeA and ehly* were the most commonly detected virulence factors amongst the STEC *strains of* dairy products. Dehkordi et al. [7] reported that the prevalence of stx1, stx2, eaeA and ehly genes amongst the STEC strains of fermented dairy products were 44%, 30%, 36% and 28%, respectively. We found that AEEC subtypes had the higher prevalence than EHEC subtype. This finding had also been reported by other researchers [5–7, 17, 18, 28, 29]. All of the previously

Table 3 Prevalence of pathogenic subtypes and related virulence factors in *Escherichia coli* strains isolated from raw milk and traditional dairy product samples

Samples (No. positive)	Subtypes	No. positive samples	Virulence genes
Raw bovine milk (30)	Non detected	7 (43.75)	–
	EHEC	4 (25)	*stx1, eae, ehly*: 4 (100)
	AEEC	5 (31.25)	*stx1*: 5 (100) *stx2*: 3 (60) *eaeA*: 5 (100) *stx1, eaeA*: 3 (60) *stx2, eaeA*: 2 (40) *stx1, stx2, eaeA*: 1 (20)
	Total	16 (53.33)	
Raw ovine milk (21)	Non detected	4 (44.44)	–
	EHEC	2 (22.22)	*stx1, eae, ehly*: 2 (100)
	AEEC	3 (33.33)	*stx1*: 3 (100) *stx2*: 1 (33.33) *eaeA*: 3 (100) *stx1, eaeA*: 1 (33.33) *stx2, eaeA*: 1 (33.33) *stx1, stx2, eaeA*: 1 (33.33)
	Total	9 (42.85)	
Raw caprine milk (23)	Non detected	4 (36.36)	–
	EHEC	3 (27.27)	*stx1, eae, ehly*: 2 (100)
	AEEC	4 (36.36)	*stx1*: 4 (100) *stx2*: 2 (50) *eaeA*: 4 (100) *stx1, eaeA*: 2 (50) *stx2, eaeA*: 1 (25) *stx1, stx2, eaeA*: 1 (25)
	Total	11 (47.82)	
Raw buffalo milk (20)	Non detected	4 (28.57)	–
	EHEC	5 (35.71)	*stx1, eae, ehly*: 5 (100)
	AEEC	5 (35.71)	*stx1*: 5 (100) *stx2*: 3 (60) *eaeA*: 5 (100) *stx1, eaeA*: 3 (60) *stx2, eaeA*: 1 (20) *stx1, stx2, eaeA*: 1 (20)
	Total	14 (70)	
Raw camel milk (2)	Non detected	1 (100)	–
	EHEC	–	–
	AEEC	–	*stx1*: *stx2*: - *eaeA*: *stx1, eaeA*: *stx2, eaeA*: - *stx1, stx2, eaeA*: -
	Total	1 (50)	
Cheese (40)	Non detected	8 (32)	–
	EHEC	8 (32)	*stx1, eae, ehly*: 8 (100)
	AEEC	9 (36)	*stx1*: 9 (100) *stx2*: 5 (55.55) *eaeA*: 8 (88.88) *stx1, eaeA*: 5 (66.66) *stx2, eaeA*: 2 (22.22) *stx1, stx2, eaeA*: 2 (22.22)
	Total	25 (62.50)	

Table 3 Prevalence of pathogenic subtypes and related virulence factors in *Escherichia coli* strains isolated from raw milk and traditional dairy product samples *(Continued)*

Samples (No. positive)	Subtypes	No. positive samples	Virulence genes
Yoghurt (5)	Non detected	1 (33.33)	–
	EHEC	1 (33.33)	*stx1, eae, ehly*: 1 (100)
	AEEC	1 (33.33)	*stx1*: 1 (100) *stx2*: 1 (100) *eaeA*: 1 (100) *stx1, eaeA*: 1 (100) *stx2, eaeA*: 1 (100) *stx1, stx2, eaeA*: 1 (100)
	Total	3 (60)	
Butter (10)	Non detected	2 (33.33)	–
	EHEC	1 (16.66)	*stx1, eae, ehly*: 1 (100)
	AEEC	3 (50)	*stx1*: 3 (100) *stx2*: 1 (33.33) *eaeA*: 3 (100) *stx1, eaeA*: 1 (33.33) *stx2, eaeA*: 1 (33.33) *stx1, stx2, eaeA*: 1 (33.33)
	Total	6 (60)	
Cream (15)	Non detected	2 (25)	–
	EHEC	2 (25)	*stx1, eae, ehly*: 2 (100)
	AEEC	4 (50)	*stx1*: 4 (100) *stx2*: 2 (50) *eaeA*: 3 (75) *stx1, eaeA*: 2 (50) *stx2, eaeA*: 1 (25) *stx1, stx2, eaeA*: 1 (25)
	Total	8 (53.33)	
Ice-cream (15)	Non detected	2 (22.22)	–
	EHEC	2 (22.22)	*stx1, eae, ehly*: 2 (100)
	AEEC	5 (55.55)	*stx1*: 5 (100) *stx2*: 3 (60) *eaeA*: 5 (100) *stx1, eaeA*: 2 (40) *stx2, eaeA*: 2 (40) *stx1, stx2, eaeA*: 1 (20)
	Total	9 (60)	

published articles in this field [5–7, 17, 18, 28, 29] found that EHEC strains harbored all stx1, eae and ehly genes together which was similar to our findings. Simultaneous presence of stx1 and eaeA and also stx1 and ehly virulence factors in the STEC strains is another important finding of the present study which was supported by previous researches [5–7, 17, 18, 28, 29].

We found that both O157 and non-O157 (especially O26, O111 and O121) serogroups had a considerable prevalence in *STEC strains isolated from* raw milk and traditional dairy product samples. These serogroups were also predominant in the STEC strains isolated from ground beef (Argentina) [30], hospital foods (Iran) [31], dairy products (France) [32] and milk (Spain) [33].

Table 4 Prevalence of O-serogroups in the STEC strains isolated from raw milk and traditional dairy product samples

Samples (No. STEC strains)	Distribution of O-serogroups (%)									
	O157	O26	O103	O111	O145	O45	O91	O113	O121	O128
Raw bovine milk (9)	4 (44.44)	3 (33.33)	–	1 (11.11)	–	–	–	–	1 (11.11)	–
Raw ovine milk (5)	2 (40)	2 (40)	–	1 (20)	–	–	–	–	–	–
Raw caprine milk (7)	3 (42.85)	2 (28.57)	–	–	–	1 (14.28)	–	–	1 (14.28)	–
Raw buffalo milk (10)	5 (50)	4 (40)	–	1 (10)	–	–	–	–	–	–
Cheese (17)	8 (47.05)	6 (35.29)	–	1 (5.88)	–	–	–	1 (5.88)	1 (5.88)	–
Yoghurt (2)	1 (50)	1 (50)	–	–	–	–	–	–	–	–
Butter (4)	1 (25)	2 (50)	–	1 (25)	–	–	–	–	–	–
Cream (6)	2 (33.33)	2 (33.33)	–	1 (16.66)	–	–	–	–	1 (16.66)	–
Ice-cream (4)	2 (50)	2 (50)	–	–	–	–	–	–	–	–
Total (64)	28 (43.75)	24 (37.50)	–	6 (9.37)	–	1 (1.56)	–	1 (1.56)	4 (6.25)	–

Hemmatinezhad et al. (2015) [34] reported that the prevalence of O103, O121 and O128 serogroups in STEC strains isolated from poultry meat samples were 3.84%, 11.53% and 5.76%, respectively. Their findings revealed that O26 (30.76%) and O157 (25.96%) were the most commonly detected O-serogroups. High prevalence of O157 serogroup in the STEC strains of our research and also those of other investigations showed that collected samples were contaminated with animal sources and especially feces. Previous studies which were conducted in Turkey [35], Canada [36] and Africa [37] had similar conclusions.

Majority of the STEC strains of our research harbored the high prevalence of resistance against commonly used antibiotics. We found that phenotypic resistance pattern of STEC strains was supported by the genotypic resistance pattern. In the other hand, high prevalence of resistance of STEC strains isolated from raw milk and traditional dairy product samples was accompanied with high prevalence of antibiotic resistance genes. Multi-drug resistance was also seen for some of the STEC strains isolated from raw milk and traditional dairy product samples. Illegal and inaccurate prescription of antibiotics especially in veterinary medicine is may be the main reason for the high prevalence of antibiotic resistance in the STEC strains isolated from raw milk and traditional dairy product samples. Dehkordi et al. (2014) [7] revealed that the STEC strains isolated from fermented dairy products showed a high prevalence of resistance against tetracycline (84%), penicillin (46%), cephalothin (42%), ampicillin (38%) and streptomycin (36%). They showed that high prevalence of resistance against commonly used antibiotics was also accompanied with high prevalence of the genes that encode resistance to tetracycline (*tetA* (76%) and *tetB* (70%)), cephalothin (*blaSHV* (38%)), ampicillin (*CITM* (36%)) and gentamicin (*aac(3)-IV* (32%)). Previous study [31] showed that the prevalence of *aac(3)-IV*, *CITM*, *tetA*, *dfrA1* and *sul1* antibiotic resistance genes amongst the STEC strains isolated from food samples were 100%, 100%, 62.50%, 56.25% and 56.25%, respectively. Tark et al.

Table 5 Prevalence of antibiotic resistance genes in the STEC strains isolated from raw milk and traditional dairy product samples

Samples (No. STEC strains)	Distribution of antibiotic resistance genes (%)										
	aadA1	*tetA*	*tetB*	*dfrA1*	*qnr*	*aac(3)-IV*	*sul1*	*blaSHV*	*CITM*	*cat1*	*cmlA*
Raw bovine milk (9)	3 (33.33)	7 (77.77)	1 (11.11)	5 (55.55)	1 (11.11)	9 (100)	4 (44.44)	3 (33.33)	9 (100)	1 (11.11)	–
Raw ovine milk (5)	3 (60)	4 (80)	1 (20)	3 (60)	1 (20)	5 (100)	2 (40)	1 (20)	5 (100)	1 (20)	–
Raw caprine milk (7)	4 (57.14)	5 (71.42)	2 (28.57)	4 (57.14)	2 (28.57)	7 (100)	2 (28.57)	2 (28.57)	7 (100)	1 (14.28)	–
Raw buffalo milk (10)	3 (30)	8 (80)	2 (20)	6 (60)	3 (30)	10 (100)	5 (50)	3 (30)	9 (90)	2 (20)	–
Cheese (17)	7 (41.17)	12 (70.58)	4 (23.52)	8 (47.05)	4 (23.52)	17 (100)	7 (41.17)	5 (29.41)	16 (94.11)	4 (23.52)	1 (755.88
Yoghurt (2)	1 (50)	2 (100)	–	1 (50)	–	2 (100)	1 (50)	1 (50)	2 (100)	–	–
Butter (4)	3 (75)	3 (75)	1 (25)	2 (50)	1 (25)	4 (100)	2 (50)	1 (25)	4 (100)	1 (25)	–
Cream (6)	4 (66.66)	5 (83.33)	1 (16.66)	3 (50)	1 (16.66)	6 (100)	2 (33.33)	2 (33.33)	6 (100)	1 (16.66)	–
Ice-cream (4)	3 (75)	3 (75)	1 (25)	3 (75)	1 (25)	4 (100)	2 (50)	2 (50)	4 (100)	1 (25)	–
Total (64)	31 (48.43)	49 (76.56)	13 (20.31)	35 (54.68)	14 (21.87)	64 (100)	27 (42.18)	20 (31.25)	62 (96.87)	12 (18.75)	1 (1.56)

Table 6 Pattern of antibiotic resistance for STEC strains isolated from raw milk and traditional dairy product samples

Antibiotic resistance	Samples (No. STEC strains)									
	Raw bovine milk (9)	Raw ovine milk (5)	Raw caprine milk (7)	Raw buffalo milk (10)	Cheese (17)	Yoghurt (2)	Butter (4)	Cream (6)	Ice-cream (4)	Total (64)
Tetracycline	9 (100)	5 (100)	7 (100)	9 (90)	16 (94.11)	2 (100)	4 (100)	6 (100)	4 (100)	62 (96.87)
Ampicillin	9 (100)	5 (100)	7 (100)	10 (100)	17 (100)	2 (100)	4 (100)	6 (100)	4 (100)	64 (100)
Gentamicin	9 (100)	5 (100)	7 (100)	10 (100)	17 (100)	2 (100)	4 (100)	6 (100)	4 (100)	64 (100)
Amikacin	6 (66.66)	3 (60)	5 (71.42)	5 (50)	12 (70.58)	1 (50)	3 (75)	3 (50)	2 (50)	40 (62.50)
Imipenem	1 (11.11)	–	–	1 (10)	2 (11.76)	–	–	–	–	4 (6.25)
Sulfamethoxazole	5 (55.55)	3 (60)	2 (28.57)	5 (50)	7 (41.17)	1 (50)	2 (50)	3 (50)	2 (50)	30 (46.87)
Cefotaxime	4 (44.44)	2 (40)	1 (14.28)	3 (30)	3 (41.17)	–	1 (25)	1 (16.66)	1 (25)	16 (25)
Ciprofloxacin	5 (55.55)	3 (60)	4 (57.14)	4 (40)	12 (70.58)	1 (50)	3 (75)	3 (50)	2 (50)	37 (57.81)
Enrofloxacin	5 (55.55)	3 (60)	5 (42.85)	4 (40)	13 (76.47)	1 (50)	3 (75)	3 (50)	3 (75)	40 (62.50)
Cotrimoxazole	4 (44.44)	3 (60)	2 (28.57)	3 (30)	6 (35.29)	–	2 (50)	2 (33.33)	2 (50)	24 (37.50)
Ceftazidime	4 (44.44)	2 (40)	1 (14.28)	3 (30)	4 (23.52)	–	2 (50)	2 (33.33)	1 (25)	19 (29.68)
Trimethoprim	4 (44.44)	3 (60)	2 (28.57)	5 (50)	8 (47.05)	1 (50)	2 (50)	3 (50)	2 (50)	30 (46.87)
Streptomycin	4 (44.44)	3 (60)	4 (57.14)	4 (40)	8 (47.05)	–	2 (50)	2 (33.33)	1 (25)	29 (45.31)
Chloramphenicol	2 (22.22)	1 (20)	–	2 (20)	–	–	–	1 (16.66)	1 (25)	3 (4.68)

(2017) [38] determined that *E. coli* strains isolated from raw milk samples harbored the high prevalence of resistance against tetracycline (23.3%), streptomycin (17.10%), ampicillin (16.60%), neomycin (11.80%), and trimethoprim/sulfamethoxazole (11.20%). Fifteen percent of their isolates had resistance against more than three classes of antibiotics. Study in Ethiopia [39] showed that STEC strains isolated from raw milk samples harbored the highest prevalence of resistance against streptomycin (81.80%), trimethoprim-sulfamethoxazole (27.30%), cefoxitin (54. 50%), kanamycin (63.60%), gentamicin (36.40%), tetracycline (81.80%) and norfloxacin (51.50%) which was similar to our findings. An Italian investigation [22] reported that STEC strains isolated from dairy products exhibited the highest levels of resistance against ampicillin, gentamicin, tetracycline, sulfamethoxazole and ciprofloxacin antibiotics.

The most significant finding obtained from our study and also those of other researches were the high prevalence of resistance against human-based antibiotics such as amikacin, imipenem, cefotaxime, ciprofloxacin, cotrimoxazole and ceftazidime. This finding showed that STEC strains isolated from raw milk and traditional dairy product samples may be transferred from infected humans. Therefore, some of the STEC strains of our study may be had anthropogenic origin and derived from infected staffs of the milking halls and also dairy producing factories. This finding was also supported by previous studies [5–7, 29, 31, 34].

We also found a considerable prevalence of resistance of STEC strains against chloramphenicol (4.68%). However, chloramphenicol was listed as a forbidden antibiotic, but its highly irregular and excessive prescription may be cause its high prevalence of resistance. High prevalence of resistance against chloramphenicol was also reported by other

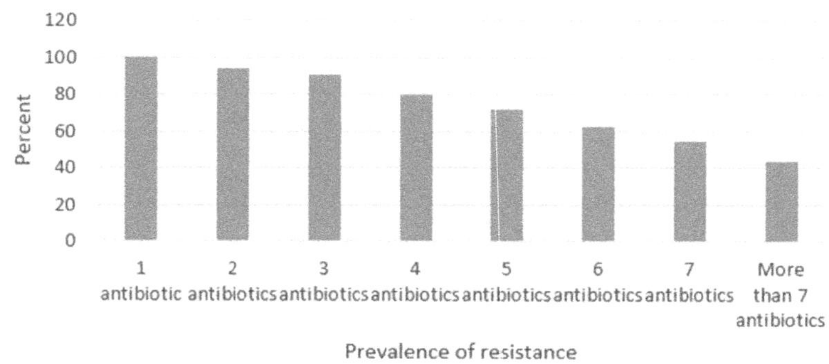

Fig. 2 Prevalence of multi-drug resistant STEC bacteria isolated from raw milk and traditional dairy product samples

studies [5–7, 17, 18, 29, 31, 40]. Findings of other investigations revealed that the STEC strains isolated from food samples harbored the high prevalence of resistance against chloramphenicol (1 to 50%) [5–7, 17, 18, 29, 31, 40]. Differences in the prevalence of resistance against various types of antibiotics observed in our study and also other researches are may be due to the differences in the availability of antibiotics, their costs and finally idea of veterinarian for antibiotic prescription in various parts of the world.

High presence of virulent and resistant *E. coli* and also other foodborne pathogens have been reported from different types of food samples [41–58]. Findings of these researchers and also those of our investigation showed that pathogenic bacteria such as *E. coli* are not limited to health-care centers. In the other hand, community and especially foods may play an important role in transmission of pathogenic bacteria such as *E. coli* to humans. Furthermore, they are mainly act as reservoir of pathogenic bacteria such as *E. coli* in the community. Raw milk and traditional dairy product samples are not exception from this important regulation. Therefore, further studies are needed to determine the role of different types of food samples as risk factor for survival and transmission of pathogenic bacteria such as *E. coli* in the community. In addition to food, presence of *E. coli* strains have been reported previously from different types of clinical infections [59–74].

Conclusions

In conclusions, we recognized a considerable prevalence of O26 and O157 serogroups, *stx1* and *eaeA* virulence factors, resistance against ampicillin, gentamicin and tetracycline and *aac(3)-IV, CITM* and *tetA* antibiotic resistance genes in the STEC strains isolated from raw milk and traditional dairy products. These characters besides the high prevalence of multi-drug resistant STEC strains represented an important public health issue regarding the consumption of raw milk and traditional dairy products. High prevalence of O157 serogroup which was accompanied with simultaneous presence of two or more putative virulence factors together showed their high pathogenicity. We found that kashk and dough were safe from contamination with *E. coli* strains. In addition, the prevalence of *E. coli* strains in raw camel milk samples was only 6.6%. Presence of O157 serogroups, EHEC strains, human-based antibiotics and even antibiotic resistance genes which encode resistance against human-based antibiotics in dairy products showed insufficiency of cooking time and temperature and transmission of pathogenic bacteria from infected staffs into the dairy samples. It seems that there were no strict supervisions on the principles of food hygiene in Iranian factories. Due to the low prevalence of STEC resistance against imipenem antibiotic, occurrence of food poisonings due to the STEC strains in tested samples can be treated with its regular prescription. Attentions to the principles of Hazard Analysis and Critical Control Point (HACCP) system can reduce the risk of STEC strains in raw milk and traditional dairy products. Complete boiling of raw milk before consumption and using from pasteurized dairy products were recommended to decrease the transmission of STEC strains to human. Attentions to the results of disk diffusion and principles of antibiotic prescription can decrease the risk of resistant STEC strains in raw milk and traditional dairy products.

Abbreviations

AEEC: Attaching and effacing *E. coli*; *E. coli*: *Escherichia coli*; *Eae*: Intimin; EHEC: Enterohemolysin or Enterohaemorrhagic *Escherichia coli*; *Ehly*: Hemolysin; HC: Hemorrhagic colitis; HUS: Hemolytic Uremic Syndrome; PCR: Polymerase Chain Reaction; SPSS: Statistical Package for the Social Sciences; STEC: Shiga toxin producing *Escherichia coli*.; *Stx*: Shiga toxin

Acknowledgements

The authors would like to thank from the Islamic Azad University of Shahrekord, Shahrekord Iran for its important technical support.

Funding

This work was supported by the Molecular Biology Research Center, Baqiyatallah University of Medical Sciences, Tehran, Iran (Grant No. 96/114).

Authors' contributions

RR and FSD carried out the culture-based identification of bacteria and PCR genetic alignment. MSS and ER carried out the samples collection, disk diffusion, statistical analysis, writing and drafting of manuscript. All authors road and approved the final manuscript.

Consent for publication

There was no consent for publication.

Competing interests

The authors declare that they have no competing interests.

Author details

[1]Molecular Biology Research Center, Systems Biology and Poisonings Institute, Baqiyatallah University of Medical Sciences, Tehran, Iran. [2]Young Researchers and Elites Club, Shahrekord Branch, Islamic Azad University, Shahrekord, Iran. [3]Doctor Veterinary Medicine, Faculty of Veterinary Medicine, Shahrekord Branch, Islamic Azad University, Shahrekord, Iran. [4]Department of Food Hygiene and Public health, Faculty of Veterinary Medicine, Shahrekord Branch, Shahrekord, Iran. [5]Department of Food Hygiene and Quality Control, Faculty of Veterinary Medicine, Shahrekord Branch, Islamic Azad University, Shahrekord, Iran.

References

1. Rozenberg S, Body J-J, Bruyère O, Bergmann P, Brandi ML, Cooper C, Devogelaer J-P, Gielen E, Goemaere S, Kaufman J-M. Effects of dairy products consumption on health: benefits and beliefs—a commentary from the Belgian bone Club and the European Society for Clinical and Economic Aspects of osteoporosis, osteoarthritis and musculoskeletal diseases. Calcif Tissue Int. 2016;98:1–17.
2. Dehkordi FS, Haghighi Borujeni MR, Rahimi E, Abdizadeh R. Detection of *Toxoplasma gondii* in raw caprine, ovine, buffalo, bovine, and camel milk using cell cultivation, cat bioassay, capture ELISA, and PCR methods in Iran. Foodborne Pathog Dis. 2013;10:120–5.

3. Mousavi S, Dehkordi FS, Rahimi E. Virulence factors and antibiotic resistance of *Helicobacter pylori* isolated from raw milk and unpasteurized dairy products in Iran. J Venom Anim Toxins Incl Trop Dis. 2014;20:51.
4. Noori A, Keshavarzian F, Mahmoudi S, Yousefi M, Nateghi L. Comparison of traditional Doogh (yogurt drinking) and Kashk characteristics (two traditional Iranian dairy products). European Journal of Experimental Biology. 2013;3:252–5.
5. Momtaz H, Farzan R, Rahimi E, Safarpoor Dehkordi F, Souod N. Molecular characterization of Shiga toxin-producing *Escherichia coli* isolated from ruminant and donkey raw milk samples and traditional dairy products in Iran. Sci World J. 2012;2012:1-13.
6. Momtaz H, Dehkordi FS, Rahimi E, Ezadi H, Arab R. Incidence of Shiga toxin-producing Escherichia coli serogroups in ruminant's meat. Meat Sci. 2013;95:381–8.
7. Dehkordi FS, Yazdani F, Mozafari J, Valizadeh Y. Virulence factors, serogroups and antimicrobial resistance properties of Escherichia coli strains in fermented dairy products. BMC research notes. 2014;7:217.
8. Bai X, Zhang W, Tang X, Xin Y, Xu Y, Sun H, Luo X, Pu J, Xu J, Xiong Y. Shiga toxin-producing Escherichia coli in plateau pika (Ochotona curzoniae) on the Qinghai-Tibetan plateau, China. Front Microbiol. 2016;7:375.
9. Dhaka P, Vijay D, Vergis J, Negi M, Kumar M, Mohan V, Doijad S, Poharkar KV, Malik SS, Barbuddhe SB. Genetic diversity and antibiogram profile of diarrhoeagenic Escherichia coli pathotypes isolated from human, animal, foods and associated environmental sources. Infection Ecol & Epidemiol. 2016;6:31055.
10. Wang J, Stanford K, McAllister TA, Johnson RP, Chen J, Hou H, Zhang G, Niu YD. Biofilm formation, virulence gene profiles, and antimicrobial resistance of nine serogroups of non-O157 Shiga toxin–producing Escherichia coli. Foodborne Pathog Dis. 2016;13:316–24.
11. Farshad S, Ranijbar R, Japoni A, Hosseini M, Anvarinejad M, Mohammadzadegan R. Microbial susceptibility, virulence factors, and plasmid profiles of uropathogenic Escherichia coli strains isolated from children in Jahrom, Iran. Archives of Iranian Medicine (AIM). 2012;15:312-6.
12. Amézquita-López BA, Quiñones B, Soto-Beltrán M, Lee BG, Yambao JC, Lugo-Melchor OY, Chaidez C. Antimicrobial resistance profiles of Shiga toxin-producing Escherichia coli O157 and non-O157 recovered from domestic farm animals in rural communities in northwestern Mexico. Antimicrob Resist Infect Control. 2016;5:1.
13. Abdi S, Ranjbar R, Vala MH, Jonaidi N, Bejestany OB, Bejestany FB. Frequency of bla TEM, bla SHV, bla CTX-M, and qnrA Among Escherichia coli Isolated From Urinary Tract Infection. Arch Clin Infect Dis. 2014;9:e18690.
14. IDF IDF. Milk and milk products - guidance on methods of sampling. In: IDF standard 50C, vol. Brussels, Belgium; 1995.
15. Woo PC, Cheung EY. Leung K-w, Yuen K-y: identification by 16S ribosomal RNA gene sequencing of an Enterobacteriaceae species with ambiguous biochemical profile from a renal transplant recipient. Diagn Microbiol Infect Dis. 2001;39:85–93.
16. Sambrook J, Russell D. Molecular cloning: a laboratory manual, (pp3. 17-3. 32). Cold Spring Harbor: Cold Spring Harbor Laboratory Press; 2001.
17. Momtaz H, Karimian A, Madani M, Dehkordi FS, Ranjbar R, Sarshar M, Souod N. Uropathogenic Escherichia coli in Iran: serogroup distributions, virulence factors and antimicrobial resistance properties. Ann Clin Microbiol Antimicrob. 2013;12:8.
18. Momtaz H, Dehkordi FS, Hosseini MJ, Sarshar M, Heidari M. Serogroups, virulence genes and antibiotic resistance in Shiga toxin-producing Escherichia coli isolated from diarrheic and non-diarrheic pediatric patients in Iran. Gut pathogens. 2013;5:1.
19. Wayne P. Clinical and laboratory standards institute (CLSI) performance standards for antimicrobial disk diffusion susceptibility tests 19th ed. approved standard. *CLSI document M100-S19*, vol. 29; 2009.
20. Ombarak RA, Hinenoya A, Awasthi SP, Iguchi A, Shima A, Elbagory A-RM, Yamasaki S. Prevalence and pathogenic potential of Escherichia coli isolates from raw milk and raw milk cheese in Egypt. Int J Food Microbiol. 2016;221: 69–76.
21. Elhadidy M, Mohammed M. Shiga toxin–producing Escherichia coli from raw milk cheese in Egypt: prevalence, molecular characterization and survival to stress conditions. Lett Appl Microbiol. 2012;56:120–7.
22. Stephan R, Schumacher S, Corti S, Krause G, Danuser J, Beutin L. Prevalence and characteristics of Shiga toxin-producing Escherichia coli in Swiss raw milk cheeses collected at producer level. J Dairy Sci. 2008;91:2561–5.
23. Mohammadi P, Abiri R, Rezaei M, Salmanzadeh-Ahrabi S. Isolation of Shiga toxin-producing Escherichia coli from raw milk in Kermanshah, Iran. *Iranian journal of microbiology*. 2013;5:233.
24. Nobili G, Franconieri I, Basanisi M, La Bella G, Tozzoli R, Caprioli A, La SG. Isolation of Shiga toxin-producing Escherichia coli in raw milk and mozzarella cheese in southern Italy. J Dairy Sci. 2016;99:7877–80.
25. Zeinhom MM, Abdel-Latef GK. Public health risk of some milk borne pathogens. Beni-Suef University Journal of Basic and Applied Sciences. 2014; 3:209–15.
26. Öksüz Ö, Arici M, Kurultay S, Gümüs T. Incidence of Escherichia coli O157 in raw milk and white pickled cheese manufactured from raw milk in Turkey. Food Control. 2004;15:453–6.
27. Xi M, Feng Y, Li Q, Yang Q, Zhang B, Li G, Shi C, Xia X. Prevalence, distribution, and diversity of Escherichia coli in plants manufacturing goat milk powder in Shaanxi, China. J Dairy Sci. 2015;98:2260–7.
28. Quinto E, Cepeda A. Incidence of toxigenic Escherichia coli in soft cheese made with raw or pasteurized milk. Lett Appl Microbiol. 1997;24:291–5.
29. Momtaz H, Safarpoor Dehkordi F, Taktaz T, Rezvani A, Yarali S. Shiga toxin-producing Escherichia coli isolated from bovine mastitic milk: serogroups, virulence factors, and antibiotic resistance properties. Sci World J. 2012;2012
30. Llorente P, Barnech L, Irino K, Rumi MV, Bentancor A. Characterization of Shiga toxin-producing Escherichia coli isolated from ground beef collected in different socioeconomic strata markets in Buenos Aires. Argentina *BioMed research international*. 2014;2014
31. Ranjbar R, Masoudimanesh M, Dehkordi FS, Jonaidi-Jafari N, Rahimi E. Shiga (Vero)-toxin producing Escherichia coli isolated from the hospital foods; virulence factors, o-serogroups and antimicrobial resistance properties. Antimicrobial Resistance & Infection Control. 2017;6:4.
32. Farrokh C, Jordan K, Auvray F, Glass K, Oppegaard H, Raynaud S, Thevenot D, Condron R, De Reu K, Govaris A. Review of Shiga-toxin-producing Escherichia coli (STEC) and their significance in dairy production. Int J Food Microbiol. 2013;162:190–212.
33. Caro I, Mateo J, Rúa J, del Rosario García-Armesto M. Occurrence of Escherichia coli O157, O111 and O26 in raw ewe's milk and performance of two enrichment broths and two plating media used for its assessment. Int J Food Microbiol. 2011;146:84–7.
34. Hemmatinezhad B, Khamesipour F, Mohammadi M, Safarpoor Dehkordi F, Mashak Z. Microbiological investigation of O-serogroups, virulence factors and antimicrobial resistance properties of Shiga toxin-producing Escherichia Coli isolated from ostrich, Turkey and quail meats. J Food Saf. 2015;35:491–500.
35. Ayaz ND, Copuroglu G, Ormeci E, Oz B. Presence of Staphylococcus aureus and Shiga toxigenic Escherichia coli O157: H7 in raw meat in Ağrı Turkey. Int J Enteric Pathog. 2016;4:e36523.
36. Neher S, Hazarika A, Barkalita L, Borah P, Bora D, Sharma R. Isolation and characterization of Shiga toxigenic Escherichia coli of animal and bird origin by multiplex polymerase chain reaction. Veterinary world. 2016;9:123.
37. Mamza SA, Egwu GO, Mshelia GD. Antibiotic susceptibility patterns of beta-lactamase-producing Escherichia coli and Staphylococcus aureus isolated from chickens in Maiduguri (arid zone), Nigeria. Veterinarski Arhiv. 2010;80:283–97.
38. Tark D-S, Moon DC, Kang HY, Kim S-R, Nam H-M, Lee H-S, Jung S-C, Lim S-K. Antimicrobial susceptibility and characterization of extended-spectrum β-lactamases in Escherichia coli isolated from bovine mastitic milk in South Korea from 2012 to 2015. J Dairy Sci. 2017;100:3463–9.
39. Disassa N, Sibhat B, Mengistu S, Muktar Y, Belina D: Prevalence and Antimicrobial Susceptibility Pattern of *E. coli* O157: H7 Isolated from Traditionally Marketed Raw Cow Milk in and around Asosa Town, Western Ethiopia. Veterinary medicine international 2017, 2017.
40. Colello R, Etcheverría AI, Conza JAD, Gutkind GO, Padola NL. Antibiotic resistance and integrons in Shiga toxin-producing Escherichia coli (STEC). Braz J Microbiol. 2015;46:1–5.
41. Atapoor S, Dehkordi FS, Rahimi E. Detection of *Helicobacter pylori* in various types of vegetables and salads. Jundishapur J Microbiol. 2014;7:e10013.
42. Momtaz H, Dehkordi FS, Rahimi E, Asgarifar A, Momeni M. Virulence genes and antimicrobial resistance profiles of *Staphylococcus aureus* isolated from chicken meat in Isfahan province, Iran. *J Appl Poultry Res*. 2013;22:913–21.
43. Dehkordi FS, Parsaei P, Saberian S, Moshkelani S, Hajshafiei P, Hosseini SR, Babaei M, Ghorbani MN. Prevalence study of *Theileria annulata* by comparison of four diagnostic techniques in Southwest Iran. Bulgar J Vet Med. 2012;15:123–30.
44. Madahi H, Rostami F, Rahimi E, Dehkordi FS. Prevalence of enterotoxigenic *Staphylococcus aureus* isolated from chicken nugget in Iran. Jundishapur J

Microbiol. 2013;7:e10237.

45. Rahimi E, Sepehri S, Dehkordi FS, Shaygan S, Momtaz H. Prevalence of Yersinia species in traditional and commercial dairy products in Isfahan Province. *Jundishapur J Microbiol.* 2014;7:e9249.
46. Momtaz H, Davood Rahimian M, Safarpoor DF. Identification and characterization of *Yersinia enterocolitica* isolated from raw chicken meat based on molecular and biological techniques, Iran. J Appl Poult Res. 2013; 22:137–45.
47. Safarpoor Dehkordi F, Barati S, Momtaz H, Hosseini Ahari SN, Nejat DS. Comparison of shedding, and antibiotic resistance properties of *Listeria monocytogenes* isolated from milk, feces, urine, and vaginal secretion of bovine, ovine, caprine, buffalo, and camel species in Iran. Jundishapur J Microbiol. 2013;6:284–94.
48. Ghorbani F, Gheisari E, Dehkordi FS. Genotyping of *vacA* alleles of *Helicobacter pylori* strains recovered from some Iranian food items. Trop J Pharm Res. 2016;15:1631–6.
49. Dehkordi FS, Khamesipour F, Momeni M. *Brucella abortus* and *Brucella melitensis* in Iranian bovine and buffalo semen samples: the first clinical trial on seasonal, senile and geographical distribution using culture, conventional and real-time polymerase chain reaction assays. Kafkas Univ Vet Fak Dergisi. 2014;20:821–8.
50. Dehkordi FS, Haghighi N, Momtaz H, Rafsanjani MS, Momeni M. Conventional vs real-time PCR for detection of bovine herpes virus type 1 in aborted bovine, buffalo and camel foetuses. Bulgar J Vet Med. 2013;16: 102–11.
51. Dehkordi AH, Khaji L, Shahreza MHS, Mashak Z, Dehkordi FS, Safaee Y, Hosseinzadeh A, Alavi I, Ghasemi E, Rabiei-Faradonbeh M. One-year prevalence of antimicrobial susceptibility pattern of methicillin-resistant *Staphylococcus aureus* recovered from raw meat. Trop Biomed. 2017;34:396–404.
52. Safarpoor FD, Gandomi H, Basti AA, Misaghi A, Rahimi E. Phenotypic and genotypic characterization of antibiotic resistance of methicillin-resistant *Staphylococcus aureus* isolated from hospital food. Antimicrob Res Infect Control. 2017;6:104.
53. Dormanesh B, Dehkordi FS, Hosseini S, Momtaz H, Mirnejad R, Hoseini MJ, Yahaghi E, Tarhriz V, Khodaverdi DE. Virulence factors and o-serogroups profiles of uropathogenic *Escherichia coli* isolated from Iranian pediatric patients. Iran Red Cres Med J. 2014;16:e14627.
54. Shahrani M, Dehkordi FS, Momtaz H. Characterization of *Escherichia coli* virulence genes, pathotypes and antibiotic resistance properties in diarrheic calves in Iran. Biol Res. 2014;47:28.
55. Nejat S, Momtaz H, Yadegari M, Nejat S, Safarpour Dehkordi F, Khamesipour F. Seasonal, geographical, age and breed distributions of equine viral arteritis in Iran. Kafkas Univ Vet Fak Dergisi. 2015;21:111–6.
56. Dehkordi FS, Valizadeh Y, Birgani TA, Dehkordi KG. Prevalence study of *Brucella melitensis* and *Brucella abortus* in cow's milk using dot enzyme linked immuno sorbent assay and duplex polymerase chain reaction. J Pure Appl Microbiol. 2014;8:1065–9.
57. Rahimi E, Yazdanpour S, Dehkordi FS. Detection of *Toxoplasma gondii* antibodies in various poultry meat samples using enzyme linked immuno sorbent assay and its confirmation by polymerase chain reaction. J Pure Appl Microbiol. 2014;8:421–7.
58. Yahaghi E, Khamesipour F, Mashayekhi F, Safarpoor Dehkordi F, Sakhaei MH, Masoudimanesh M, Khayyat Khameneie M. Helicobacter pylori in vegetables and salads: genotyping and antimicrobial resistance properties. BioMed Res Int. 2014;2014:1-11.
59. Ranjbar R, Karami A, Farshad S, Giammanco GM, Mammina C. Typing methods used in the molecular epidemiology of microbial pathogens: a how-to guide. New Microbiol. 2014;37:1-15.
60. Jahandeh N, Ranjbar R, Behzadi P, Behzadi E. Uropathogenic Escherichia coli virulence genes: invaluable approaches for designing DNA microarray probes. Cent European J Urol. 2015;68:452-8.
61. Tajbakhsh E, Khamesipour F, Ranjbar R, Ugwu IC. Prevalence of class 1 and 2 integrons in multi-drug resistant Escherichia coli isolated from aquaculture water in Chaharmahal Va Bakhtiari province, Iran. Ann Clin Microbiol Antimicrob. 2015;14:37.
62. Farshad S, Ranjbar R, Japoni A, Hosseini M, Anvarinejad M, Mohammadzadegan R. Microbial susceptibility, virulence factors, and plasmid profiles of uropathogenic Escherichia coli strains isolated from children in Jahrom, Iran. Arch Iran Med. 2012;15:312-6.
63. Anvarinejad M, Farshad Sh, Ranjbar R, Giammanco GM, Alborzi A, Japoni A. Genotypic Analysis of E. coli Strains Isolated from Patients with Cystitis and Pyelonephritis. Iran Red Crescent Med J. 2012;14:408-16.
64. Ranjbar, R, Haghi-Ashtiani, MT, Jafari, NJ, Abedini, M. The prevalence and antimicrobial susceptibility of bacterial uropathogens isolated from pediatric patients. Iran J Publ Health. 2009;38:134-8.
65. Khademestarki NS, Ranjbar R. The Phylogenetic Study of Escherichia coli Strains Isolated from Clinical Cases. J Pure Appl Microbiol. 2016;10:351-4.
66. Ranjbar R, Hosseini S, Zahraei-Salehi T, Kheiri R, Khamesipour F. Investigation on prevalence of Escherichia coli strains carrying virulence genes ipaH, estA, eaeA and bfpA isolated from different water sources. Asian Pacific J Trop Dis. 2016;6:278-83.
67. Behzadi P, Najafi A, Behzadi E, Ranjbar R. Microarray long oligo probe designing for Escherichia coli: An in-silico DNA marker extraction. Central Eur J Urol. 2016;69:105-11.
68. Ranjbar R, Ahmadnezhad B, Jonaidi N. The prevalence of beta lactamase producing Escherichia coli strains isolated from the urine samples in Valiasr Hospital. Biomed Pharmacol J. 2014;7:425-431.
69. Farshad S, Anvarinejad M, Tavana AM, Ranjbar R, Japoni A, Zadegan RM, Alborzi A. Molecular epidemiology of Escherichia coli strains isolated from children with community acquired urinary tract infections. Afr J Microbiol Res. 2011;5:4476-83.
70. Anvarinejad M, Farshad S, Alborzi A, Ranjbar R, Giammanco GM, Japoni A. Integron and genotype patterns of quinolones-resistant uropathogenic Escherichia coli. Afr J Microbiol Res. 2011;5:3765-70.
71. Ranjbar R, Behzadi P, Najafi A, Roudi R. DNA microarray for rapid detection and identification of food and water borne bacteria: from dry to wet lab. Open Microbiol J. 2017;11:330-8.
72. Ranjbar R, Sami M. Genetic Investigation of beta-lactam associated antibiotic resistance among Escherichia coli strains isolated from water sources. Open Microbiol J. 2017;11:203-10.
73. Ranjbar R, Farahani O. The Prevalence of plasmid-mediated quinolone resistance genes in Escherichia coli isolated from hospital wastewater sources in Tehran, Iran. Iran J Public Health. 2017;46:1285-91.
74. Ranjbar R, Pezeshknejad P, Khamesipour F, Amini K, Kheiri R. Genomic fingerprints of Escherichia coli strains isolated from surface water in Alborz province, Iran. BMC Res Notes. 2017;10:295.

10

The effect of antibiotic use on prevalence of nosocomial vancomycin-resistant enterococci

Cornelius Remschmidt*, Michael Behnke, Axel Kola, Luis A. Peña Diaz, Anna M. Rohde, Petra Gastmeier and Frank Schwab

Abstract

Background: Vancomycin-resistant enterococci (VRE) are among the most common antimicrobial-resistant pathogens causing nosocomial infections. Although antibiotic use has been identified as a risk factor for VRE, it remains unclear which antimicrobial agents particularly facilitate VRE selection. Here, we assessed whether use of specific antimicrobial agents is independently associated with healthcare-associated (HA) VRE rates in a university hospital setting in Berlin, Germany.

Methods: We conducted the study between January 2014 and December 2015 at the Charité-university hospital of Berlin, Germany. From the hospital pharmacy, we extracted data for all antibacterials for systemic use (anatomical therapeutic chemical (ATC)-classification J01) and calculated ward specific antibiotic consumption in defined daily doses (DDDs) per 100 patient-days (PD). We used the microbiology laboratory database to identify all patients with isolation of invasive or non-invasive VRE and calculated HA-VRE incidence as nosocomial VRE-cases per 100 patients and HA-VRE incidence density as nosocomial VRE-cases per 1000 PD. We defined VRE isolates as hospital-acquired if they were identified three days or later after hospital admission and otherwise as community-acquired (CA-VRE). We performed univariable and multivariable regression analyses to estimate the association of the frequency of HA-VRE per month with antibiotic use and other parameters such as length of stay, type of ward or presence of at least one CA-VRE on ward. In a second analysis, we considered only patients with VRE infections.

Results: We included data from 204,054 patients with 948,380 PD from 61 wards. Overall, 1430 VRE-cases were identified of which 409 (28.6%) were considered hospital-acquired (HA). We found that carbapenem use in the current month and prior-month use of glycopeptides increased the risk for HA-VRE by 1% per 1 DDD/100 PD and 3% per 1 DDD/100 PD, respectively. However, when only VRE from clinical samples were considered, only glycopeptide use showed a statistically significant association. In both models, detection of at least one patient with CA-VRE on a ward in the current month significantly increased the risk of HA-VRE, thereby indicating nosocomial spread of VRE.

Conclusions: Our findings suggest that the risk of HA-VRE is associated with specific antimicrobial agents. Prudent use of these antimicrobial agents might reduce nosocomial VRE rates. That appearance of at least one CA-VRE case on the ward increased the risk of HA-VRE detection highlights the importance of strict hand hygiene practices to interrupt person-to-person transmission of VRE.

Keywords: Vancomycin-resistant enterococcus, Transmission, Antibiotic use, Carbapenems, Glycopeptides

* Correspondence: cornelius.remschmidt@charite.de
Institute of Hygiene and Environmental Medicine, Charité-Universitätsmedizin Berlin, Hindenburgdamm 27, 12203 Berlin, Germany

Background

Vancomycin-resistant enterococci (VRE) are emerging worldwide and are among the most common antimicrobial-resistant pathogens causing nosocomial infections [1–4]. Since infections with VRE are associated with prolonged in-hospital stay and excess mortality [5, 6], increasing VRE rates pose a serious threat to global health. In fact, the World Health Organization (WHO) judged VRE to be of high importance in the "Global Priority list of antibiotic-resistant bacteria to guide research, discovery and development of new antibiotics" [7].

So far, several risk factors for VRE colonization or infection have been identified, such as long periods of hospitalization, immunosuppression, serious comorbid conditions, close proximity to patients infected or colonized with VRE as well as antibiotic use [2, 8–12]. Although antibiotic use has been advocated as a major modifiable risk factor [8, 13], controversies remain regarding the impact of specific antimicrobial agents or antimicrobial groups on the selection process of VRE [8, 12].

Therefore, the primary objective of the study was to investigate whether use of specific antimicrobial agents is independently associated with nosocomial VRE rates in a university hospital setting in Berlin, Germany. Secondary objective was to identify other risk factors that are associated with nosocomial VRE rates.

Methods

This study was conducted at the Charité-university hospital of Berlin, between January 2014 and December 2015. The Charité is a tertiary care center with more than 3000 beds and more than 140,000 inpatient cases per year.

From the microbiology laboratory database of Charité we prospectively identified patients with vancomycin-resistant Enterococcus (*E.*) *faecium*- or *E. faecalis*-isolates from intensive care units (ICUs) and surgical, medical and hemato-oncological wards. In case of screening samples, selective chromogenic medium (chromID® VRE, bioMérieux) and VITEK 2 system (bioMérieux) were used, while clinical samples were processed following standard procedures dependent on specimen type. Results were interpreted according to European Committee on Antimicrobial Susceptibility Testing definitions (EUCAST, http://www.eucast.org). A molecular characterization of the VRE isolates was not performed.

We defined VRE isolates as hospital-acquired (HA-VRE) if they were identified three days or later after hospital admission and otherwise as community-acquired (CA-VRE). In patients with multiple VRE isolates during the same hospital stay, only the first identified isolate was considered. We included isolates irrespective whether they were obtained for infection control surveillance or recovered from clinical specimen and irrespective whether they were associated with colonization or infection.

Performance of screening

At the Charité, a targeted risk adjusted screening policy is implemented: in patients in whom a VRE has been isolated within the previous three years, a rectal swab is obtained at admission. However, during the study period eight (non-ICU) wards performed an intensified admission screening that involved all patients irrespective of underlying risk factors. In this ecologic study, we did not collect data on compliance with the screening policy or compliance with hand hygiene or cleaning procedures on the respective wards.

Systemic antibiotic use

Antimicrobial agents were classified according to the anatomical therapeutic chemical (ATC) system (34). From the pharmacy of Charité, ward specific data on antibiotic consumption were converted into defined daily doses (DDDs) and reported as DDD/100 patient-days (PD) at monthly intervals. We collected data for all antibacterials for systemic use (ATC-code J01). Data on antifungal or antiviral medication were not considered.

Ethics and data protection

For this ecologic study, we analyzed aggregated and anonymous data that were collected by the hospital in accordance with the German "Protection against Infection Act", §23. Therefore, ethical approval and informed consent were not required and institutional review boards were not consulted.

Statistical analysis

We calculated median and interquartile range (IQR) for the total study period (24 months) for the following variables: number of patients, patient-days (PD), average length of stay (LOS), number of beds per ward, bed occupancy rate, month of VRE-detection, HA-VRE rates and antibiotic use. HA-VRE incidence was calculated as nosocomial VRE-cases per 100 patients and HA-VRE incidence density as nosocomial VRE-cases per 1000 PD. We reported data for all wards as well as stratified by type of ward (i.e. surgical, medical, ICU, hemato-oncological). Differences in baseline characteristics between different types of wards were compared by using the Kruskal-Wallis test. Univariable and multivariable regression using generalized linear models was performed to estimate the association of the frequency of HA-VRE per month with different antimicrobial groups in the current month and the month before the current month and further confounding parameters such as length of stay (LOS), bed occupancy (patient days/bed places on ward available), type of ward and at least one patient with community-acquired VRE on ward in the current month. In addition, we added a variable that took the different screening policies (screening of all patients on admission irrespective of underlying risk factors on eight wards) into account. Since observations within a ward are not statistically independent due to the diagnostic and management policies (particularly the frequency of microbiological tests and screening), adjusted incidence rate ratios (IRR) with 95% confidence intervals (CI) were estimated. They were based on generalized estimating equation (GEE) models which account for this clustering effect by using an exchangeable correlation structure (35).

We used negative-binomial distribution instead of Poisson distribution because the variance exceeds the mean and overdispersion was observed. The Lagrange multiplier test was used to test whether the negative binomial model significantly differs from the Poisson model. The log number of patient days during each month was used as an offset in the model. All parameter with $p < 0.2$ in the univariable regression model were included in a full model and then non-significant parameters were excluded stepwise. The selection criterion was the smallest Chi-square value and $p \geq 0.05$ in the type III score statistic. The quasi-likelihood information criterion (QIC) as a modification of the Akaike information criterion (AIC) was used as goodness-of-fit measure in the GEE model. We calculated two models. The first model considered all identified HA-VRE isolates (clinical and screening samples) the second model considered only clinical specimen. Antimicrobial agents that are relevant for the treatment of VRE, such as daptomycin, linezolid and tigecyclin were excluded from the analysis. Additionally, spearman correlation coefficients were calculated between the antibiotic use and the incidence density of HA-VRE for the entire study period (24 months). *P*-values less than 0.05 were considered significant. All analyses were performed using SPSS [IBM SPSS statistics, Somer, NY, USA] and SAS 9.4 [SAS Institute, Cary, NC, USA].

Results

From 61 wards (20 surgical, 18 medical, 14 ICUs, 9 hemato-oncological) we included data from 204,054 patients with 948,380 patient-days. Median length of stay was 4.7 days (IQR, 3.9–5.8) and was statistically significant higher in ICUs and hemato-oncological wards as compared to surgical wards (see Table 1).

Rates of HA-VRE

Overall, 1430 VRE-cases were identified of which 409 (28.6%) were considered hospital-acquired. Of those, 238 (58.2%) HA-VRE were identified in 2015. The median HA-VRE incidence and HA-VRE incidence density in all 61 wards was 0.11 (IQR, 0.03–0.32) and 0.24 (0.07–0.54), respectively (Table 1); however, rates of HA-VRE differed significantly between types of ward. Highest HA-VRE rates were observed on ICUs (incidence density: 1.17 (0.71–1.75)) and lowest HA-VRE rates on medical wards (incidence density: 0.07 (0–0.22)).

Systemic antibiotic use

Between 2014 and 2015 median antibiotic use among all wards was 76.8 (IQR, 61.6–131.9) DDD/100 PD. Antibiotic use ranged from 64.1 DDD/100 PD on medical wards to 163.2 DDD/100 PD on ICUs (see Table 1). Particularly, the use of broad-spectrum antibiotics such as third-generation cephalosporins, glycopeptides and carbapenems was 3 to 13-fold higher on ICUs as compared to medical or surgical wards. For example, median carbapenem use on medical wards was 3.2 (1.5–8.4) DDD/100 PD, whereas it was 42.3 (22.5–49.4) DDD/100 PD on ICUs.

Associations between HA-VRE and antibiotic use

According to Spearmans correlation, several antimicrobial groups were associated with HA-VRE incidence density. For example, carbapenem use ($r = 0.801$, $p < 0.001$, ATC code J01DH), glycopeptide use ($r = 0.76$, p < 0.001, ATC code J01XA) and use of third-generation cephalosporines ($r = 0.57$, p < 0.001, ATC code J01DD) showed a strong correlation with HA-VRE incidence density (see Fig. 1).

The first multivariable regression model (screening and clinical specimen) indicated that carbapenem use in the current month independently increased the risk for HA-VRE by 1% per 1 DDD/100 patient-days (incidence rate ratio (IRR), 1.01; 95% confidence interval (CI) 1.00–1.02, $p < 0.01$), see Table 2. Glycopeptide use in the previous month but not in the current month was also associated with an increased risk of HA-VRE (IRR 1.03; 95% CI, 1.01–1.05, $p < 0.01$). In addition, type of hospital ward (ICU and hemato-oncological ward vs. surgical ward), detection of at least one patient with CA-VRE in the current month, an intensified screening policy and the year 2015 were independently associated with higher VRE rates.

The second multivariable regression model considering only VRE from clinical specimen showed that glycopeptide use in the previous month (IRR 1.03, 95% CI 1.01–1.05, p < 0.01) were the only antimicrobial agent that was statistically significant associated with HA-VRE (see Table 3). Furthermore, being hospitalized on an ICU, detection of at least one patient with CA-VRE in the current month and the year 2015 increased the risk for HA-VRE.

In both multivariable models, size of ward, length of stay and bed occupancy rate were no independent risk factors for HA-VRE in the final models.

Table 1 Descriptive data, VRE cases and antibiotic use of the 61 wards considered in the analysis in total and by type of ward

Characteristic	Type of hospital ward				
Baseline characteristics	All (n = 61) Median (IQR)	Surgical (n = 20) N (%)/median (IQR)	Medical (n = 18) N (%)/median (IQR)	Intensive Care Unit (n = 14) N (%)/median (IQR)	Hemato-oncological (n = 9) N (%)/median (IQR)
Patients, N = 204,054	3260 (1886–4478)	4180 (2642–5002)	3849 (3486–4909)	1483 (1252–1899)	2031 (1576–2268)
Patient-days, N = 948,380	14,773 (10,642–19,154)	16,488 (13,488–19,819)	17,912 (15,018–20,758)	8949 (6961–10,642)	13,722 (10,849–14,430)
Average length of stay, d	4.7 (3.9–5.8)	4.4 (3.7–5.0)	4.3 (3.7–5.1)	5.6 (5.1–7.0)	6.4 (4.8–8.2)
Beds, N = 1604	27 (18–32)	32 (30–33)	31.5 (26–36)	13 (10–16)	21 (18–21)
Bed occupancy rate (bed-days/patient-days*100)	81.1 (77.4–92.6)	77.2 (67.0–81.5)	79.1 (78.0–82.4)	94.9 (94.0–97.2)	89.5 (81.1–93.1)
VRE rates					
VRE cases (all[a]), N = 1430	12 (5–24)	5.5 (4.5–12.5)	7 (3–15)	20 (13–70)	48 (33–69)
Screening cases, N = 939 (65.7%)	4 (2–12)	3.5 (1.5–5)	3.5 (2–4)	9 (0–26)	42 (31–63)
Clinical cases, N = 491 (34.3%)	4 (2–10)	4 (1.5–6.5)	3 (1–8)	12.5 (8–23)	3 (2–6)
VRE cases (nosocomial), N = 409 (28.6%)	3 (1–7)	2 (1–4)	1 (0–4)	11.5 (5–21)	5 (3–8)
VRE incidence (nosocomial VRE/100 patients)	0.11 (0.03–0.32)	0.05 (0.02–0.14)	0.03 (0–0.11)	0.68 (0.32–1.22)	0.29 (0.14–0.53)
VRE incidence density (nosocomial VRE/ 1000 patient-days)	0.24 (0.07–0.54)	0.11 (0.06–0.27)	0.07 (0–0.22)	1.17 (0.71–1.75)	0.35 (0.24–0.54)
Systemic antibiotic use (ATC-code) in DDD/100 patient-days					
All antibacterials for systemic use (J01)	76.8 (61.6–131.9)	72.8 (58.1–83.6)	64.1 (39.2–72.8)	163.2 (144.1–200.7)	115.0 (65.4–123.8)
- Beta-lactam antibacterials, penicillins (J01C)	19.5 (13.8–34.4)	15.6 (12.1–38.7)	17.0 (11.5–28.6)	34.1 (30.1–46.2)	17.6 (16.1–20.4)
- Combinations of penicillins, incl. Beta-lactamase inhibitors (J01CR)	14.2 (10.6–26.8)	12.2 (9.5–34.3)	10.7 (8.4–16.4)	21.4 (15.9–31.0)	15.2 (13.7–18.3)
- Ampicillin and enzyme inhibitor (J01CR01)	5.3 (2.5–16.5)	5.7 (2.8–25.4)	3.8 (2.4–9.7)	11.2 (6.5–17.9)	2.3 (1.0–3.8)
- Piperacillin and enzyme inhibitor (J01CR05)	6.0 (2.6–9.2)	2.7 (1.6–4.1)	3.1 (2.0–5.8)	10.2 (7.2–12.9)	10.4 (7.4–11.5)
- Other beta-lactam antibacterials (J01D)	21.6 (16.9–37.5)	18.6 (14.2–29.2)	18.5 (10.3–22.8)	57.5 (45.7–68.5)	20.5 (18.2–34.5)
- Second-generation cephalosporins (J01 DC)	4 (2.6–11.7)	9.0 (3.4–20.0)	3.3 (1.9–8.2)	4.3 (2.7–17.1)	2.8 (2.1–3.5)
- Third-generation cephalosporins (J01DD)	3.9 (2.2–6.7)	2.4 (1.2–3.4)	3.1 (2.0–6.4)	9.0 (6.6–12.6)	4.3 (3.5–6.3)
- Ceftriaxone (J01DD04)	2.6 (1.2–4.7)	1.6 (0.7–2.8)	2.8 (1.5–5.6)	4.7 (2.8–5.8)	1.6 (0.9–2.8)
- Carbapenems (J01DH)	8.4 (2.3–19.0)	4.6 (1.0–7.5)	3.2 (1.5–8.4)	42.3 (22.5–49.4)	11.8 (10.7–25.7)
- Meropenem (J01DH02)	7.8 (2.2–16.8)	3.3 (0.8–6.8)	2.5 (1.5–7.8)	40.3 (22.1–45.0)	11.5 (10.4–25.4)
- Sulfonamides and Trimethoprim (J01E)	2.7 (1.4–5.0)	2.7 (1.4–3.3)	1.1 (0.6–2.0)	4.3 (3.1–7.1)	13.5 (2.7–15.8)
- Makrolides, lincosamides and streptogramins (J01F)	7.3 (4.5–9.4)	6.4 (3.4–8.4)	6.2 (4.2–7.8)	8.8 (6.4–10.5)	8.0 (7.0–10.4)
- Aminoglycosides (J01G)	0.4 (0.2–1.3)	0.2 (0.1–0.4)	0.2 (0.1–0.6)	3.5 (1.4–7.9)	0.3 (0.2–0.4)
- Quinolones (J01M)	11.2 (6.8–20.7)	8.3 (6.1–16.0)	7.4 (3.7–12.4)	23.3 (17.9–27.3)	13.5 (10.2–43.6)
- Ciprofloxacin (J01MA02)	10.5 (6.0–19.0)	8.0 (5.7–14.1)	6.9 (3.1–11.0)	21.6 (17.4–25.2)	11.1 (9.2–41.9)
- Other antibacterials (J01X)	7.5 (3.5–12.9)	6.1 (3.2–9.3)	3.7 (1.7–6.3)	29.2 (20.8–36.7)	8.8 (5.1–11.0)
- Glycopeptide antibacterials (J01XA)	3.0 (1.5–8.7)	1.8 (1.4–3.1)	1.7 (0.8–2.2)	12.8 (8.7–19.0)	5.6 (3.7–9.4)
- Vancomycin (J01XA01)	2.6 (1.5–6.7)	1.8 (1.4–3.1)	1.6 (0.8–2.2)	12.4 (8.7–16.6)	2.8 (2.6–4.0)

IQR, interquartile range; VRE, vancomycin-resistant enterococci; ATC, Anatomical Therapeutic Chemical classification system
[a]nosocomial and community acquired VRE

Discussion

Antibiotic use is one of the most important risk factors for VRE occurrence within the hospital setting [13]. Although specific antimicrobial agents such as piperacillin/tazobactam [14] or ceftriaxone [15] or antimicrobial groups such as glycopeptides, third-generation cephalosporines and fluoroquinolones [16–18] have been found to be associated with increasing VRE prevalence, controversies remain. For example, although a large prospective study found that vancomycin was strongly associated with increased prevalence of VRE [18], a systematic review that assessed the impact of reducing vancomycin use on the prevalence and incidence of VRE colonization in the US did not find a positive effect of such

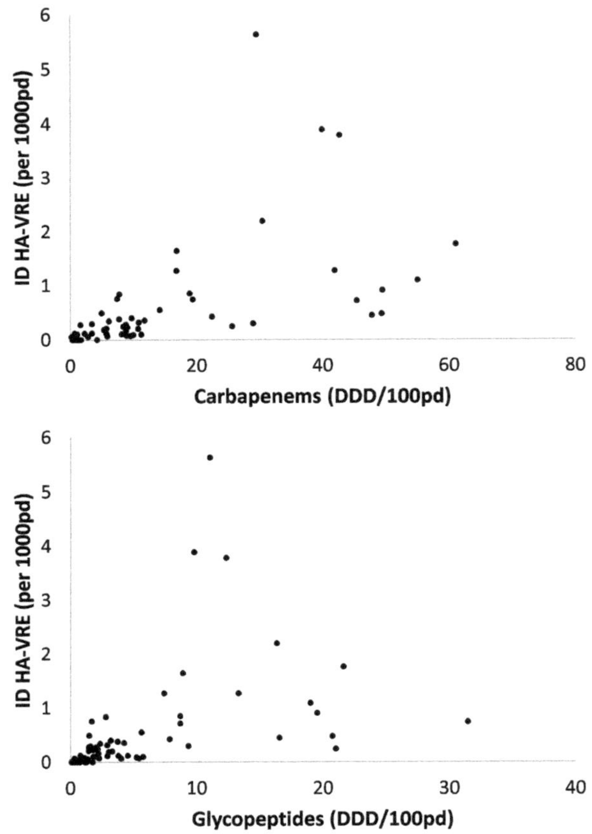

Fig. 1 Association between incidence density of hospital-acquired vancomycin resistant enterococci (ID HA-VRE) and antibiotic use density (DDD/100pd) of carbapenems (ATC-code J01DH, Spearman correlation coefficient r = 0.801, p < 0.001) and glycopeptides (ATC code J01XA, r = 0.76, p < 0.001) on 61 wards, 2014–2015, Berlin, Germany

interventions [19]. Interestingly, Kritsotakis et al. found that the effect of antibiotic use might influence VRE rates with a time lag, ranging from 2 month for vancomycin to 6 months for third-generation cephalosporins. Studies that did not account statistically for such a time delay might therefore miss a possible association.

It is unclear, why among antimicrobial groups only glycopeptides but not carbapenems were associated in both models with HA-VRE rates. A possible explanation is that glycopeptide use constitutes only a first step in the selection process of VRE: Although glycopeptide exposure does not promote emergence of VRE through genetic mutations in individual patients, it might facilitate selection of intestinal VRE [8, 13]. In a second step, use of specific antimicrobial agents further influences the microbial balance leading to high-density colonization with VRE at detectable levels [2, 8, 20].

In fact, Donskey et al. showed that in patients colonized with VRE exposure to antimicrobial agents with activity against Gram-negative bacteria or with anti-anaerobic activity leads to a rapid increase of intestinal VRE density, whereas discontinuation of these antibiotics decreased VRE density [21]. Since fecal density of VRE directly affects the sensitivity of screening results, active surveillance (i.e. rectal screening) for VRE at hospital admission might lead to false-negative results in patients with low VRE densities [22, 23]. In case that VRE-related precaution measures are not implemented, this may contribute to increased spread of VRE within hospitals, particularly if antibiotic therapy is initiated [21]. However, for clinical infections other factors such as immunosuppression or hygiene practices might be more important, factors that were only indirect (ward type ICU; presence of at least one CA-VRE on ward) assessed in our study.

It is also unclear, why carbapenem use in the current but not in the prior month was associated

Table 2 (including HA-VRE from screening and clinical specimen). Results of multivariable analysis for hospital-acquired VRE cases with antibiotic use by antibiotic group (ATC-code 5-digit)

Parameter/category	IRR	95% CI	*p*-value
Ward			
Medical ward	1 = reference		
Hematological/oncological ward	4.90	1.8–13.3	0.002
Intensive care unit	5.97	2.83–12.60	<.0001
Surgical ward	1.25	0.59–2.63	0.554
At least one patient with community-acquired VRE on ward in the current month	1.69	1.32–2.16	<.0001
Screening of all patients on admission irrespective of underlying risk factors (1 = yes)	2.27	1.01–5.08	0.047
Carbapenem (J01DH) use in the current month (per 1 DDD/100 patient-days)	1.01	1.00–1.02	0.01
Glycopetide (J01XA) use in the previous month (per 1 DDD/100 patient-days)	1.02	1.01–1.04	0.002
Year 2015 (compared to 2014)	1.45	1.17–1.79	<.0001

DDD Defined daily dose; *IRR* Incidence rate ratio; *CI* Confidence interval

Table 3 (including only HA-VRE from clinical specimen). Results of multivariable analysis for the frequency of hospital-acquired vancomycin resistant enterococci cases with antibiotic use by antibiotic group (ATC-code 5-digit)

Parameter/category	IRR	95% CI	*p*-value
Ward			
Medical ward	1 = reference		
Hematological/oncological ward	1.38	0-60-3.19	0.451
Intensive care unit	4.7	2.02–10.96	<.0001
Surgical ward	1.24	0.55–2.83	0.594
Patient with community-acquired VRE on warc in the current month	1.77	1.19–2.63	0.005
Glycopetide (J01XA) use in the previous month (per 1 DDD/100 patient-days)	1.03	1.01–1.05	0.0038
Year 2015 (compared to 2014)	1.40	1.05–1.86	0.005

DDD Defined daily dose; *IRR* Incidence rate ratio; *CI* Confidence interval

with HA-VRE-rates when screening and clinical specimen were considered. However, given the available evidence it seems unlikely that a single antimicrobial agent is responsible for the multifactorial process of VRE selection. It is rather an interaction of different antimicrobial agents with the competing intestinal microbiota and might differ from individual to individual [8].

Regarding antibiotics, the use of broad-spectrum antibiotics such as glycopeptides and carbapenems was 3 to 13-fold higher on ICUs as compared to medical or surgical wards. Although interpreting these results without individual patient data is challenging, this rates might indicate inappropriate use of these antibiotics on ICUs. Antibiotic stewardship could limit unnecessary or inappropriate use of antibiotics, thereby improving the quality of antibiotic use in hospitals [24].

In addition to glycopeptides and carbapenems, we found that hospitalization on an ICU as well as detection of CA-VRE increased the risk of HA-VRE acquisition. These results are in line with other studies that found that hospitalization on ICUs or severe underlying comorbidities and immunosuppression are risk factors for VRE colonization or infection [2, 12, 25]. That appearance of at least one CA-VRE case on the ward almost doubled the risk of HA-VRE detection highlights the importance of strict hand hygiene practices for health care workers to interrupt person-to-person transmission [26–28].

The fact that HA-VRE cases increased from 2014 to 2015 might indicate an epidemiological trend that has been already observed in other studies [16, 17, 29, 30]; however, the situation regarding spread of VRE in Europe is diverse [1]. Since data in our study were collected for only two years, these results have to be interpreted with caution.

Our study has several limitations. First, we used an ecological study design, which can give valuable insights in understanding the association between antibiotic use and VRE selection; however, causality cannot be proven. Second, we analyzed aggregated data on ward level and had no data on individual patients. Therefore, controlling for important confounders, such as duration of antibiotic therapy, history of antibiotic exposure or severity of underlying illness was not possible. Since it has been shown that group-level and individual-patient-level analyses might yield different results when the association between antibiotic exposure and resistance is assessed [31], our results have to be interpreted with caution. Third, routine screening for VRE at hospital admission was implemented only on some wards at Charité. Patients from other wards may have been colonized on admission or may have acquired VRE in outside hospitals. Therefore, the proportion of HA-VRE might be overestimated [32]. Fourth, the DDD is the assumed average maintenance dose per day for a drug used for its main indication in adults and does not necessarily reflect the recommended or prescribed daily dose [33]. Fifth, a molecular characterization of the identified VRE was not performed and we could not exclude clonal dissemination on the respective wards; however, since we did not identify VRE cluster on ward level during the study period, large outbreaks seems unlikely. Finally, data on compliance with hand hygiene and cleaning procedures were not measured, therefore confounding effects of these factors on our results are unknown.

Conclusions

In conclusion, we found a positive correlation between prior-month use of glycopeptides and current use of carbapenems and the incidence of HA-VRE on ward level when invasive and non-invasive VRE were considered. In addition, detection of at least one patient with CA-VRE in the current month significantly increased the risk of nosocomial acquisition of VRE, thereby indicating the risk of person-to-person transmission of VRE. To this end, a multifaceted approach to lower HA-VRE rates is required including prudent use of antimicrobial agents as well as implementation of and strict compliance to infection control measures to prevent VRE transmission.

Abbreviations

95% CI: 95% confidence interval; ATC: Anatomical therapeutic chemical (classification system); CA: Community-acquired; DDD: Defined daily dose; HA: Hospital-acquired; ICU: Intensive care unit; IQR: Interquartile range; IRR: Incidence rate ratio; LOS: Length of stay; PD: Patient-days; VRE: Vancomycin-resistant enterococcus

Acknowledgements

Not applicable.

Funding

No external funding was received for this study.

Authors' contributions

CR, PG and FS were responsible for the study design. PG supervised the study. MB, LPD and AR were responsible for data collection and data cleaning. AK analyzed the microbiological isolates and/or interpreted the results on antimicrobial susceptibility testing. FS conducted the statistical analysis. All authors interpreted the data, gave important intellectual content and revised the manuscript critically. All authors read and approved the final manuscript.

Consent for publication

Not applicable.

Competing interests

The authors declare that they have no competing interests.

References

1. Werner G, Coque TM, Hammerum AM, Hope R, Hryniewicz W, Johnson A, Klare I, Kristinsson KG, Leclercq R, Lester CH, Lillie M, Novais C, Olsson-Liljequist B, Peixe LV, Sadowy E, Simonsen GS, Top J, Vuopio-Varkila J, Willems RJ, Witte W, Woodford N. Emergence and spread of vancomycin resistance among enterococci in Europe. Euro Surveill. 2008;13(47):pii=19046.
2. Arias CA, Murray BE. The rise of the enterococcus: beyond vancomycin resistance. Nat Rev Microbiol. 2012;10(4):266–78.
3. Weiner LM, Webb AK, Limbago B, Dudeck MA, Patel J, Kallen AJ, Edwards JR, Sievert DM. Antimicrobial-resistant pathogens associated with healthcare-associated infections: summary of data reported to the National Healthcare Safety Network at the Centers for Disease Control and Prevention, 2011-2014. Infect Control Hosp Epidemiol. 2016;37(11):1288–301.
4. Gastmeier P, Schroder C, Behnke M, Meyer E, Geffers C. Dramatic increase in vancomycin-resistant enterococci in Germany. J Antimicrob Chemother. 2014;69(6):1660–4.
5. Chiang HY, Perencevich EN, Nair R, Nelson RE, Samore M, Khader K, Chorazy ML, Herwaldt LA, Blevins A, Ward MA, et al. Incidence and outcomes associated with infections caused by Vancomycin-resistant enterococci in the United States: systematic literature review and meta-analysis. Infect Control Hosp Epidemiol. 2017;38(2):203–15.
6. DiazGranados CA, Zimmer SM, Klein M, Jernigan JA. Comparison of mortality associated with vancomycin-resistant and vancomycin-susceptible enterococcal bloodstream infections: a meta-analysis. Clin Infect Dis. 2005;41(3):327–33.
7. World Health Organization (WHO): Global priority list of antibiotic-resistant bacteria to guide research, discovery, and development of new antibiotics. Available at http://www.who.int/medicines/publications/WHO-PPL-Short_Summary_25Feb-ET_NM_WHO.pdf?ua=1. Accessed on March 03, 2017. 2017.
8. Harbarth S, Cosgrove S, Carmeli Y. Effects of antibiotics on nosocomial epidemiology of vancomycin-resistant enterococci. Antimicrob Agents Chemother. 2002;46(6):1619–28.
9. Vergis EN, Hayden MK, Chow JW, Snydman DR, Zervos MJ, Linden PK, Wagener MM, Schmitt B, Muder RR. Determinants of vancomycin resistance and mortality rates in enterococcal bacteremia. A prospective multicenter study. Ann Intern Med. 2001;135(7):484–92.
10. Tornieporth NG, Roberts RB, John J, Hafner A, Riley LW. Risk factors associated with vancomycin-resistant enterococcus faecium infection or colonization in 145 matched case patients and control patients. Clin Infect Dis. 1996;23(4):767–72.
11. DiazGranados CA, Jernigan JA. Impact of vancomycin resistance on mortality among patients with neutropenia and enterococcal bloodstream infection. J Infect Dis. 2005;191(4):588–95.
12. O'Driscoll T, Crank CW. Vancomycin-resistant enterococcal infections: epidemiology, clinical manifestations, and optimal management. Infect Drug Resist. 2015;8:217–30.
13. Murray BE. Vancomycin-resistant enterococcal infections. N Engl J Med. 2000;342(10):710–21.
14. Stiefel U, Paterson DL, Pultz NJ, Gordon SM, Aron DC, Donskey CJ. Effect of the increasing use of piperacillin/tazobactam on the incidence of vancomycin-resistant enterococci in four academic medical centers. Infect Control Hosp Epidemiol. 2004;25(5):380–3.
15. McKinnell JA, Kunz DF, Chamot E, Patel M, Shirley RM, Moser SA, Baddley JW, Pappas PG, Miller LG. Association between vancomycin-resistant enterococci bacteremia and ceftriaxone usage. Infect Control Hosp Epidemiol. 2012;33(7):718–24.
16. Kritsotakis EI, Christidou A, Roumbelaki M, Tselentis Y, Gikas A. The dynamic relationship between antibiotic use and the incidence of vancomycin-resistant enterococcus: time-series modelling of 7-year surveillance data in a tertiary-care hospital. Clin Microbiol Infect. 2008;14(8):747–54.
17. Forstner C, Diab-Elschahawi M, Kivaranovic D, Graninger W, Mitteregger D, Macher M, Wrba T, Presterl E. Non-linear significant relationship between use of glycopeptides and isolation of vancomycin-resistant Enterococcus species in a university hospital setting. Antimicrob Resist Infect Control. 2015;4:25.
18. Fridkin SK, Edwards JR, Courval JM, Hill H, Tenover FC, Lawton R, Gaynes RP, McGowan JE Jr. Intensive care antimicrobial resistance epidemiology P, the National Nosocomial Infections Surveillance System H: the effect of vancomycin and third-generation cephalosporins on prevalence of vancomycin-resistant enterococci in 126 U.S. adult intensive care units. Ann Intern Med. 2001;135(3):175–83.
19. de Bruin MA, Riley LW. Does vancomycin prescribing intervention affect vancomycin-resistant enterococcus infection and colonization in hospitals? A systematic review. BMC Infect Dis. 2007;7:24.
20. Fuller RE, Harrell LJ, Meredith FT, Sexton DJ, Colvin LG. Vancomycin-resistant enterococci: risk related to the use of intravenous vancomycin in a university hospital. Infect Control Hosp Epidemiol. 1998;19(11):821–3.
21. Donskey CJ, Chowdhry TK, Hecker MT, Hoyen CK, Hanrahan JA, Hujer AM, Hutton-Thomas RA, Whalen CC, Bonomo RA, Rice LB. Effect of antibiotic therapy on the density of vancomycin-resistant enterococci in the stool of colonized patients. N Engl J Med. 2000;343(26):1925–32.
22. Wijesuriya TM, Perry P, Pryce T, Boehm J, Kay I, Flexman J, Coombs GW, Ingram PR. Low vancomycin MICs and fecal densities reduce the sensitivity of screening methods for vancomycin resistance in enterococci. J Clin Microbiol. 2014;52(8):2829–33.
23. D'Agata EM, Gautam S, Green WK, Tang YW. High rate of false-negative results of the rectal swab culture method in detection of gastrointestinal colonization with vancomycin-resistant enterococci. Clin Infect Dis. 2002; 34(2):167–72.
24. Schuts EC, Hulscher ME, Mouton JW, Verduin CM, Stuart JW, Overdiek HW, van der Linden PD, Natsch S, Hertogh CM, Wolfs TF, et al. Current evidence on hospital antimicrobial stewardship objectives: a systematic review and meta-analysis. Lancet Infect Dis. 2016;16(7):847–56.
25. Ostrowsky BE, Trick WE, Sohn AH, Quirk SB, Holt S, Carson LA, Hill BC, Arduino MJ, Kuehnert MJ, Jarvis WR. Control of vancomycin-resistant enterococcus in health care facilities in a region. N Engl J Med. 2001; 344(19):1427–33.
26. Sydnor ER, Perl TM. Hospital epidemiology and infection control in acute-care settings. Clin Microbiol Rev. 2011;24(1):141–73.
27. LeDell K, Muto CA, Jarvis WR, Farr BM. SHEA guideline for preventing nosocomial transmission of multidrug-resistant strains of Staphylococcus Aureus and enterococcus. Infect Control Hosp Epidemiol. 2003;24(9):639–41.
28. Siegel JD, Rhinehart E, Jackson M, Chiarello L. Healthcare infection control practices advisory C: management of multidrug-resistant organisms in health care settings, 2006. Am J Infect Control. 2007;35(10 Suppl 2):S165–93.
29. Lai CC, Chu CC, Cheng A, Huang YT, Hsueh PR. Correlation between antimicrobial consumption and incidence of health-care-associated infections due to methicillin-resistant Staphylococcus Aureus and vancomycin-resistant enterococci at a university hospital in Taiwan from 2000 to 2010. J Microbiol Immunol

Infect. 2015;48(4):431–6.

30. Meyer E, Gastmeier P, Deja M, Schwab F. Antibiotic consumption and resistance: data from Europe and Germany. Int J Med Microbiol. 2013;303(6–7):388–95.
31. Harbarth S, Harris AD, Carmeli Y, Samore MH. Parallel analysis of individual and aggregated data on antibiotic exposure and resistance in gram-negative bacilli. Clin Infect Dis. 2001;33(9):1462–8.
32. Erb S, Frei R, Dangel M, Widmer AF. Multidrug-resistant organisms detected more than 48 hours after hospital admission are not necessarily hospital-acquired. Infect Control Hosp Epidemiol. 2017;38(1):18–23.
33. (WHO) WHO: Defined Daily Dose - Definition and general considerations. Available at: https://www.whocc.no/ddd/definition_and_general_considera/. Acessed on 20 July 2017. 2015.

11

Co-existence of bla_{OXA-23} and bla_{NDM-1} genes of *Acinetobacter baumannii* isolated from Nepal: antimicrobial resistance and clinical significance

Prabhu Raj Joshi[1], Mahesh Acharya[1], Trishna Kakshapati[2], Udomluk Leungtongkam[3], Rapee Thummeepak[3] and Sutthirat Sitthisak[3,4*]

Abstract

Background: Molecular analysis of carbapenem-resistant genes in *Acinetobacter baumannii*, an emerging pathogen, is less commonly reported from Nepal. In this study we determined the antibiotic susceptibility profile and genetic mechanism of carbapenem resistance in clinical isolates of *A. baumannii*.

Methods: *A. baumannii* were isolated from various clinical specimens and identified based on Gram staining, biochemical tests, and PCR amplification of organism specific 16S rRNA and bla_{OXA-51} genes. The antibiotic susceptibility testing was performed using disc diffusion and E-test method. Multiplex PCR assays were used to detect the following β-lactamase genes: four class D carbapenem hydrolyzing oxacillinases (bla_{OXA-51}, bla_{OXA-23}, bla_{OXA-24} and bla_{OXA-58}). Uniplex PCRs were used to detect three class B metallo-β-lactamases genes (bla_{IMP}, bla_{VIM} and bla_{NDM-1}), class C cephalosporin resistance genes (bla_{ADC}), aminoglycoside resistance gene (*aphA6*), and IS*Aba1* of all isolates. Insertion sequence IS*Aba125* among NDM-1 positive strains was detected. Clonal relatedness of all isolates were analyzed using repetitive sequence-based PCR (rep-PCR).

Results: Of total 44 analyzed isolates, 97.7% ($n = 43$) were carbapenem-resistant *A. baumannii* (CR-AB) and 97.7% ($n = 43$) were multidrug resistant *A. baumannii* (MDR-AB). One isolate was detected to be extremely drug resistant *A. baumannii* (XDR-AB). All the isolates were fully susceptible to colistin (MICs < 2 μg/ml). The bla_{OXA-23} gene was detected in all isolates, while bla_{NDM-1} was detected in 6 isolates (13.6%). Insertion sequence, IS*Aba1* was detected in all of bla_{OXA-23} positive isolates. IS*Aba125* was detected in all bla_{NDM-1} positive strains. The bla_{ADC} and *aphA6* genes were detected in 90.1 and 40.1%, respectively. The rep-PCR of all isolates represented 7 different genotypes.

Conclusion: We found high prevalence of CR-AB and MDR-AB with bla_{OXA-23} gene in a tertiary care hospital in Nepal. Systemic network surveillance should be established for monitoring and controlling the spread of these resistant strains.

Keywords: *Acinetobacter baumannii*, Carbapenem resistance, bla_{OXA-23} and bla_{NDM-1} carbapenemase genes

* Correspondence: sutthirats@nu.ac.th
[3]Department of Microbiology and Parasitology, Faculty of Medical Science, Naresuan University, Phitsanulok, Thailand
[4]Centre of Excellence in Medical Biotechnology, Faculty of Medical Science, Naresuan University, Phitsanulok, Thailand
Full list of author information is available at the end of the article

Background

Acinetobacter baumannii, an emerging pathogen of healthcare centers, shows intrinsic as well as acquired drug-resistance mechanisms [1]. Multidrug-resistant *A. baumannii* can be resistant to all of the currently available antibiotics, and in its deadliest form these are only susceptible to potentially toxic polymyxins and colistins, leaving limited options for treatment [2]. Infections with carbapenem- and colistin-resistant *A. baumannii* are emerging globally [3].

Carbapenem resistance in *A. baumannii* encompasses production of class B, C and class D carbapenemase, decreased membrane permeability, altered penicillin-binding proteins, and overexpression of efflux pumps [4, 5]. Most commonly, *Acinetobacter* spp. develop carbapenem resistance by production of OXA-type carbapenemase and metallo-β-lactamases (MBLs) [6, 7]; bla_{OXA-23}-like, bla_{OXA-40}-like, bla_{OXA-58}-like and bla_{OXA-51}-like carbapenemases are broadly reported, where bla_{OXA-51}-like β-lactamases, intrinsic to *A. baumannii*, is used for species identification [8–10]. Among multiple MBL genes, bla_{IMP} and bla_{VIM} types (chromosomal or plasmid encoded) encode carbapenemase in *A. baumannii* [9]. *A. baumannii* harboring plasmid encoded New Delhi metallo-β-lactamase-1 (NDM-1), a novel carbapenemase gene, is reported from many countries [11, 12]. In addition, detection of class C β-lactamase genes (bla_{ADC}) which mediated cephalosporin resistances and aminoglycoside resistant genes (*aphA6*) has increased in recent years in *A. baumannii* clinical isolates [13, 14].

A. baumannii remains a critical problem in many healthcare settings throughout the world despite the implementation of infection control practices. There are limited data on carbapenem-resistant *A. baumannii* in Nepal. The objective of this study was to determine antibiotic susceptibility profile, antibiotic resistance genes and genetic mechanism of carbapenem resistance of *A. baumannii* in clinical isolates at a tertiary care hospital, Nepal.

Methods

Bacterial isolation and identification

A. baumannii isolates were collected from inpatient units of a tertiary hospital, Nepal. Forty-four non-duplicate isolates were collected (24 male and 20 female; age range between 24 to 80 years) over 9 months periods (October 2014 to June 2015). All isolates were identified by classical biochemical methods and confirmed by PCR method for detecting 16S rRNA gene and bla_{OXA-51} gene [15, 16]. Isolates were identified as *A. baumannii* by PCR result of positive for both PCRs.

Antibiotic susceptibility testing

The antibiotic susceptibility of amikacin (30), cefotaxime (30), ceftazidime (30), ceftriaxone (30), cefepime (30), ciprofloxacin (5), gentamicin (10), imipenem (10), meropenem (10), trimethoprim/sulfamethoxazole (1.25/23.75), tetracycline (30), and piperacillin/tazobactam (100/10) (Oxoid) was determined on Mueller Hinton Agar (High Media, India) according to the antibiotic disk diffusion method [17]. The plates were incubated at 37 °C for 24 h. The zones of inhibition were determined whether the microorganism was susceptible, intermediately resistant, or resistant to each antibiotic according to Clinical and Laboratory Standards Institute (CLSI) guidelines. E-test was performed to determine the Minimum inhibitory concentration (MIC) of ceftazidime, imipenem, tigecycline and colistin (High Media, India) according to manufacturer instructions and interpreted as per CLSI guidelines except for tigecycline. Multidrung-resistant *A. baumannii* (MDR-AB) was defined when *A. baumannii* resistant to multiple antibiotics, often defined as three or more antibiotic classes. Extensively drug resistant *A. baumannii* (XDR-AB) was defined when *A. baumannii* was resistant to all antimicrobial agents except polymyxins (colistin) [18].

PCR amplification of antibiotic resistance genes

PCR assays to detect bla_{OXA-23}, bla_{OXA-24}, bla_{OXA-51}, bla_{OXA-58}, bla_{IMP}, bla_{VIM}, bla_{NDM}, bla_{ADC} and *ahpA6* genes were performed using primers as describe previously (Table 1). The amplification reaction was performed using *A. baumannii* cell lysate as DNA template. Each PCR was performed in triplicate in a thermocycler with a PCR condition as described previously [14, 16, 19–21]. All PCR assays used 16S rRNA or bla_{OXA-51} genes as the internal control. The IS*Aba1* of bla_{OXA-23} gene was detected using combination of primers IS*Aba1*-F/IS*Aba1*-R and IS*Aba1*-F/bla_{OXA-23}-R (Table 1) [22]. The IS*Aba125* of bla_{NDM-1} gene were determined in all bla_{NDM-1} positive strains using combination of primers ISA125-F/ISA125-R and ISA125-F/bla_{NDM}-R (Table 1). PCR products of the bla_{NDM-1} genes were purified and sequenced. BLAST was used to compare the sequences of bla_{NDM-1} genes against the GenBank Database. PCR products were analyzed by electrophoresis in 1% agarose gel containing 0.5 μg/ml ethidium bromides.

IPM-EDTA combined disk test

All bla_{NDM-1} positive strains were tested for MBL production by IPM-EDTA combined disk test. The test was performed as previously described [23]. After 24 h incubation, the difference of inhibition zone diameter between IPM-EDTA disk and IPM disk alone (≥7 mm) was considered the positive criteria for the presence of MBL.

Table 1 List of primer for detection of genes used in this study

Target genes	Primer name	Sequence 5'-3'	Size/ Annealing temp.	References
16S rRNA	16S rRNA-F	AGAGTTTGATCCTGGCTCAG	1500/58	[15]
	16S rRNA-R	ACGGCTACCTTGTTACGACTT		
bla_{OXA-23}	bla_{OXA-23}-F	GATCGGATTGGAGAACCAGA	501/52	[16]
	bla_{OXA-23}-R	ATTTCTGACCGCATTTCCAT		
bla_{OXA-51}	bla_{OXA-51}-F	TAATGCTTTGATCGGCCTTG	353/52	[16]
	bla_{OXA-51}-R	TGGATTGCACTTCATCTTGG		
bla_{OXA-24}	bla_{OXA-24}-F	GGTTAGTTGGCCCCCTTAAA	246/52	[16]
	bla_{OXA-24}-R	AGTTGAGCGAAAAGGGGATT		
bla_{OXA-58}	bla_{OXA-58}-F	AAGTATTGGGGCTTGTGCTG	599/52	[16]
	bla_{OXA-58}-R	CCCCTCTGCGCTCTACATAC		
bla_{IMP}	bla_{IMP} –F	GGAATAGAGTGGCTTAAYTCTC	232/52	[20]
	bla_{IMP} –R	GGTTTAAYAAAACAACCACC		
bla_{VIM}	bla_{VIM} –F	GATGGTGTTTGGTCGCATA	390/52	[20]
	bla_{VIM} –R	CGAATGCGCAGCACCAG		
bla_{NDM}	bla_{NDM}–F	GGTTTGGCGATCTGGTTTTC	621/52	[21]
	bla_{NDM}–R	CGGAATGGCTCATCACGATC		
bla_{ADC}	bla_{ADC}-F	TAAACACCACATATGTTCCG	663/56	[19]
	bla_{ADC}-F	ACTTACTTCAACTCGCGACG		
aphA6	*aphA6*-F	ATGGAATTGCCCAATATTATTC	736/55	[14]
	aphA6-R	TCAATTCAATTCATCAAGTTTTA		
IS*Aba1*	IS*Aba1*-F	CATTGGCATTAAACTGAGGAGAAA	451/52	[22]
	IS*Aba1*-R	TTGGAAATGGGGAAAACGAA		
IS*Aba125*	ISA125-F	TGTTGAAGCGATCCGTTGTT	755/57	This study
	ISA125-R	GTGCGACAGTTTCAAAAGCCA		
Rep-PCR	ERIC-2	AAGTAAGTGACTGGGGTGAGCG	variable length/45	[24]

Repetitive element PCR-mediated DNA fingerprinting (rep-PCR)

Genomic DNA of each isolates was extracted from the overnight cultures using GF-1 bacterial DNA extraction kit (Vivantis, Malaysia). Rep-PCR was performed by using genomic DNA as a template for PCR amplification with the ERIC-2 primer (Table 1) using condition as describe previously [24, 25]. PCR-banding patterns and rep-PCR types were analyzed and interpreted as previously described [25].

Results

Demographic characteristic of patients

Demographic characteristics of the inpatients with *A. baumannii* infection were analyzed; 24 (54.5%) were male and 20 (45.5%) were female. Most of the specimens were from ICU wards ($n = 27$, 61.4%) (Fig. 1). Isolates were collected from sputum ($n = 26$, 59.1%), tracheal aspirates ($n = 9$, 20.4%), catheter tip, ($n = 4$, 9.1%), pus ($n = 4$, 9.1%) and urine ($n = 1$, 2.3%) (Fig. 1).

Antibiotic susceptibility

Of the 44 isolates, resistance was found against ciprofloxacin ($n = 43$, 97.7%), cefotaxime ($n = 43$, 97.7%), ceftazidime ($n = 42$, 95.4%), ceftriaxone ($n = 41$, 93.2%), cefepime ($n = 39$, 88.6%), amikacin ($n = 19$, 43.2%), gentamicin ($n = 23$, 52.3%), trimethoprim/sulfamethoxazole ($n = 41$, 93.2%), tetracycline ($n = 21$, 47.7%) and piperacillin/tazobactam ($n = 43$, 97.7%). Only one isolate of *A.baumannii* was susceptible to all tested antibiotics. Most isolates (97.7%, $n = 43$) were carbapenem resistant *A. baumannii* (CR-AB); all CR-AB were MDR-AB. One isolate was detected to be XDR-AB. All the isolates were fully susceptible to colistin (MICs < 2 μg/ml) and MIC of tigecycline was determined to be <2.5 μg/ml (Table 2).

Antibiotic resistance genes and IS element in *A. baumannii*

Aminoglycoside resistance gene, *aphA6* and cephalosporin resistance genes, bla_{ADC} were detected in 40.1% (18/44) and 90.1% (40/44), respectively. The bla_{OXA-23} was present in all isolates. Other class D β-lactamase

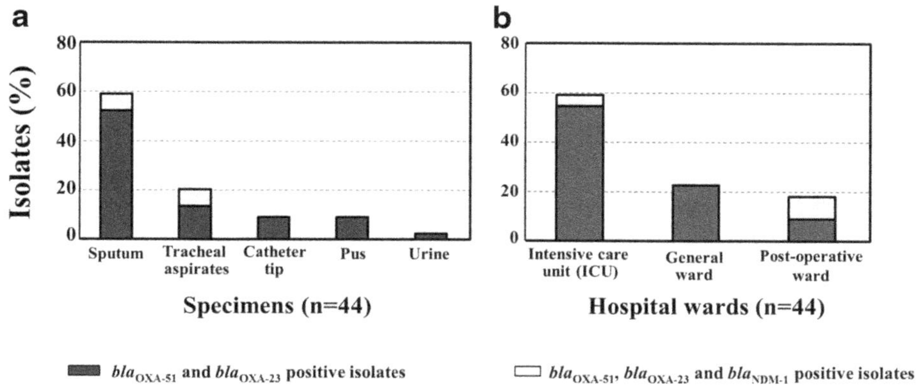

Fig. 1 Distribution of *A. baumannii* carrying carbapenemase genes in different specimen types **a** and wards **b**

genes, including bla_{OXA-24} and bla_{OXA-58}, markers of carbapenem resistance in *A. baumannii,* were not detected in analyzed isolates. IS*Aba1* was detected in all of bla_{OXA-23} positive isolates (100%). Of total analyzed isolates, 6 (13.6%) also harbored bla_{NDM-1} gene in addition to bla_{OXA-23} and bla_{OXA-51}. All NDM-1 positive strains exhibited insertion sequence IS*Aba125* detecting with primers ISA125-F/ISA125-R. All isolates also detected a band of 1.6 kb in a PCR using ISA125-F/bla_{NDM}-R primers. Metallo-β-lactamase (MBL) genes, including bla_{VIM} and bla_{IMP}, were not detected in all isolates. The sequences of the bla_{NDM-1} gene yielded 99-100% sequence identity to the bla_{NDM-1} gene from *Acinetobacter lwoffii* strain WJ10621 plasmid pNDM-BJ01 (Accession: JQ001791) obtained from the GenBank Database.

MBL production

Six *A. baumannii* isolates harbored bla_{NDM-1} gene were detected for MBL production. All of bla_{NDM-1} positive strains were positive for MBL production. MBL positive strains showed resistance to fluoroquinolones and β-lactam.

Epidemiological typing

Clonal relationship among isolates were studied using rep-PCR typing. The fingerprinting represented 7 different DNA patterns consisting of 2 to 5 DNA fragment sizes. The amplicons size for ERIC-2 PCR was 500–4000 bp. The genotype was named A-G as shown in Fig. 2. The high prevalence genotype was type C (n = 14; 31.8%) and D (n = 12; 27.3%). Genotype A, B, C and D were disseminated in all isolated ward (ICU, general ward and post-operative ward). Among 44 isolates, one isolate of type F (2.3%) and G (2.3%) was found. Type F was obtained from a catheter tip specimen from the ICU ward. Type G was obtained from sputum of a patient from a general ward. All NDM-1 positive strains exhibited genotype A (n = 1), B (n = 1), C (n = 3) and D (n = 1).

Discussions

A. baumannii harboring bla_{OXA-51}-like gene has been identified as a marker for species identification. An intrinsic bla_{OXA-51}-like gene detected in all isolates in this study supports the use of this gene as a surrogate marker of *A. baumannii* identification [8–10]. High prevalence of cephalosporin resistance genes, bla_{ADC} (90.1%) was found in this study. In addition, we found a high rate of cepharosporin resistant antibiotics (cefotaxime, ceftazidime, ceftriaxone) using the disk diffusion method. These data indicated that cephalosporins no longer work to treat *A. baumannii* isolated from Nepal. Carbapenem resistance in *A. baumannii* is a major concern and is most often associated with class D

Table 2 The carbapenemases gene patterns, rep-PCR types and MIC determination of *A. baumannii* isolated from difference wards

Sites	β-lactamase gene patterns	No. of isolates	Rep-PCR Types (n)	MIC (μg/ml) range			
				CAZ	IMP	TG	CL
Intensive care unit	$bla_{OXA-51/\ OXA-23}$	25	A (2), B (6), C (8), D (6), E (2), F (1)	4– > 256	1– > 32	1.6–3.9	0.13–2
	$bla_{OXA-51/\ OXA-23/\ NDM-1}$	2	B (1), C (1)	>256	>32	1.7–3.2	0.61–0.79
General ward	$bla_{OXA-51/\ OXA-23}$	9	A (1), B (1), C (1), D (5), G (1)	>256	>24–>32	2–3.4	0.32–0.88
Post-operative ward	$bla_{OXA-51/\ OXA-23}$	4	A (1), B (1), C (2)	>256	>32	2.3–3.3	0.54–0.78
	$bla_{OXA-51/\ OXA-23/\ NDM-1}$	4	A (1), C (2) D (1)	>256	>32	2.1–3.2	0.23–0.51

Abbreviations: *CAZ* ceftazidime, *IPM* imipenem, *TG* tigecycline, *CL* colistin

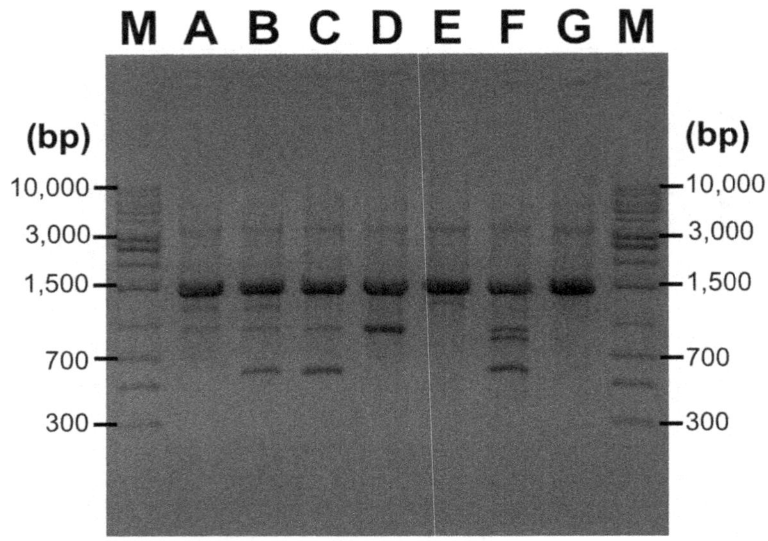

Fig. 2 Rep-PCR-based DNA fingerprint patterns of *A. baumannii* isolates. The *lanes* marked M contain molecular markers. Each lane represents genotype patterns of *A–G*

β-lactamases and MBLs. The full susceptibility of all CR-AB to colistin in this study indicates that colistin is still an option of drug for the treatment of infections caused by *A. baumannii* in Nepal hospital.

OXA-type carbapenemases are predominant in *A. baumannii* [6, 7]. In agreement with this finding, high prevalence of $bla_{OXA\text{-}23}$ carrying *A. baumannii* strains has been reported in Nepalese patients [26]. The acquired $bla_{OXA\text{-}23}$ is the dominant genetic determinant in Asia. The $bla_{OXA\text{-}23}$ gene located on plasmid can be transferred between *A. baumannii* through conjugation. Thus, antibiotic resistant bacteria have been rapidly increasing worldwide [27]. The $bla_{OXA\text{-}24}$ and $bla_{OXA\text{-}58}$ were not detected in any isolates from this study. The $bla_{OXA\text{-}24/40}$ and $bla_{OXA\text{-}58}$ genes were common in *A. baumannii* isolated from Europe [2, 28]. Recently, $bla_{OXA\text{-}143}$ and $bla_{OXA\text{-}235}$, which are novel class D β-lactamase genes in *A. baumannii* have been identified. To date, these determinants were detected only in Brazil, Mexico and the USA [29, 30]. IS*Aba1* was detected in widespread clones of *A. baumannii* worldwide. Our study found IS*Aba1* upstream of $bla_{OXA\text{-}23}$ in all *A. baumannii* isolates. A correlation between *A. baumannii* clusters carrying the IS*Aba1*/$bla_{OXA\text{-}23}$ gene and increased minimal inhibitory concentrations for carbapenems was reported [31]. One isolate (AB-13) that was recovered from catheter tips of long-stay hospital patients showed an extreme drug resistance pattern (Additional file 1: Table S1). This isolate represented $bla_{OXA\text{-}23}$, bla_{ADC} and *aphA6* genes. Further molecular study to detect other antibiotic resistance genes is needed to explain what factors correlated with extreme drug resistance. We also found one isolate (AB-25) harboring $bla_{OXA\text{-}23}$, bla_{ADC} and *aphA6* genes was sensitive to all tested drugs (Additional file 1: Table S1). This may be due to the lack of promoter or mutation of IS*Aba1* or $bla_{OXA\text{-}23}$ gene. Further study is needed to warrant the conclusion.

The $bla_{NDM\text{-}1}$ carrying *A. baumannii* has recently been emerged in many countries, including Germany, Spain, Israel, Egypt, Switzerland, Libya, India, Pakistan and Nepal [11, 26, 32, 33]. The $bla_{NDM\text{-}1}$ gene has been identified as a chimeric gene constructed by the fusion of the aminoglycoside-resistance gene *aphA6* with a mannose-binding lectin gene. This event most likely occurs in *Acinetobacter* spp., indicating that these bacteria are likely the origin of this gene [34]. In this study, we identified 13.6% of *A. baumannii* carrying $bla_{NDM\text{-}1}$ gene. Previous study has identified high prevalence (24.6%) of the *A. baumannii* harbored the $bla_{NDM\text{-}1}$ gene in Nepal in 2013–2014 [26]. Taking into consideration the relationship between India, China and Nepal, the spread of $bla_{NDM\text{-}1}$ is likely to occur rapidly, mostly through *A. baumannii* rather than Enterobacteriaceae. *A. baumannii* able to transfer the $bla_{NDM\text{-}1}$ gene via conjugation to the recipients and Tn*125* appears to be the main vehicle for dissemination of the $bla_{NDM\text{-}1}$ genes in *A. baumannii* [35]. Poirel et al. reported that the $bla_{NDM\text{-}1}$ gene was located within the composite transposon Tn*125* bracketed by two copies of a strong promoter of $bla_{NDM\text{-}1}$ gene called IS*Aba125* [11]. This report was correlated with our finding that found IS*Aba125* in 100% of NDM-1 producing *A. baumannii*.

The previous study reported that the most of *A. baumannii* isolates harboring $bla_{NDM\text{-}1}$ belonged to ST85 and ST25 [35–37]. In Libyan hospital, Libya, the main clone of imipenem-resistant NDM-1-producing *A. baumannii* belonged to ST2 [33]. We used rep-PCR typing to determine the clonal relationship in NDM-1 producing *A. baumannii*. Our study highlighted that most of NDM-1-producing *A. baumannii* isolates belonged to 4 genotypes using rep-PCR. Rep-PCR is a method that generates DNA fingerprints to discriminate between bacterial strains, and has been used to characterize *A. baumannii* isolates from hospitalized patients [38]. Our rep-PCR typing represented a high genetic diversity (A-G) among *A. baumannii* isolates from Nepal. Some clonally related groups (A, B, C and D) were observed in the all wards represented the disseminated of these clones in the hospital. Four genotypes (A, B, C, and D) of co-existence of bla_{OXA-23} and bla_{NDM-1} *A. baumannii* isolates were found. In addition, dissemination of these four genotypes into different wards also confirms as a major epidemic. Since rep-PCR is less discriminatory for molecular typing of bacterial strains, further study using multi-locus sequence typing could be useful for epidemiological investigations.

Conclusion

Antibiotic resistance in *A. baumannii* is considered to be a major future challenge in Nepal. Beyond OXA-type carbapenemase, there is no doubt the emergence and spreads of NDM-1 encoding *A. baumannii*–a superbug–will further limit chemotherapeutic options and threaten the public health of Nepal. The mechanism of hospital adaptiveness beyond antibiotic resistance will be more demanded in order to fully understand and combat MDR and XDR *A. baumannii*.

Abbreviations

CR-AB: Carbapenem-resistant *Acinetobacter baumannii*; ICU: Intensive care unit; IPM-EDTA: Imipenem-ethylenediaminetetraacetic acid; MBL: Metallo-beta-lactamase; MDR-AB: Multidrug-resistant *Acinetobacter baumannii*; MIC: Minimum inhibitory concentration; NDM: New Delhi metallo-beta-lactamase; PCR: Polymerase chain reaction; XDR-AB: Extremely drug resistant *Acinetobacter baumannii*

Acknowledgements

We thank Dr. Basant Pant, Neurosurgeon, Annapurna Neurological Institute and Allied Sciences for providing laboratory facility and moral support. We also acknowledge Nepal Health Research Council for approving this study.

Funding

This study was partial funding by Thailand Research Fund (RSA5780015).

Authors' contributions

PRJ and MA designed the study, collected data, analyzed the data and prepared the manuscript, TK supervised the study, UL and RT collected data, SS, analyzed the data, supervised the study and prepared the manuscript. All authors read and approved the manuscript.

Competing interests

The authors declare that they have no competing interests.

Consent for publication

Not applicable.

Author details

[1]Central Department of Microbiology, Tribhuvan University, Kirtipur, Kathmandu, Nepal. [2]Annapurna Neurological Institute and Allied Sciences, Maitighar, Kathmandu, Nepal. [3]Department of Microbiology and Parasitology, Faculty of Medical Science, Naresuan University, Phitsanulok, Thailand. [4]Centre of Excellence in Medical Biotechnology, Faculty of Medical Science, Naresuan University, Phitsanulok, Thailand.

References

1. Yamamoto M, Nagao M, Matsumura Y, Matsushima A, Ito Y, Takakura S, et al. Interspecies dissemination of a novel class 1 integron carrying bla_{IMP-19} among *Acinetobacter* species in Japan. J Antimicrob Chemother. 2011;66:2480–3.
2. Villalon P, Valdezate S, Medina-Pascual MJ, Carrasco G, Vindel A, Saez-Nieto JA. Epidemiology of the *Acinetobacter*-derived cephalosporinase, carbapenem-hydrolysingoxacillinase and metallo-beta-lactamase genes, and of common insertion sequences, in epidemic clones of *Acinetobacter baumannii* from Spain. J Antimicrob Chemother. 2013;68:550–3.
3. Agodi A, Voulgari E, Barchitta M, Quattrocchi A, Bellocchi P, Poulou A, et al. Spread of a carbapenem- and colistin-resistant *Acinetobacter baumannii* ST2 clonal strain causing outbreaks in two Sicilian hospitals. J Hosp Infect. 2014;86:260–6.
4. Heritier C, Poirel L, Lambert T, Nordmann P. Contribution of acquired carbapenem-hydrolyzing oxacillinases to carbapenem resistance in *Acinetobacter baumannii*. Antimicrob Agents Chemother. 2005;49:3198–202.
5. Quale J, Bratu S, Landman D, Heddurshetti R. Molecular epidemiology and mechanisms of carbapenem resistance in *Acinetobacter baumannii* endemic in New York City. Clin Infect Dis Off Publ Infect Dis Soc Am. 2003;37:214–20.
6. Amudhan MS, Sekar U, Kamalanathan A, Balaraman S. bla_{IMP} and bla_{VIM} mediated carbapenem resistance in *Pseudomonas* and *Acinetobacter* species in India. J Infect Develop Ctries. 2012;6:757–62.
7. Thomson JM, Bonomo RA. The threat of antibiotic resistance in Gram negative pathogenic bacteria: beta-lactams in peril! Curr Opin Microbiol. 2005;8:518–24.
8. Cicek AC, Saral A, Iraz M, Ceylan A, Duzgun AO, Peleg AY, et al. OXA- and GES-type beta-lactamases predominate in extensively drug-resistant *Acinetobacter baumannii* isolates from a Turkish University Hospital. Clin Microbiol Infect. 2014;20:410–5.
9. Tsakris A, Ikonomidis A, Pournaras S, Tzouvelekis LS, Sofianou D, Legakis NJ, et al. VIM-1 metallo-beta-lactamase in *Acinetobacter baumannii*. Emerg Infect Dis. 2006;12:981–3.
10. Kusradze I, Diene SM, Goderdzishvili M, Rolain JM. Molecular detection of OXA carbapenemase genes in multidrug-resistant *Acinetobacter baumannii* isolates from Iraq and Georgia. Int J Antimicrob Agents. 2011;38:164–8.
11. Poirel L, Bonnin RA, Boulanger A, Schrenzel J, Kaase M, Nordmann P. Tn125-related acquisition of *bla*NDM-like genes in *Acinetobacter baumannii*. Antimicrob Agents Chemother. 2012;56:1087–9.
12. Abbas M, Cherkaoui A, Fankhauser C, Schrenzel J, Harbarth S. Epidemiology and clinical implications of carbapenemase-producing bacteria in Switzerland. Rev Med Suisse. 2012;8:882–4.
13. Sarhaddi N, Soleimanpour S, Farsiani H, Mosavat A, Dolatabadi S, Salimizand H, et al. Elevated prevalence of multidrug-resistant *Acinetobacter baumannii* with extensive genetic diversity in the largest burn centre of northeast Iran. J Glob Antimicrob Resist. 2016;8:60–6.
14. Hujer KM, Hujer AM, Hulten EA, Bajaksouzian S, Adams JM, Donskey CJ, et al. Analysis of antibiotic resistance genes in multidrug-resistant *Acinetobacter* sp. isolates from military and civilian patients treated at the Walter Reed Army Medical Center. Antimicrob Agents Chemother. 2006;50:4114–23.
15. Misbah S, Hassan H, Yusof MY, Hanifah YS, Abu-Bakar S. Genomic species identification of *Acinetobacter* of clinical isolates by 16S rDNA sequencing. Singapore. Med J. 2005;46:461–4.
16. Woodford N, Ellington MJ, Coelho JM, Turton JF, Ward ME, Brown S, et al. Multiplex PCR for genes encoding prevalent OXA carbapenemases in *Acinetobacter* spp. Int J Antimicrob Agents. 2006;27:351–3.
17. Clinical and Laboratory Standards Institute. Performance standards for

antimicrobial susceptibility testing, document M100-24. Wayne: Clinical and Laboratory Standards Institute; 2014.

18. Magiorakos AP, Srinivasan A, Carey RB, Carmeli Y, Falagas ME, Giske CG, et al. Multidrug-resistant, extensively drug-resistant and pandrug-resistant bacteria: an international expert proposal for interim standard definitions for acquired resistance. Clin Microbiol Infect. 2012;18:268–81.
19. Liu Y, Liu X. Detection of AmpC β-lactamases in *Acinetobacter baumannii* in the Xuzhou region and analysis of drug resistance. Exp Ther Med. 2015;10:933–6.
20. Ellington MJ, Kistler J, Livermore DM, Woodford N. Multiplex PCR for rapid detection of genes encoding acquired metallo-beta-lactamases. J Antimicrob Chemother. 2007;59:321–2.
21. Poirel L, Walsh TR, Cuvillier V, Nordmann P. Multiplex PCR for detection of acquired carbapenemase genes. Diagn Microbiol Infect Dis. 2011;70:119–23.
22. Ruiz M, Marti S, Fernandez-Cuenca F, Pascual A, Vila J. Prevalence of IS (*Aba1*) in epidemiologically unrelated *Acinetobacter baumannii* clinical isolates. FEMS Microbiol Lett. 2007;274:63–6.
23. Yong D, Lee K, Yum JH, Shin HB, Rossolini GM, Chong Y. Imipenem-EDTA disk method for differentiation of metallo-beta-lactamase-producing clinical isolates of *Pseudomonas* spp. and *Acinetobacter* spp. J Clin Microbiol. 2002; 40:3798–801.
24. Vila J, Marcos MA, Jiminez de Anta MT. A comparative study of different PCR-based DNA fingerprinting techniques for typing of the *Acinetobacter calcoaceticus-A. baumannii* complex. J Med Microbiol. 1996;44:482–9.
25. Grundmann HJ, Towner KJ, Dijkshoorn L, Gerner-Smidt P, Maher M, Seifert H, et al. Multicenter study using standardized protocols and reagents for evaluation of reproducibility of PCR-based fingerprinting of *Acinetobacter* spp. J Clin Microbiol. 1997;35:3071–7.
26. Shrestha S, Tadab T, Miyoshi-Akiyamac T, Oharad H, Shimadab K, Satoue K, et al. Molecular epidemiology of multidrug-resistant *Acinetobacter baumannii* isolates in a university hospital in Nepal reveals the emergence of a novel epidemic clonal lineage. Int J Antimicrob Agents. 2015;46:526–31.
27. Bertini A, Poirel L, Mugnier PD, Villa L, Nordmann P, Carattoli A. Characterization and PCR-based replicon typing of resistance plasmids in *Acinetobacter baumannii*. Antimicrob Agents Chemother. 2010;54:4168–77.
28. Cherkaoui A, Emonet S, Renzi G, Schrenzel J. Characteristics of multidrug-resistant *Acinetobacter baumannii* strains isolated in Geneva during colonization or infection. Ann Clin Microbiol Antimicrob. 2015;11:14–42.
29. Higgins PG, Pérez-Llarena FJ, Zander E, Fernández A, Bou G, Seifert H. OXA-235, a novel class D β-lactamase involved in resistance to carbapenems in *Acinetobacter baumannii*. Antimicrob Agents Chemother. 2013;57:2121–6.
30. Zander E, Bonnin RA, Seifert H, Higgins PG. Characterization of $bla_{\text{OXA-143}}$ variants in *Acinetobacter baumannii* and *Acinetobacter pittii*. Antimicrob Agents Chemother. 2014;58:2704–8.
31. Viana GF, Zago MC, Moreira RR, Zarpellon MN, Menegucci TC, Cardoso CL, et al. IS*Aba1*/$bla_{\text{OXA-23}}$: A serious obstacle to controlling the spread and treatment of *Acinetobacter baumannii* strains. Am J Infect Control. 2016;44:593–5.
32. Decousser JW, Jansen C, Nordmann P, Emirian A, Bonnin RA, Anais L, et al. Outbreak of NDM-1-producing *Acinetobacter baumannii* in France, January to May 2013. Eurosurveillance. 2013;18. doi:10.2807/1560-7917.ES2013.18.31.20547
33. Mathlouthi N, El Salabi AA, Ben Jomàa-Jemili M, Bakour S, Al-Bayssari C, Zorgani AA, et al. Early detection of metallo-β-lactamase NDM-1- and OXA-23 carbapenemase-producing *Acinetobacter baumannii* in Libyan hospitals. Int J Antimicrob Agents. 2016;48:46–50.
34. Toleman MA, Spencer J, Jones L, Walsh TR. $bla_{\text{NDM-1}}$ is a chimera likely constructed in *Acinetobacter baumannii*. Antimicrob Agents Chemother. 2012;56:2773–76.
35. Ramoul A, Loucif L, Bakour S, Amiri S, Dekhil M, Rolain JM. Co-occurrence of $bla_{\text{NDM-1}}$ with $bla_{\text{OXA-23}}$ or $bla_{\text{OXA-58}}$ in clinical multidrug-resistant *Acinetobacter baumannii* isolates in Algeria. J Glob Antimicrob Resist. 2016;6:136–41.
36. Rafei R, Pailhoriès H, Hamze M, Eveillard M, Mallat H, Dabboussi F, et al. Molecular epidemiology of *Acinetobacter baumannii* in different hospitals in Tripoli, Lebanon using $bla_{\text{OXA-51-like}}$ sequence based typing. BMC Microbiol. 2015;15:11–7.
37. Bakour S, Touati A, Bachiri T, Sahli F, Tiouit D, Naim M, et al. First report of 16S rRNA methylase ArmA-producing *Acinetobacter baumannii* and rapid spread of metallo-β-lactamase NDM-1 in Algerian hospitals. 2014. J Infect Chemother. 2014;20:696–701.
38. Pasanen T, Koskela S, Mero S, Tarkka E, Tissari P, Vaara M, et al. Rapid molecular characterization of *Acinetobacter baumannii* clones with rep-PCR and evaluation of carbapenemase genes by new multiplex PCR in hospital district of Helsinki and Uusimaa. Plos One. 2014;9:e85854.

12

The prevalence, antibiotic resistance and *mecA* characterization of coagulase negative staphylococci recovered from non-healthcare settings in London, UK

Zhen Xu[1,2], Haroun N. Shah[3], Raju Misra[4], Jiazhen Chen[5], Wenhong Zhang[5], Yuting Liu[6], Ronald R. Cutler[2] and Hermine V. Mkrtchyan[2,7*]

Abstract

Background: Coagulase negative staphylococci (CoNS) are important reservoirs of antibiotic resistance genes and associated mobile genetic elements and are believed to contribute to the emergence of successful methicillin resistant *Staphylococcus aureus* (MRSA) clones. Although, these bacteria have been linked to various ecological niches, little is known about the dissemination and genetic diversity of antibiotic resistant CoNS in general public settings.

Methods: Four hundred seventy-nine samples were collected from different non-healthcare/general public settings in various locations ($n = 355$) and from the hands of volunteers ($n = 124$) in London UK between April 2013 and Nov 2014.

Results: Six hundred forty-three staphylococcal isolates belonging to 19 staphylococcal species were identified. Five hundred seventy-two (94%) isolates were resistant to at least one antibiotic, and only 34 isolates were fully susceptible. Sixty-eight (11%) *mecA* positive staphylococcal isolates were determined in this study. SCC*mec* types were fully determined for forty-six isolates. Thirteen staphylococci (19%) carried SCC*mec* V, followed by 8 isolates carrying SCC*mec* type I (2%), 5 SCC*mec* type IV (7%), 4 SCC*mec* type II (6%), 1 SCC*mec* type III (2%), 1 SCC*mec* type VI (2%), and 1 SCC*mec* type VIII (2%). In addition, three isolates harboured a new SCC*mec* type 1A, which carried combination of class A *mec* complex and *ccr* type 1.
MLST typing revealed that all *S. epidermidis* strains possess new MLST types and were assigned the following new sequence types: ST599, ST600, ST600, ST600, ST601, ST602, ST602, ST603, ST604, ST605, ST606, ST607 and ST608.

Conclusions: The prevalence of antibiotic resistant staphylococci in general public settings demonstrates that antibiotics in the natural environments contribute to the selection of antibiotic resistant microorganisms. The finding of various SCC*mec* types in non-healthcare associated environments indicates the complexity of SCC*mec*. We also report on new MLST types that were assigned for all *S. epidermidis* isolates, which demonstrates the genetic variability of these isolates.

Keywords: CoNS, Antibiotic resistance, SCC*mec*, MLST

* Correspondence: h.mkrtchyan@uel.ac.uk
[2]School of Biological and Chemical Sciences, Queen Mary University of London, London, UK
[7]School of Health, Sport and Biosciences, University of East London, E1 4NS, London, UK
Full list of author information is available at the end of the article

Background

Staphylococci are the most frequently isolated nosocomial pathogens, accounting for 30% of hospital associated infections [1]. Despite, that the high virulence of *S. aureus* has been evidenced in many studies [2], it is believed that coagulase-negative staphylococci (CoNS) act as an important reservoir of antimicrobial resistance genes and resistance-associated mobile genetic elements, which can transfer between staphylococcal species. Among other CoNS, *S. epidermidis, S. hominis* and *S. haemolyticus* are often reported to be resistant to multiple antibiotics [3, 4].

The *mecA* gene responsible for methicillin resistance was first determined in *S. aureus*, however, many other staphylococcal species were found to also harbour it [5]. The *mecA* gene encodes an additional penicillin-binding protein 2a (PBP 2a), which mediates cell wall synthesis in the presence of β-lactam antibiotics [6]. Together with its regulators *mecI-mecR1* and site specific recombination genes *ccrA* and *ccrB*, the *mecA* gene, is located on a mobile genetic element known as staphylococcal cassette chromosome *mec* (SCC*mec*) [7]. A number of studies have demonstrated the transfer of *mecA* gene from coagulase-negative staphylococcal species to *S. aureus* in vivo, and thus contributing to more successful *S. aureus* clones [8]. To date 11 SCC*mec* types have been reported based on combinations of *mec* (A, B, C1, C2 and D) and *ccr* (AB1, AB2, AB3, AB4 and *ccrC*) complexes and so called J regions (1, 2, 3) [9].

Traditionally recognised as hospital associated pathogens, methicillin resistant coagulase negative staphylococci (MR-CoNS) have recently been linked with a range of ecological niches (community, wildlife and environmental sources) [10–12]. As a result, today increasing attention is being paid to the rapid spread of MR-CoNS and their role in transmission within the community and non - hospital settings [13].

In this study we demonstrate the dissemination of antibiotic resistance in CoNS isolated from various environmental sites in London, UK. The characterization of *mecA* gene and the SCC*mec* elements provide insights into the diversity of environmental CoNS clones.

Methods

Isolation

Four hundred seventy-nine samples were collected from different environmental sites in various locations (n = 355) and from the hands of volunteers (n = 124) in London UK between April 2013 and Nov 2014. Environmental sites included hotels (n = 100), baby care facilities (n = 65), handbags (n = 43), supermarkets (n = 37), restaurants (n = 36), public transport (n = 54), and a public library (n = 20). All specimens were plated on Mannitol Salt Agar (Oxoid, Basingstoke, UK), and then incubated aerobically at 37 °C for 24–72 h). One or two colonies for each site were selected based on staphylococci morphology [4]. The colonies were then purified on Nutrient Agar (Oxoid, Basingstoke, UK).

Identification

All isolates were initially screened using Gram staining, catalase and coagulase tests. Those that demonstrated potential staphylococci characteristics were identified by Matrix-assisted laser desorption ionization time flight mass-spectroscopy (MALDI-TOF-MS, Microflex LT, Bruker Daltonics, Coventry, UK) in a positive linear mode (2000–20,000 m/z range) as described previously [12]. The resulting spectra were compared with reference spectra by using the Biotyper 3.0 software (Bruker Daltonics, Coventry, UK). *Escherichia. coli* DH5α (Bruker Daltonics, Coventry, UK) was used as a standard for calibration and quality control.

Antimicrobial susceptibility test

A panel of 11 antibiotics was used to determine the antibiotic susceptibility of all the isolates. The standard disk diffusion method was used to test AM: amoxicillin (10 μg); CEP: cefepime (30 μg); CHL: chloramphenicol (30 μg); ERY: erythromycin (5 μg); FC: fusidic acid (10 μg); GEN: gentamicin (10 μg); MUP: mupirocin (20 μg); OX: oxacillin (1 μg); PEN: penicillin (1 unit); STR: streptomycin (10 μg); TET: tetracycline (10 μg);. The susceptible, intermediate resistant or resistant were determined by the Guidelines for Susceptibility Testing [14]. The Minimum Inhibitory Concentrations (MIC) for oxacillin were additionally evaluated using "M.I.C. evaluators" (Oxoid Ltd., Basingstoke, UK).

Detection of *mecA* gene and staphylococcal cassette chromosome *mec* (SCC*mec*) typing

The *mecA* gene was determined by using PCR method as described previously [15]. For *mecA* positive isolates, SCC*mec* types were determined by evaluating *mec* and *ccr* complexes [15].

MLST typing of *Staphylococcus epidermidis*

Multi-locus sequence typing (MLST) was used to determine the sequence types of *S. epidermidis* [16]. Sequence types were assigned using the *S. epidermidis* database (www.mlst.net).

Results

Purification of isolates

A total of 643 staphylococci isolates were recovered in this study, including those from hotels (n = 74), baby care facilities (n = 46), handbags (n = 17), supermarkets (n = 89), restaurants (n = 96), public transportation (n = 94), human hands (n = 192) and public libraries (n = 35) (Additional file 1: Table S1).

Species determination

Six hundred forty-three staphylococcal isolates belonging to 19 staphylococcal species were identified in this study. This included: *S. epidermidis* (*n* = 193), *S. hominis* (*n* = 161), *S. capitis* (*n* = 77), *S. warneri* (*n* = 63), *S. haemolyticus* (*n* = 45), *S. pasteuri* (*n* = 33), *S. saprophyticus* (*n* = 20), *S. aureus* (*n* = 12), *S. simiae* (*n* = 10), *S. cohnii* (*n* = 9), *S. sciuri* (*n* = 5), *S. pettenkoferi* (*n* = 3), *S. auricularis* (*n* = 2), *S. caprae* (*n* = 2), *S. equorum* (*n* = 2), *S. lugdunensis* (*n* = 2), *S. xylosus* (*n* = 2), *S. arlettae* (*n* = 1), and *S. simulans* (*n* = 1). *S. epidermidis* was the predominant species, followed by *S. hominis, S. capitis, S. warneri, S. haemolyticus, S. pasteuri,* and *S. saprophyticus* However, the occurrence of the species varied for different sites. *S. epidermidis* was predominant among the isolates recovered from restaurants, public transport, hands and handbags, whereas *S. hominis* was predominant among the isolates recovered from supermarkets, baby care facilities and hotels and *S. haemolyticus* was predominantly isolated from the library (Table 1).

Antibiotic susceptibility test results

The disc diffusion method was used to test 606 isolates against a panel of 11 antibiotics. 572 (94%) isolates were resistant to at least one antibiotic, and only 34 isolates were fully susceptible. Resistance to penicillin, and fusidic acid was observed in more than 65% of all staphylococcal isolates tested. 202 (33%) isolates were resistant to streptomycin, 190 (31%) to erythromycin, 161 (27%) to amoxicillin, 98 (16%) to tetracycline, 87 (14%) to mupirocin, 59 (10%) to gentamicin, 48 (8%) cefepime, 36 (6%) oxacillin, and 21(3%) chloramphenicol (Table 2).

mecA gene determination and SCC*mec* typing results

Sixty-eight (11%) *mecA* positive staphylococcal isolates were determined, however, no MRSA was determined in this study. *S. sciuri* had the highest *mecA* gene carriage (80%) among all 19 staphylococcal species, followed by *S. cohnii* (33%), *S. haemolyticus* (22%), and *S. saprothyticus* (20%). Other isolates demonstrated relatively lower carriage of *mecA* gene, including *S.hominis* (3%), *S.capitis* (8%), *S. epidermidis* (11%), *S.warneri* (11%), *S.pasteuri* (13%). No *mecA* gene was found in the remaining 10 species, including *S. aureus, S. simiae, S. equorum, S. caprae, S. xylosus, S. auricularis, S. simulans, S. arlettae S.pettenkoferi,* and *S. lugdunensis.*

SCC*mec* types were fully determined in forty-six isolates. Twenty-two out of 68 isolates lacked either the *mec* gene complex or the *ccr* gene complex. Thirteen staphylococci (19%) carried SCC*mec* type V, followed by 8 isolates carrying SCC*mec* type I (2%), 5 isolates SCC*mec* type IV (7%), 4 isolates SCC*mec* type II (6%), 1 isolate SCC*mec* type III (2%), 1 isolate SCC*mec* type VI (2%), and 1 isolate SCC*mec* type VIII (2%). In addition, three isolates harboured a new SCC*mec* type 1A, which carried combination of class A *mec* complex and *ccr* type 1. Of the ten isolates that were non-typeable, three carried a combination of class A *mec* complex and *ccrC*, six carried a combination of class B *mec* and *ccrC*, and one carried class B *mec* and *ccr* type 3 (Table 3).

Multi-locus sequence typing of *S. epidermidis*

MLST was performed to determine the housekeeping genes of 13 oxacillin resistant and *mecA* positive *S. epidermidis*. MLST typing revealed that all *S. epidermidis* strains possess new MLST types. MLST types of *S. epidermidis* isolates with in house numbers of 279, 133, 134, 135, 126, 259, 124, 127, 234, 187, 308, 153 and 191 were respectively assigned as ST599, ST600, ST600, ST600, ST601, ST602, ST602, ST603, ST604, ST605, ST606, ST607 and ST608 (Table 4). Three *S. epidermidis* isolates shared the same sequence types (ST), including *S. epidermidis* 133, 134 and 135 that were isolated from different sites of a library (DSL) possessed ST600 whereas *S. epidermidis* 259, and *S. epidermidis* 124 that had ST602 sequence type were isolated from the human hands (HH) and different sites of hotels (DSH) respectively.

Table 1 Predominant and common staphylococcal species recovered from the human hands and different environmental sites

Sites	Predominant species (%)	Commonly isolated species (%)
BCF	*S. hominis* (17%)	*S. warneri* (17%)
DSH	*S. hominis* (30%)	*S. haemolyticus* (18%)
DSL	*S. haemolyticus* (29%)	*S. epidermidis* (26%)
DSR	*S. epidermidis* (38%)	*S. hominis* (35%)
DSS	*S. hominis* (44%)	*S. epidermidis* (29%)
DST	*S. epidermidis* (35%)	*S. capitis* (15%)
HB	*S. epidermidis* (40%)	*S. capitis* (27%)
HH	*S. epidermidis* (36%)	*S. hominis* (23%)

BCF baby care facilities, *DSH* different sites of hotels, *DSL* different sites of a library, *DSR* different sites of restaurants, *DSS* different sites of supermarkets; *DST* different sites of transportation facilities, *HB* handbags, *HH* human hand

Discussion

Environmental staphylococcal species

Although antibiotic resistance is commonly linked to the clinic, recent studies from different ecological niches revealed multidrug resistant bacteria is widespread in the environment [11, 12, 17].

We have previously reported on high levels of antibiotic resistance in staphylococci isolated from different environmental/public settings [11, 12]. In this study we evaluated the dissemination of antibiotic resistant staphylococci recovered from a wide range of environmental settings, and characterised the carriage of the *mecA* gene and the diversity of SCC*mec* elements in these isolates.

Table 2 Antibiotic susceptibility profile of staphylococci isolates recovered from general public settings

Isolates	No of isolates	Resistance to a panel of 11 antibiotics (%)										
		OX	PG	MUP	CEF	GM	FC	S	A	E	T	C
S. epidermidis	176	8	72	16	9	7	64	22	26	43	16	2
S. hominis	152	2	68	9	5	7	66	24	17	38	21	3
S. capitis	73	4	58	15	4	1	60	47	23	14	10	5
S. haemolyticus	40	10	50	13	23	15	68	73	45	0	25	10
S. warneri	63	3	54	17	10	22	59	51	40	27	16	2
S. pasteuri	31	6	69	13	6	9	69	25	31	44	17	3
S. saprophyticus	20	15	90	25	5	10	100	10	25	35	15	10
S. aureus	12	0	83	17	0	58	83	33	50	25	0	8
S. simiae	10	0	10	0	0	0	40	0	0	0	0	0
S. cohnii	9	24	67	11	33	0	78	78	22	56	11	0
S. sciuri	5	60	60	80	0	20	80	80	40	0	0	0
S. pettenkoferi	3	0	33	0	0	0	67	67	33	0	0	0
S. lugdunensis	2	0	50	0	0	0	50	0	0	0	0	0
S. equorum	2	0	50	50	0	0	50	50	50	0	50	0
S. caprae	2	0	100	0	100	100	100	50	50	0	0	0
S. xylosus	2	0	100	50	50	50	100	100	0	0	50	0
S. auricularis	2	0	50	0	50	0	50	0	50	0	0	0
S. arlettae	1	0	100	0	0	0	100	100	100	100	0	0
S. simulans	1	0	100	0	0	0	100	0	0	0	0	0

OX oxacillin (1 µg), *PG* penicillin G (1 unit), *MUP* mupirocin (20 µg), *CEF* cefepime (30 µg), *GM* gentamicin (10 µg), *FC* fusidic acid (10 µg), *S* streptomycin (10 µg), *A* amoxicillin (10 µg), *E* erythromycin (5 µg), *T* tetracycline (10 µg), *C* chloramphenicol (30 µg)

Six hundred and forty-three staphylococci isolates belonging to 19 species, including *S. epidermidis, S. hominis, S. haemolyticus, S. capitis, S. warneri, S. pasteuri, S. saprophyticus, S. cohnii, S. aureus, S. simiae, S. sciuri, S. pettenkoferi, S. lugdunensis, S. equorum, S. caprae, S. xylosus, S. auricularis, S. simulans,* and *S. arlettae,* were identified in this study. Interestingly, many of the staphylococci species recovered in our study have previously been associated with the community, preserved food, and wildlife [4, 10].

Antibiotic resistance

Antibiotic resistance of staphylococci associated with healthcare settings is well documented, however, little is known about the antibiotic resistance in staphylococci isolated from different ecological niches [4]. In this study, the majority of staphylococci were resistant to penicillin (65%) and fusidic acid (66%) (Fig. 1). Despite that 80% of hospital associated CoNS (across Europe) were reported to be resistant to oxacillin [18], only 6% of CoNS were resistant to oxacillin in this study. In addition, the levels of resistance to chloramphenicol (3%), cefepime (8%), gentamicin (10%), mupirocin (14%), tetracycline (16%), and erythromycin (31%) were lower compared to those reported in clinical settings [19–22]. In contrast, the rates of resistance to fusidic acid (66%), amoxicillin (27%) and streptomycin (33%) in environmental staphylococcal isolates were higher than those reported in clinical staphylococci isolates [21, 23, 24]. It is widely accepted that higher levels of antibiotic resistance in clinical isolates are due to consistent antibiotic exposure [25]. The environment may also contribute to the development of antibiotic resistance in microorganisms due to human/ animal therapeutics, sewage, agriculture and industrial use of antibiotics [26]. Therefore, the wide dissemination of multidrug resistant CoNS in non-healthcare associated environments is a disturbing finding. In our study, 94% of staphylococcal isolates were phenotypically resistant to at least 1 antibiotic, 18% were resistant to five or more antibiotics and only 6% staphylococcal isolates were fully susceptible. The study also revealed that the number of isolates resistant to multiple antibiotics varied between the different isolation sites. The least number of multiple antibiotic resistant CoNS isolates were recovered from the public transport (58%), the highest was isolated from hotels (78%).

Methicillin-resistant staphylococci

Methicillin resistant staphylococci pose a major public health threat, and cause severe economic and health consequences [27]. Methicillin resistance is determined by the *mecA* gene, which encodes for penicillin binding protein 2a (PBP2a) that has a low affinity to β-lactam antibiotics [28]. Hussain et al. assessed the correlation between *mecA*

Table 3 Molecular characterisation and antibiotic resistance of *mecA* gene positive staphylococci

ID	Sites	Species	PG	MUP	CEF	GM	FC	S	A	E	T	C	*mecA*	*mec*	*ccr*	SCC*mec*	MIC/OX (mg l^{-1})
71	HH	*S. capitis*	S	S	S	S	S	R	S	S	S	S	+	–	–	I	0.5
100	DSH	*S. cohnii*	R	R	S	S	S	S	R	R	S	S	+	Class A	5	5A	1
97	BCF	*S. cohnii*	R	S	R	S	R	R	S	R	S	S	+	Class B	1	I	**0.25**
279	HH	*S. epidermidis*	R	S	S	S	R	S	S	R	S	S	+	Class B	2	IV	2
127	DSH	*S. epidermidis*	R	S	I	S	S	S	R	R	R	S	+	Class C	5	V	2
139	DSR	*S. epidermidis*	R	R	R	S	R	S	R	R	R	S	+	Class C	5	V	2
191	DSS	*S. epidermidis*	R	S	S	S	R	S	R	S	S	S	+	Class B	4	VI	2
153	DSH	*S. epidermidis*	R	S	S	S	R	S	S	S	S	S	+	Class C	5	V	1
187	DSS	*S. epidermidis*	R	S	S	S	S	S	S	R	S	S	+	Class C	5	V	1
134	DSL	*S. epidermidis**	R	S	S	S	R	R	R	R	R	S	+	Class B	1	I	1
259	HH	*S. epidermidis*	R	S	R	S	R	R	R	R	S	S	+	Class C	5	V	1
135	DSL	*S. epidermidis**	R	S	S	S	R	R	R	R	R	S	+	Class B	2	IV	0.5
124	DSH	*S. epidermidis*	R	S	R	S	R	R	R	S	R	S	+	Class B	2	IV	0.5
133	DSL	*S. epidermidis**	R	S	S	S	R	R	R	R	R	S	+	Class B	3	3B	0.5
126	HH	*S. epidermidis*	R	S	I	S	S	R	R	R	S	S	+	–	–	III	0.5
119	DSH	*S. epidermidis*	R	S	S	S	S	S	R	I	R	S	+	Class C	5	V	**0.12**
111	BCF	*S. epidermidis*	R	S	S	S	S	S	S	S	S	S	+	Class A	2	II	**0.12**
202	DST	*S. epidermidis*	S	R	S	S	R	I	S	S	S	S	+	Class B	5	5B	**0.12**
264	HH	*S. epidermidis*	S	R	S	S	R	R	S	S	S	S	+	Class B	2	IV	**0.06**
129	DSL	*S. epidermidis*	R	S	S	S	R	R	R	R	R	S	+	Class B	1	I	**0.03**
362	DSL	*S. haemolyticus*	R	S	I	S	S	R	R	S	S	S	+	Class C	5	V	2
367	DSL	*S. haemolyticus*	R	S	R	S	S	R	R	S	S	S	+	Class C	5	V	2
355	DSH	*S. haemolyticus*	R	S	R	R	R	R	R	S	R	S	+	Class C	5	V	2
384	HH	*S. haemolyticus*	R	R	S	S	R	R	S	S	S	S	+	Class C	5	V	2
322	DSH	*S. haemolyticus*	R	S	S	S	S	I	R	S	R	S	+	Class A	1	1A	**0.25**
382	HH	*S. haemolyticus*	R	S	I	S	R	R	S	R	S	S	+	–	–	II	**0.25**
323	DSH	*S. haemolyticus*	S	S	S	R	S	R	R	I	R	S	+	Class A	2	II	**0.12**
381	HH	*S. haemolyticus*	S	S	I	S	S	R	S	S	S	S	+	Class B	5	5B	**0.12**
360	DSH	*S. haemolyticus*	S	S	S	S	R	S	S	S	S	R	+	Class B	5	5B	**0.06**
369	DSL	*S. haemolyticus*	R	S	S	S	R	R	S	R	S	R	+	Class B	1	I	**0.03**
413	DSH	*S. hominis*	S	R	S	S	R	R	S	S	S	S	+	Class C	5	V	2
506	DSS	*S. hominis*	S	S	S	S	R	S	S	S	S	S	+	Class B	1	I	0.5
400	DSH	*S. hominis*	R	R	S	S	R	S	R	R	R	S	+	Class A	1	1A	**0.12**
326	DSH	*S. hominis*	S	S	S	S	S	S	R	I	S	S	+	Class A	1	1A	**0.06**
589	HB	*S. pasteuri*	R	S	S	S	R	R	S	R	S	S	+	Class A	5	5A	**0.25**
592	HH	*S. pasteuri*	S	R	S	S	R	R	S	S	S	S	+	Class B	5	5B	**0.25**
627	HH	*S. saprophyticus*	R	I	S	S	R	S	S	S	R	S	+	Class B	5	5B	0.5
621	DSS	*S. saprophyticus*	R	R	R	S	R	S	R	S	R	S	+	Class B	2	IV	**0.25**
630	HH	*S. sciuri*	R	R	I	S	R	R	S	S	S	S	+	Class A	4	VIII	2
632	DSH	*S. sciuri*	R	S	I	S	R	R	R	S	S	S	+	Class A	5	5A	1
633	DSH	*S. sciuri*	R	R	I	R	R	R	R	S	S	S	+	Class B	5	5B	1
629	HH	*S. sciuri*	S	R	S	S	S	S	S	S	S	S	+	–	–	II	0.25
704	HH	*S. warneri*	R	S	I	S	R	R	R	R	S	S	+	Class C	5	V	0.5
662	DSH	*S. warneri*	R	S	S	R	R	R	R	S	R	S	+	Class C	5	V	**0.25**

Table 3 Molecular characterisation and antibiotic resistance of *mecA* gene positive staphylococci *(Continued)*

ID	Sites	Species	PG	MUP	CEF	GM	FC	S	A	E	T	C	*mecA*	*mec*	*ccr*	SCC*mec*	MIC/OX (mg l^{-1})
694	HH	*S. warneri*	R	S	S	S	S	S	S	S	R	S	+	–	–	I	**0.25**
655	BCF	*S. warneri*	S	R	S	R	R	R	S	I	S	S	+	Class B	1	I	**0.12**

Note: * *S. epidermidis* isolates with similar MLST types
R: resistant, *S* sensitive. *I* intermediate
BCF baby care facility, *DSH* different sites of hotels, *DSL* different sites of a library, *DSR* different sites of restaurants, *DSS* different sites of supermarkets, *DST* different sites of transportation facilities, *HB* handbags, *HH* human hands
A amoxicillin (10 μg), *CEF* cefepime (30 μg), *C* chloramphenicol (30 μg), *E* erythromycin (5 μg), *FC* fusidic acid (10 μg), *GM* gentamicin (10 μg), *MUP* mupirocin (20 μg), *OX* oxacillin (1 μg), *PG* penicillin G (1 unit), *S* streptomycin (10 μg), *T* tetracycline (10 μg)

gene and oxacillin susceptibility breakpoints (0.5 mg l^{-1}) of 493 clinical CoNS belonging to and classified into 4 categories [29]. The *mecA* gene positive staphylococci were categorized into groups I and II, and demonstrated that group I (*S. haemolyticus* (83.3%), *S. epidermidis* (61.9%), *S. hominis* (51.8%)) differs from group II (*S. cohnii* (28.5%), *S. warneri* (27.3%), *S. saprophyticus* (9.0%)) by their high levels of *mecA*-carriage [29]. Interestingly, *S. hominis* (38%), *S. haemolyticus* (22%), and *S. epidermidis* (7%) isolated in this study harboured significantly lower levels of the *mecA* gene. Moreover, in this study *S. cohnii* (33%) and *S. saprophyticus* (10%) showed higher *mecA* gene carriage than clinical isolates reported by Hussain, et al. [29], whereas the levels of *mecA* gene carriage in *S. warneri* (6%) were lower than in clinical isolates. No *mecA* gene was detected in staphylococcal species of groups III and IV, which included *S. xylosus*, *S. lugdunensis*, *S. capitis*, *S.simulans*, and *S. schleiferi* [29]. Similarly, in this study *S. lugdunensis*, *S. xylosus* and *S. simulans* were determined to be susceptible to oxacillin and lacked *mecA* gene. However, in contrast to the reports by Hussain, et al. [29] we found that *mecA* gene was present in 8% of *S. capitis* isolates.

Oxacillin susceptible *mecA* gene positive *S. aureus* (OS-MRSA) has been reported worldwide, and the risk of induced high levels of oxacillin resistance was determined in OS-MRSA [30, 31]. In this study, 68 (46%) staphylococcal isolates were confirmed by PCR to carry the *mecA* gene, however, they were phenotypically susceptible to oxacillin with the MICs (oxacillin) varying from 0.015 to 2 mg l^{-1}. This study demonstrates the prevalence of *mecA* positive but oxacillin susceptible CoNS (OS-CoNS) in the environment. Little is known about OS-CoNS isolates recovered from the environment and their epidemiological data are limited. Additional studies are necessary to further our understanding of the prevalence and molecular epidemiology of OS-CoNS in the environment.

SCC*mec* elements

SCC*mec* is a mobile genetic element with two essential components: the *mec* gene complex, and the cassette chromosome recombinase (*ccr*) gene complex [32]. The combination of the *mec* gene complex and *ccr* gene complex confers different SCC*mec* types [32]. SCC*mec* type I, II, III are reported to be associated with MRSA recovered from healthcare settings, whereas SCC*mec* type IV and V are mainly associated with the community [32]. Moreover, it has been shown that the size of SCC*mec* types IV and V are smaller than SCC*mec* types I, II and III, thus conferring

Table 4 MLST types of 13 oxacillin resistant and *mecA* positive *S. epidermidis*

ID	Sites	Species	*arcC*	*aroE*	*gtr*	*mutS*	*pyrR*	*tpiA*	*yqiL*	MLST types
279	HH	*S. epidermidis*	57	17	5	5	3	4	31	ST599
133	DSL	*S. epidermidis*	57	1	2	2	4	1	4	ST600
134	DSL	*S. epidermidis*	57	1	2	2	4	1	4	ST600
135	DSL	*S. epidermidis*	57	1	2	2	4	1	4	ST600
126	HH	*S. epidermidis*	57	25	9	5	6	1	8	ST601
259	HH	*S. epidermidis*	57	1	2	2	4	1	1	ST602
124	DSH	*S. epidermidis*	57	1	2	2	4	1	1	ST602
127	DSH	*S. epidermidis*	57	10	5	5	10	16	21	ST603
234	HB	*S. epidermidis*	57	1	1	1	2	41	1	ST604
187	DSS	*S. epidermidis*	57	1	1	2	2	1	1	ST605
308	HH	*S. epidermidis*	57	1	2	2	4	7	1	ST606
153	DSH	*S. epidermidis*	57	1	22	2	2	16	1	ST607
191	DSS	*S. epidermidis*	57	3	5	5	7	14	11	ST608

HH human hands, *DSL* different sites of a library, *DSH* different sites of hotels, *DSS* different sites of supermarkets
MLST Multi-locus sequence typing

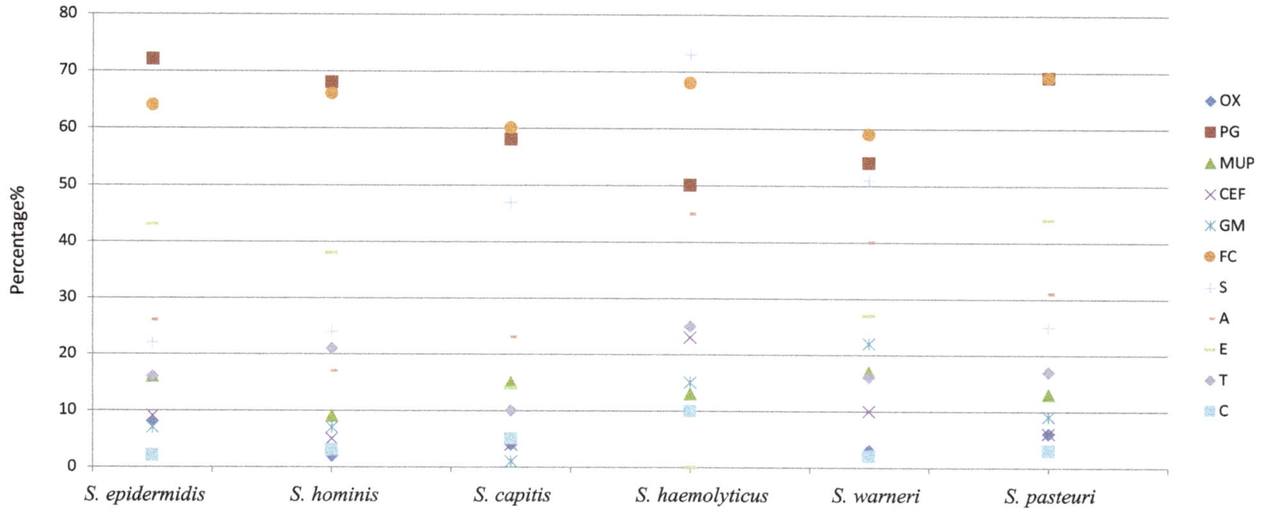

Fig. 1 The scatter plot of staphylococcal (> 30 isolates) susceptibility profile. Legend: OX: oxacillin (1 μg); PG: penicillin G (1 unit); MUP: mupirocin (20 μg); CEF: cefepime (30 μg); GM: gentamicin (10 μg); FC: fusidic acid (10 μg); S: streptomycin (10 μg);A: amoxicillin (10 μg); E: erythromycin (5 μg); T: tetracycline (10 μg); C: chloramphenicol (30 μg)

increased mobility by their smaller size and contributing the spread of these smaller SCC*mec* elements [33] . In this study, SCC*mec* type I, II or III were found in 19% ($n = 13$) of *mecA*-positive CoNS, whereas 27% ($n = 18$) of CoNS were determined to harbour SCC*mec* type IV or V. SCC*mec* type VI and VIII were previously identified in Portugal (2006) and Canada (2009) in hospital associated MRSA (HA-MRSA) [33, 34]. In this study, we identified one of each type, however, we did not detect SCC*mec* types IX.

Becker et al., have previously summarized the community and livestock associated staphylococcal species and their SCC*mec* types, which included *S. capitis* (I, IA, II, III, IV, IVa, V, non-typeable: (NT)), *S. cohnii* (NT), *S. epidermidis* (I, IIa, IIb, III, III (variant), IV, IVa, IVb, IVc, IVd, IVe, IVg, V, VI, NT), *S. haemolyticus* (I, II, II.1, III, III (variant), IV, V, NT), *S. honomis* (I, III, IV, NT), *S. pasteuri* (IVc), *S. saprophyticus* (III, NT), *S. sciuri* (I, III, IIIA, V, VII, NT) and *S. warneri* (IV, IV.1, IVb, IVE) [4]. In this study, species associated SCC*mec* types differed and included the following: *S. capitis* (I, NT), *S. haemolyticus* (I, II, V, NT) and *S. hominis* (I, V, NT), *S. cohnii* (I, V, NT), *S. pasteuri* (NT), *S. saprophyticus* (IV, NT), *S. sciuri* (II, VIII), *S. warneri* (I, V, NT). *S. epidermidis* possessed SCC*mec* types similar to those reported previously [4].

Thirteen unclassified SCC*mec* types were determined in this study, including three carrying class A *mec* complex and *ccrC*, six had a combination of class B *mec* and *ccrC*, one carried class B *mec* and *ccr3*, and three had a combination of class A *mec* complex and *ccr* type 1. The 1A was previously defined as a new SCC*mec* type 1A by others [35]. Pseudo (ψ)-SCC*mec* harbours the *mec* complex but lacks *ccr*, while, SCC*mec*12263 is reported to carry the *ccr* complex but lacks *mec* complex [36, 37]. In this study, 21 isolates (29%) were categorized as (ψ)-SCC*mec* and SCC*mec*12263 since they lacked either *mec* complex or *ccr* complexes. ψ SCC element is characterized by lacking genes for *ccr* and *mec* [4]. One of *S. saprophyticus* isolates in this study was found to possess the ψ SCC element (Table 5).

MLST of *S. epidermidis*

Whilst many studies have reported on the changing epidemiology of *S. aureus*, epidemiological data of other staphylococcal species are limited [38, 39]. In this study, 10 new MLST types were determined in 13 *S. epidermidis* isolates. Interestingly, although isolates recovered from human hands (*S. epidermidis* 259/ SCC*mec* V) and hotels (*S. epidermidis* 124/ SCC*mec* IV) harboured different *SCCmec* types, they shared the same MLST type ST602. In addition, three *S. epidermidis* isolates recovered from libraries (*S. epidermidis* 133, *S. epidermidis* 134, *S. epidermidis* 135) shared the same MLST type ST600 (Table 4). However, despite sharing the same MLST type *S. epidermidis* 133, *S. epidermidis* 134 and *S. epidermidis* 135 harbored SCC*mec* type 3B, I, IV respectively. Others reported that *S. epidermidis* ST2 was associated with type II, III, IV and non-typable SCC*mec*, and *S. epidermidis* ST22 harboured SCC*mec* type III, IV and V [40].

Conclusions

Systematic analysis of staphylococci isolated from non-healthcare environments provided insights into the diversity and antibiotic susceptibility patterns of these

Table 5 The diversity of SCC*mec* types of *mecA* gene positive staphylococci

ID	Sites	Species	PG	MUP	CEF	GM	FC	S	A	E	T	C	*mecA*	*mec*	*ccr*	SCC*mec*	MIC/OX (mg l^{-1})
75	HH	*S. capitis*	R	S	S	S	R	R	S	S	S	S	+	Class A	NT	Pseudo (ψ)-SCC*mec*	0.5
81	HH	*S. capitis*	R	S	R	S	R	R	R	R	S	S	+	NT	5	SCC*mec*12263	0.5
70	HH	*S. capitis*	R	S	S	S	S	R	S	S	R	S	+	NT	5	SCC*mec*12263	**0.25**
83	HH	*S. capitis*	S	R	S	S	R	R	S	S	S	S	+	NT	5	SCC*mec*12263	**0.12**
24	DSH	*S. capitis*	S	S	S	S	R	R	S	S	S	S	+	NT	1	SCC*mec*12263	**0.12**
108	HH	*S. cohnii*	S	S	I	S	R	R	S	R	R	S	+	Class A	NT	Pseudo (ψ)-SCC*mec*	1
308	HH	*S. epidermidis*	R	R	S	S	R	S	R	R	S	S	+	Class B	NT	Pseudo (ψ)-SCC*mec*	2
234	HB	*S. epidermidis*	S	R	S	S	R	R	S	R	R	S	+	Class A	NT	Pseudo (ψ)-SCC*mec*	1
249	DSH	*S. epidermidis*	R	S	S	S	R	R	S	S	R	S	+	NT	2	SCC*mec*12263	**0.12**
125	DSH	*S. epidermidis*	S	S	I	S	S	R	S	S	S	S	+	NT	5	SCC*mec*12263	**0.06**
185	DSS	*S. epidermidis*	R	S	S	S	S	S	S	S	S	S	+	Class C	NT	Pseudo (ψ)-SCC*mec*	**0.06**
498	DSS	*S. hominis*	R	S	S	S	R	S	S	R	S	S	+	Class A	NT	Pseudo (ψ)-SCC*mec*	0.5
426	DSH	*S. hominis*	R	S	I	S	R	R	R	R	S	S	+	Class A	NT	Pseudo (ψ)-SCC*mec*	**0.25**
412	DSH	*S. hominis*	R	S	S	S	R	S	R	R	S	S	+	NT	1	SCC*mec*12263	**0.06**
391	BCF	*S. hominis*	R	S	S	S	R	S	S	S	S	S	+	NT	5	SCC*mec*12263	**0.03**
593	HH	*S. pasteuri*	R	S	S	R	R	R	R	S	S	S	+	NT	5	SCC*mec*12263	0.5
597	HH	*S. pasteuri*	R	R	I	S	S	R	S	S	S	S	+	NT	5	SCC*mec*12263	0.5
616	BCF	*S. saprophyticus*	R	R	S	S	R	I	R	R	R	S	+	NT	5	SCC*mec*12263	256
612	BCF	*S. saprophyticus*	R	R	S	S	R	S	S	R	S	S	+	NT	NT	ψ SCC	1
659	DSH	*S. warneri*	R	R	S	S	R	R	R	S	S	S	+	NT	5	SCC*mec*12263	0.5
648	BCF	*S. warneri*	R	S	S	R	R	S	R	S	S	S	+	NT	5	SCC*mec*12263	**0.06**
645	BCF	*S. warneri*	R	S	S	S	R	S	S	S	S	S	+	NT	4	SCC*mec*12263	**0.015**

R resistant, *S* sensitive, *I* intermediate
BCF baby care facility, *DSH* different sites of hotels, *DSL* different sites of a library, *DSR* different sites of restaurants, *DSS* different sites of supermarkets; *DST* different sites of transportation facilities, *HB* handbags, *HH* human hands
A amoxicillin (10 μg), *CEF* cefepime (30 μg), *C* chloramphenicol (30 μg), *E* erythromycin (5 μg), *FC* fusidic acid (10 μg), *GM* gentamicin (10 μg), *MUP* mupirocin (20 μg), *OX* oxacillin (1 μg), *PG* penicillin G (1 unit), *S* streptomycin (10 μg), *T* tetracycline (10 μg)

isolates. Multi-drug resistance was commonly seen in each staphylococcal species. The prevalence of multiple antibiotic resistant staphylococci in this study provides evidence that antibiotics in the natural environments can contribute to the selection of antibiotic resistance in microorganisms. The finding of various SCC*mec* types in non-healthcare associated environments emphasizes the complexity of SCC*mec* elements. In addition to this, we also report on new MLST types that were assigned for all *S. epidermidis* isolates. This highlights the genetic variability of these isolates. In conclusion, the non-healthcare environments may act as a reservoir of multidrug resistant staphylococci, and current infection control measures are ineffective in limiting the spread of these bacteria.

Abbreviations

AM: Amoxicillin; BCF: Baby care facility; CEP: Cefepime; CHL: Chloramphenicol; CoNS: Coagulase-negative staphylococci; DSH: Different sites of hotels; DSL: Different sites of a library; DSR: Different sites of restaurants; DSS: Different sites of supermarkets; DST: Different sites of transportation facilities; ERY: Erythromycin; FC: Fusidic acid; GEN: Gentamicin; HB: Handbags; HH: Human hands; MALDI-TOF-MS: Matrix-assisted laser desorption ionization time flight mass-spectroscopy; MIC: Minimum Inhibitory Concentrations; MLST: Multi-locus sequence typing; MR-CoNS: Methicillin resistant coagulase negative staphylococci; MRSA: Methicillin resistant *Staphylococcus aureus*; MUP: Mupirocin; OX: Oxacillin; PEN: Penicillin; SCC*mec*: Staphylococcal cassette chromosome mec; ST: Sequence types; STR: Streptomycin; TET: Tetracycline

Funding

This work was part of Zhen Xu's PhD study funded by China Scholarship Council.

Authors' contributions

ZX: samples collection, laboratory work, data analysis, manuscript preparation. HS: study design, critically reviewing the paper. RM: Data analysis, critically reviewing the paper. JC: data analysis, critically reviewing the paper. WZ: data analysis, critically reviewing the paper. YL: data analysis, critically reviewing the paper. RRC: conception and design of the study. HVM: conception and design of the study; data analysis; writing and critically reviewing the paper. All authors read and approved the final manuscript.

Consent for publication

Not applicable.

Competing interests
The authors declare that they have no competing interests.

Author details
[1]National Demonstration Center for Experimental Preventive Medicine Education, Tianjin Medical University, Qixiang Road No. 22, Tianjin 300070, China. [2]School of Biological and Chemical Sciences, Queen Mary University of London, London, UK. [3]Department of Natural Sciences, Middlesex University, The Burroughs Hendon, Middlesex NW4 4BT, UK. [4]Natural History Museum, Cromwell Rd, London SW7 5BD, UK. [5]Department of Infectious Diseases, Huashan Hospital, Fudan University, Shanghai 200040, China. [6]Tianjin Xiqing hospital, Tianjin 300380, China. [7]School of Health, Sport and Biosciences, University of East London, E1 4NS, London, UK.

References

1. Kloos WE, Bannerman TL. Update on clinical significance of coagulase-negative staphylococci. Clin Microbiol Rev. 1994 7(1):117–40.
2. Foster TJ, Geoghegan JA, Ganesh VK, Höök M. Adhesion, invasion and evasion: the many functions of the surface proteins of *Staphylococcus aureus*. Nat Rev Microbiol. 2014;12(1):49–62.
3. Bouchami O, Achour W, Mekni MA, Rolo J, Ben HA. Antibiotic resistance and molecular characterization of clinical isolates of methicillin-resistant coagulase-negative staphylococci isolated from bacteremic patients in oncohematology. Folia Microbiol. 2011;56(2):122–30.
4. Becker K, Heilmann C, Peters G. Coagulase-negative staphylococci. Clin Microbiol Rev. 2014;27(4):870–926.
5. Ubukata K, Nonoguchi R, Song MD, Matsuhashi M, Konno M. Homology of *mecA* gene in methicillin-resistant *Staphylococcus haemolyticus* and *Staphylococcus simulans* to that of *Staphylococcus aureus*. Antimicrob Agents Chemother. 1990;34(1):170–2.
6. Pinho MG, de Lencastre H, Tomasz A. An acquired and a native penicillin-binding protein cooperate in building the cell wall of drug-resistant staphylococci. Proc Natl Acad Sci. 2001;98(19):10886–91.
7. Hiramatsu K, Cui L, Kuroda M, Ito T. The emergence and evolution of methicillin-resistant *Staphylococcus aureus*. Trends Microbiol. 2001;9(10):486–93.
8. Harrison EM, Paterson GK, Holden MTG, Ba X, Rolo J, Morgan FJE, et al. A novel hybrid SCC*mec*-*mecC* region in *Staphylococcus sciuri*. J Antimicrob Chemother. 2014;69(4):911–8.
9. IWG-SCC. Classification of staphylococcal cassette chromosome *mec* (SCC*mec*): guidelines for reporting novel SCC*mec* elements. Antimicrob Agents Chemother. 2009;53(12):4961–7.
10. Pantucek R. *Staphylococcus simiae* sp. nov., isolated from south American squirrel monkeys. Int J Syst Evol Microbiol. 2005;55(5):1953–8.
11. Xu Z, Mkrtchyan HV, Cutler RR. Antibiotic resistance and *mecA* characterization of coagulase-negative staphylococci isolated from three hotels in London, UK. Front Microbiol. 2015;6:947.
12. Mkrtchyan HV, Russell CA, Wang N, Cutler RR. Could public restrooms be an environment for bacterial Resistomes? PLoS One. 2013;8(1):e54223.
13. Boyce JM. Environmental contamination makes an important contribution to hospital infection. J Hosp Infect. 2007;65(Suppl 2):50–4.
14. Andrews JM, Howe RA. BSAC standardized disc susceptibility testing method (version 10). J Antimicrob Chemother. 2011;66:2726–57.
15. Kondo Y, Ito T, Ma XX, Watanabe S, Kreiswirth BN, Etienne J, et al. Combination of multiplex PCRs for staphylococcal cassette chromosome *mec* type assignment: rapid identification system for *mec*, *ccr*, and major differences in junkyard regions. Antimicrob Agents Chemother. 2007;51(1):264–74.
16. Thomas JC, Vargas MR, Miragaia M, Peacock SJ, Archer GL, Enright MC. Improved multilocus sequence typing scheme for *Staphylococcus epidermidis*. J Clin Microbiol. 2007;45(2):616–9.
17. Leonard FC, Markey BK. Meticillin-resistant *Staphylococcus aureus* in animals: a review. Vet J. 2008;175(1):27–36.
18. Hanberger H, Diekema D, Fluit A, Jones R, Struelens M, Spencer R, et al. Surveillance of antibiotic resistance in European ICUs. J Hosp Infect. 2001;48(3):161–76.
19. Agvald-Ohman C, Lund B, Edlund C. Multiresistant coagulase-negative staphylococci disseminate frequently between intubated patients in a multidisciplinary intensive care unit. Crit Care. 2004;8(1):R42–7.
20. Mohan U, Jindal N, Aggarwal P. Species distribution and antibiotic sensitivity pattern of coagulase negative staphylococci isolated from various clinical specimens. Indian J Med Microbiol. 2002;20(1):45–6.
21. Akinkunmi E, Lamikanra A. Species Distribution and Antibiotic resistance in coagulase-negative staphylococci colonizing the gastrointestinal tract of children in Ile-Ife, Nigeria. Trop J Pharm Res. 2010;9(1):35–43.
22. Fritsche TR, Sader HS, Jones RN. Comparative activity and spectrum of broad-spectrum β-lactams (cefepime, ceftazidime, ceftriaxone, piperacillin/tazobactam) tested against 12,295 staphylococci and streptococci: report from the SENTRY antimicrobial surveillance program (North America: 2001-2002). Diagn Microbiol Infect Dis. 2003;47(2):435–40.
23. Ferreira RBR, Nunes APF, Kokis VM, Krepsky N, de Fonseca LS, de Bastos Mdo CF, et al. Simultaneous detection of the mecA and ileS-2 genes in coagulase-negative staphylococci isolated from Brazilian hospitals by multiplex PCR. Diagn Microbiol Infect Dis. 2002;42(3):205–12.
24. Idriss SHE, Foltys V, Tančin V, Kirchnerová K, Tančinová D, Zaujec K. Mastitis pathogens and their resistance against antimicrobial agents in dairy cows in Nitra, Slovakia. Slovak J Anim Sci. 2014;47(1):33–8.
25. Antoniadou A, Kanellakopoulou K, Kanellopoulou M, Polemis M, Koratzanis G, Papademetriou E, et al. Impact of a hospital-wide antibiotic restriction policy program on the resistance rates of nosocomial gram-negative bacteria. Infect Dis (Auckl). 2013;45(6):438–45.
26. Cantas L, Shah SQA, Cavaco LM, Manaia CM, Walsh F, Popowska M, et al. A brief multi-disciplinary review on antimicrobial resistance in medicine and its linkage to the global environmental microbiota. Front Microbiol. 2013;4(10):96.
27. Stefani S, Varaldo PE. Epidemiology of methicillin-resistant staphylococci in Europe. Clin Microbiol Infect. 2003;9(12):1179–86.
28. Tulinski P, Fluit AC, Wagenaar JA, Mevius D, van de Vijver L, Duim B. Methicillin-resistant coagulase-negative staphylococci on pig farms as a reservoir of heterogeneous staphylococcal cassette chromosome *mec* elements. Appl Environ Microbiol. 2012;78(2):299–304.
29. Hussain Z, Stoakes L, Massey V, Diagre D, Fitzgerald V, El Sayed S, et al. Correlation of oxacillin MIC with *mecA* gene carriage in coagulase-negative staphylococci. J Clin Microbiol. 2000;38(2):752–4.
30. Hososaka Y, Hanaki H, Endo H, Suzuki Y, Nagasawa Z, Otsuka Y, et al. Characterization of oxacillin-susceptible *mecA*-positive *Staphylococcus aureus*: a new type of MRSA. J Infect Chemother. 2007;13(2):79–86.
31. Saeed K, Dryden M, Parnaby R. Oxacillin-susceptible MRSA, the emerging MRSA clone in the UK? J Hosp Infect. 2010;76(3):267–8.
32. Monecke S, Coombs G, Shore AC, Coleman DC, Akpaka P, Borg M, et al. A field guide to pandemic, epidemic and sporadic clones of methicillin-resistant *Staphylococcus aureus*. PLoS One. 2011;6(4):e17936.
33. Oliveira DC, Tomasz ALH. Secrets of success of a human pathogen: molecular evolution of pandemic clones of meticillin-resistant *Staphylococcus aureus*. Lancet Infect Dis. 2002;2(3):180–9.
34. Zhang K, McClure J-A, Elsayed S, Conly JM. Novel staphylococcal cassette chromosome *mec* type, tentatively designated type VIII, harboring class a *mec* and type 4 ccr gene complexes in a Canadian epidemic strain of methicillin-resistant *Staphylococcus aureus*. Antimicrob Agents Chemother. 2009;53(2):531–40.
35. Bouchami O, Ben Hassen A, de Lencastre H, Miragaia M. Molecular epidemiology of methicillin-resistant *Staphylococcus hominis* (MRSHo): low Clonality and reservoirs of SCC*mec* structural elements. Chaturvedi V, editor PLoS One. 2011;6(7):e21940.
36. Harrison EM, Paterson GK, Holden MTG, Morgan FJE, Larsen AR, Petersen A, et al. A *Staphylococcus xylosus* isolate with a new *mecC* allotype. Antimicrob Agents Chemother. 2013;57(3):1524–8.
37. Katayama Y, Takeuchi F, Ito T, Ma XX, Ui-Mizutani Y, Kobayashi I, et al. Identification in methicillin-susceptible *Staphylococcus hominis* of an active primordial mobile genetic element for the staphylococcal cassette chromosome *mec* of methicillin-resistant *Staphylococcus aureus*. J Bacteriol. 2003;185(9):2711–22.
38. Herwaldt LA, Geiss M, Kao C, Pfaller MA. The positive predictive value of isolating coagulase-negative staphylococci from blood cultures. Clin Infect Dis. 1996;22(1):14–20.
39. Wang XM, Noble L, Kreiswirth BN, Eisner W, McClements W, Jansen KU, et al. Evaluation of a multilocus sequence typing system for *Staphylococcus epidermidis*. J Med Microbiol. 2003;52(11):989–98.
40. Miragaia M, Thomas JC, Couto I, Enright MC, de Lencastre H. Inferring a population structure for *Staphylococcus epidermidis* from multilocus sequence typing data. J Bacteriol. 2007;189(6):2540–52.

13

Assessment of the potential for resistance to antimicrobial violet-blue light in *Staphylococcus aureus*

Rachael M. Tomb[1*], Michelle Maclean[1,2], John E. Coia[3], Scott J. MacGregor[1] and John G. Anderson[1]

Abstract

Background: Antimicrobial violet-blue light in the region of 405 nm is emerging as an alternative technology for hospital decontamination and clinical treatment. The mechanism of action is the excitation of endogenous porphyrins within exposed microorganisms, resulting in ROS generation, oxidative damage and cell death. Although resistance to 405 nm light is not thought likely, little evidence has been published to support this. This study was designed to establish if there is potential for tolerance development, using the nosocomial pathogen *Staphylococcus aureus* as the model organism.

Methods: The first stage of this study investigated the potential for *S. aureus* to develop tolerance to high-intensity 405 nm light if pre-cultured in low-level stress violet-blue light ($\leq$1 mW/cm^2) conditions. Secondly, the potential for tolerance development in bacteria subjected to repeated sub-lethal exposure was compared by carrying out 15 cycles of exposure to high-intensity 405 nm light, using a sub-lethal dose of 108 J/cm^2. Inactivation kinetics and antibiotic susceptibility were also compared.

Results: When cultured in low-level violet-blue light conditions, *S. aureus* required a greater dose of high-intensity 405 nm light for complete inactivation, however this did not increase with multiple (3) low-stress cultivations. Repeated sub-lethal exposures indicated no evidence of bacterial tolerance to 405 nm light. After 15 sub-lethal exposures 1.2 and 1.4 $\log_{10}$ reductions were achieved for MSSA and MRSA respectively, which were not significantly different to the initial 1.3 $\log_{10}$ reductions achieved (P = 0.242 & 0.116, respectively). Antibiotic susceptibility was unaffected, with the maximum change in zone of inhibition being $\pm$ 2 mm.

Conclusions: Repeated sub-lethal exposure of non-proliferating *S. aureus* populations did not affect the susceptibility of the organism to 405 nm light, nor to antibiotics. Culture in low-level violet-blue light prior to 405 nm light exposure may increase oxidative stress responses in *S. aureus*, however, inactivation still occurs and results demonstrate that this is unlikely to be a selective process. These results demonstrate that tolerance from repeated exposure is unlikely to occur, and further supports the potential development of 405 nm light for clinical decontamination and treatment applications.

Keywords: 405 nm light, Bacterial tolerance, Bacterial resistance, *Staphylococcus aureus*, EMRSA-15

* Correspondence: rachael.tomb.2013@uni.strath.ac.uk
[1]The Robertson Trust Laboratory for Electronic Sterilisation Technologies (ROLEST), Department of Electronic & Electrical Engineering, University of Strathclyde, Glasgow, UK
Full list of author information is available at the end of the article

Background

There is global concern surrounding antibiotic resistant organisms, such as methicillin-resistant *Staphylococcus aureus* (MRSA). These organisms negatively impact on healthcare systems by causing infections which are harder to treat due to reduced antibiotic choices, resulting in longer hospital stays and increased mortality of patients [1]. To reduce transmission of these pathogenic organisms, new technologies are being developed to aid environmental decontamination and clinical treatment.

One such antimicrobial technology is 405 nm light. Violet-blue light in this region photo-excites intracellular porphyrins within microorganisms, producing a range of reactive oxygen species (ROS) which cause oxidative damage and cell death [2–4]. Although less germicidal than ultraviolet (UV) light, 405 nm light has broad-spectrum antimicrobial action against Gram positive and negative bacteria, bacterial biofilms, endospores, yeasts, fungi and in some circumstances viruses [5–11]. When used at appropriate irradiances, these wavelengths of visible light can also exert antimicrobial effects whilst being non-detrimental to mammalian cells [12–14], giving it operational advantages over UV-light for applications such as continuous decontamination of occupied environments [15–18] and wound decontamination [12]. Additionally, it has recently been reported that 405 nm light can also have a synergistic antimicrobial effect with common chlorinated disinfectants, providing further support for its beneficial use for environmental decontamination [19].

Although 405 nm light has extensive antimicrobial action and safety advantages, little is known about the potential for the development of bacterial resistance or tolerance to violet-blue 405 nm light inactivation. It is hypothesised that tolerance is unlikely due to the mechanism of inactivation [13, 17, 20]. Similar to that of photodynamic inactivation (PDI), which makes use of an additional photosensitizer, the mechanism of inactivation is thought to be non-selective, as the ROS and $^1O_2$ produced cause unspecific damage to a wide spectrum of targets within bacterial cells [13, 17, 20, 21]. Nevertheless there is little evidence available to support this hypothesis. Several studies have investigated tolerance formation following repeated PDI in a range of microorganisms including methicillin-sensitive and methicillin-resistant *S. aureus*, *Escherichia coli*, *Pseudomonas aeruginosa*, *Peptostreptococcus micros*, *Actinobacillus actinomycetes* and *Vibrio fischeri*, in which none of the aforementioned species were found to become tolerant [21–25]. However little is known about the potential for bacterial tolerance development to antimicrobial 405 nm light alone.

This study was carried out to determine if there is potential for tolerance development in exposed organisms, using the nosocomial pathogen *S. aureus* as the model organism. The first stage of the study assessed whether preculture in low-level light-stress conditions would subsequently affect the susceptibility of the organism to 405 nm light inactivation and increase tolerance. Secondly, the study investigated the effect of repeated sub-lethal exposure to high-intensity 405 nm light on methicillin-sensitive and methicillin-resistant *S. aureus*, with the number of sub-lethal exposures being extended past those carried out in previously published studies [20, 26, 27]. To further investigate the likelihood of tolerance, the inactivation kinetics and antibiotic susceptibility of survivors after sublethal exposure were analysed and compared. The results provide novel fundamental evidence to support the hypothesis that tolerance following repeated exposure to 405 nm light is unlikely in both proliferating and nonproliferating bacteria.

Methods

Microorganisms

Two strains of *Staphylococcus aureus* were used in this study, methicillin-sensitive *S. aureus* NCTC 4135 (National Collection of Type Cultures, Collindale, UK) and epidemic methicillin-resistant *S. aureus*-15 (EMRSA-15) (Scottish Reference Laboratory, Glasgow, UK), which are referred to as MSSA and MRSA throughout the study.

Determining potential for tolerance development when cultured under different lighting conditions

Cultivation in different lighting conditions

MSSA was inoculated in 100 ml nutrient broth (NB; Oxoid, UK) and cultivated under different lighting conditions: (i) complete darkness (flasks wrapped in aluminium foil); (ii) normal laboratory fluorescent lighting, approximately 200 Lux (measured using a Light Level Meter; Labfacility, UK); and (iii) 3 levels of low-intensity 405 nm light: 0.15, 0.5 & 1 mW/cm^2 (measured using a radiant power meter and photodiode detector (LOT Oriel, USA)). The light source used was a low-power matrix of 9-light emitting diode arrays (LED) (GE Illumination, USA) with a peak wavelength in the region of 405 nm and a full width at half maximum (FWHM) of approximately 18 nm (Fig. 1). Arrays were arranged in a 3 × 3 grid pattern on a heat sink (for heat dissipation), and powered by a variable DC power supply (Velleman, Belgium). The light source and power supply were placed in the 37 °C incubator, 30 cm from the cultivation flask, and allowed to stabilise before setting the irradiance; this ensured that the current would not fluctuate during temperature increase. Utilising this light source enabled low level illumination of a large surface area (culture flask) during bacterial cultivation. Bacteria were cultured in these lighting conditions under rotary incubation (120 rpm) at 37 °C for 18–24 h. The broths were then centrifuged at 3939×*g* for 10 min and the pellets re-suspended in 100 ml phosphate buffer saline (PBS; Oxoid, UK). Bacterial suspensions were then diluted in PBS to an experimental starting

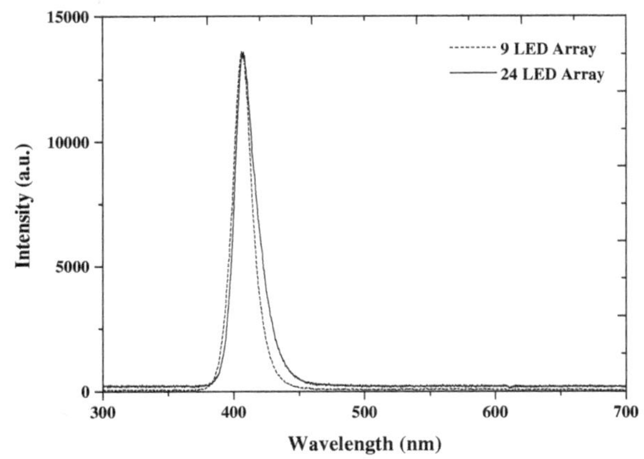

Fig. 1 Optical emission spectrum of the 9-LED and 24-LED 405 nm arrays. Measured using an HR4000 spectrometer (Ocean Optics, Germany) and Spectra Suite software version 2.0.151

population of 1–2 × 10^5 CFU/ml for exposure to high-irradiance 405 nm light.

Exposure to high-irradiance 405 nm light following cultivation under different lighting conditions

Following cultivation in the different lighting conditions, the bacteria where exposed to high-irradiance 405 nm light to establish if their susceptibility to 405 nm light had been affected. The high-power light source used for exposure was a 24-LED array (PhotonStar Technologies, UK) with peak wavelength in the region of 405 nm and 19 nm FWHM (Fig. 1). The source was connected to a heat sink and cooling fan for heat dissipation, and was powered by a 40 V Xitanium LED Driver (Phillips, Netherlands). This light source provided high-intensity illumination over a small surface area, ideal for exposure of samples in 6-well plates.

The array was held in a PVC housing approximately 6 cm above the surface of the bacterial samples. Five millileters bacterial samples were exposed to 405 nm light at an irradiance of 60 mW/cm^2, with sample plates positioned on a magnetic stirring plate to permit constant agitation. Control plates were held under identical conditions however only subjected to normal laboratory lighting. Samples were exposed to increasing doses of light, with dose (J/cm^2) calculated as irradiance (W/cm^2) × exposure time (s). During exposure, samples were taken at 15 min intervals and plated onto nutrient agar (NA; Oxoid, UK). Plates were incubated at 37 °C for 24 h and then enumerated, with results reported as colony forming units per millilitre (CFU/ml) as a function of dose (J/cm^2).

Investigating the minimum inhibitory concentration of H_2O_2

To investigate if there were any intracellular changes in catalase production following growth in low-level violet-blue light, a minimum inhibitory concentration (MIC) assay of hydrogen peroxide (H_2O_2) was performed. This was based upon methodology used by Lipovsky et al. [28]. Briefly, following 4–5 h of cultivation in fluorescent laboratory lighting, complete darkness or 1 mW/cm^2 405 nm light, 100 µl of MSSA (10^6 CFU/ml) was added to two-fold dilutions of H_2O_2 in NB. The H_2O_2 dilutions were then incubated at 37 °C for 24 h and the MIC identified as the lowest concentration of H_2O_2 which caused visible inhibition of bacterial growth.

Carotenoid (Staphyloxanthin) extraction

To investigate if carotenoid pigments protected *S. aureus* against singlet oxygen stress during growth in low-level violet-blue light, carotenoid content was measured. Carotenoid extraction was adapted from that used by Bartolomeu et al. [25]. MSSA was cultured in fluorescent laboratory lighting, complete darkness or 1 mW/cm^2 405 nm light for 24 h. After cultivation the cultures were washed thrice in sterile H_2O, re-suspended in 5 ml 99.9% methanol, and incubated in a 55 °C water bath for 15 mins until the cells had been bleached. Following extraction, the samples were centrifuged at 8000×*g* for 10 min. The supernatant was removed and re-centrifuged at 10,000×*g* for 15 mins to ensure removal of any residual biomass. The carotenoid content was then measured by recording the absorbance at 465 nm in a quartz cuvette, using a Biomate 5 Spectrophotometer (Thermo Fischer Scientific, UK).

Determining potential for tolerance development following repeated sub-lethal exposure to high-intensity 405 nm light

Repeated sub-lethal exposure

MSSA and MRSA were inoculated, in triplicate, in 100 ml NB, and cultivated at 37 °C for 18–24 h under rotary conditions (120 rpm) in the dark. Cultures were re-suspended in PBS and diluted to a 10^5 CFU/ml population. Bacterial samples were then exposed to 405 nm light at a dose of 108 J/cm^2 (60 mW/cm^2 for 30 min) using the high-intensity 24-LED array (as described in earlier section 'Exposure to High-Irradiance 405 nm Light Following Cultivation under Different Lighting Conditions').

Following exposure, samples were plated onto NA and incubated at 37 °C for 24 h. Surviving colonies were enumerated and termed as survivors from 'Run 1'. Surviving colonies from 'Run 1' were then used to inoculate NB, in triplicate, and the above process of exposure-subculture-exposure was repeated until 15 sub-lethal exposures had occurred (Fig. 2). Survivors from each run were tested using Staphaurex Plus Latex Agglutination (Thermo Fischer Scientific, UK) and Penicillin Binding Protein (PBP2') Latex (Oxoid, UK) to ensure no contamination had occurred. This

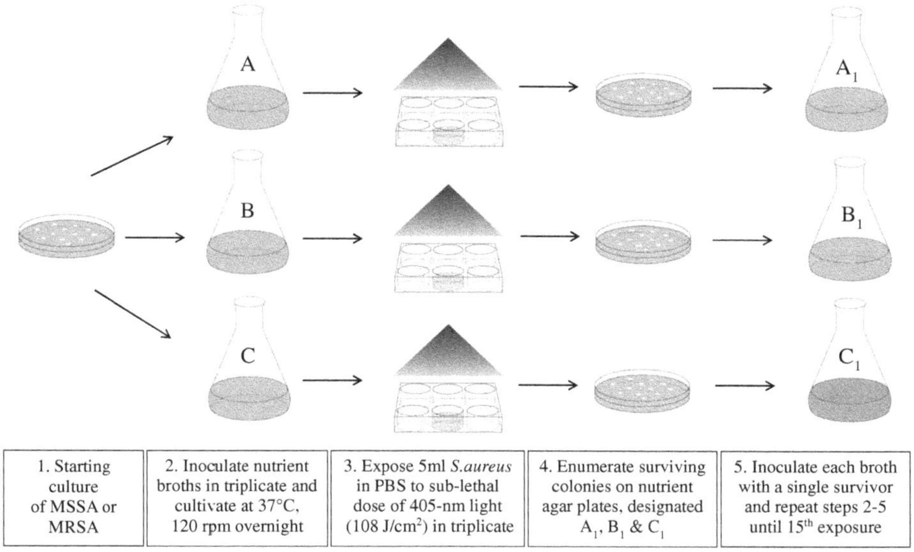

Fig. 2 Flow diagram of the experimental procedure used during repeated sub-lethal 405 nm light exposure. Methicillin-sensitive *Staphylococcus aureus* (MSSA) and methicillin-resistant *Staphylococcus aureus* (MRSA) were exposed to 15 cycles of a dose of 108 J/cm^2, at an irradiance of 60 mW/cm^2

was based on the principle that if the Staphaurex test gave a negative result, then this would indicate that the surviving isolate was not the test organism and that contamination by a rogue organism had occurred. If however, the isolate gave a positive Staphaurex result but a negative PBP2' result, then this would indicate that the MRSA cultures were likely contaminated with MSSA or that MRSA had lost the ability to produce PBP2' following exposure to 405 nm light.

Inactivation kinetics of survivors following sub-lethal exposure

Full inactivation kinetics were also established out using the initial cultures and survivors after 5, 10 and 15 sub-lethal exposures. These isolates were cultivated in 100 ml NB in the dark and exposed to 60 mW/cm^2 405 nm light, with samples taken every 15 min for 75 mins and 90 mins for MSSA and MRSA respectively (as described in earlier section 'Exposure to High-Irradiance 405 nm Light Following Cultivation under Different Lighting Conditions').

Antibiotic susceptibility testing

Antibiotic susceptibility testing was carried out following the EUCAST guidelines [29] as closely as possible (variations included the use of 90 mm plates, stacking during incubation, and inoculation with only one antibiotic disc/plate to prevent overlap if bacterial susceptibility increased). The antibiotics used were chloramphenicol, ciprofloxacin, erythromycin, fusidic acid, gentamicin, mupirocin, oxacillin, rifampicin, tetracycline and vancomycin. These 10 were selected as they represented antibiotics, with differing antimicrobial mechanisms, which are recommended clinical treatment options for *Staphylococcus aureus* infections. Fresh bacterial cultures were diluted to a 10^8 CFU/ml population, spread onto mueller-hinton (MH) agar plates (Oxoid, UK) using sterile swabs and a single antibiotic disc (Mast Group, UK) placed into the centre of the plate. The plates were immediately incubated at 35 ± 2 °C for 18–20 h after which the diameter of the zone of inhibition was measured in normal laboratory lighting and recorded to the nearest mm.

Data analysis

Data represents mean results ± standard deviation (SD), taken from triplicate independent experiments, measured in at least duplicate for 405 nm light inactivation experiments ($n \geq 6$). As samples were directly plated onto NA plates, some samples counted were below the detection limit (25 CFU/ml) however these have been included in graphs to demonstrate the near-to-complete inactivation effect achieved. Repeated sub-lethal exposure results are reported as bacterial inactivation efficiency ($\log_{10} N_0/N$), with N representing the light-exposed population, and N_0 the equivalent non-exposed control population. Significant differences were calculated using Two-Sample T-Tests or One-way ANOVA with Dunnett's post-hoc test (Minitab 17 Statistical Software), with results found to be significant when $P \leq 0.05$.

Results

Determining potential for tolerance development when cultured under different lighting conditions

Bacterial inactivation kinetics following single culture

The first stage of the study investigated 405 nm light susceptibility of methicillin-sensitive *S. aureus* (MSSA) following growth in different lighting conditions. As shown in Fig. 3, relatively linear inactivation kinetics were demonstrated for both MSSA cultivated in fluorescent laboratory light (white light) and in complete darkness, with 5 log_{10} reductions achieved after a final dose of 216 J/cm^2 405 nm light. No significant differences in inactivation between MSSA cultures cultivated in fluorescent laboratory light or in complete darkness were detected at any of the tested sampling points using a Two-Sample t-Test ($P \geq 0.05$). No significant change was seen in the equivalent non-exposed controls (P = 0.932 & 0.747 for light and dark cultures, respectively).

When cultured under low-intensity 405 nm light, some slight differences in the inactivation kinetics were observed. Although trends appeared similar (Fig. 4), differences in the susceptibility of bacteria cultured in low-intensity 405 nm light versus dark cultured can be seen at certain points during the experiment. Following exposure to 108 and 162 J/cm^2 high-intensity 405 nm light, MSSA cultured in 0.15, 0.5 and 1 mW/cm^2 405 nm light showed significantly less inactivation than that cultured in complete darkness ($P < 0.05$). By a final dose of 216 J/cm^2, the inactivation achieved between the dark cultured and low-irradiance 405 nm light cultured MSSA was similar (~4–5 log_{10} reduction), with the exception of the MSSA cultured in 1 mW/cm^2 405 nm light: when cultured under this lighting condition, only 3.3 log_{10} reduction was achieved compared to 5 log_{10} reduction for dark-cultivated MSSA (P = 0.045). No significant change was seen in the equivalent non-exposed controls (P = 1.00, 0.268 & 0.744 for 0.15, 0.5 and 1 mW/cm^2 cultures, respectively).

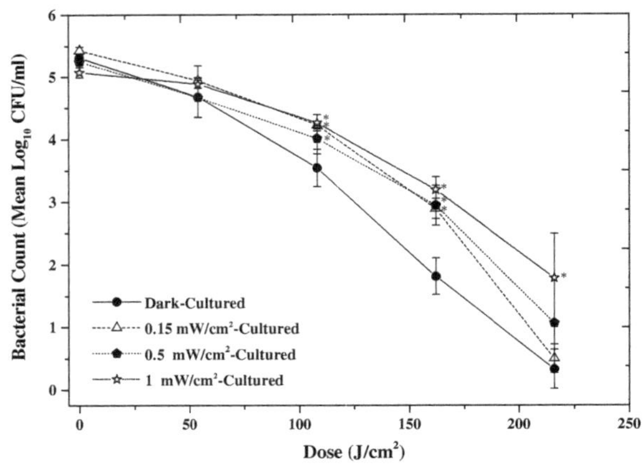

Fig. 4 Inactivation of MSSA following overnight culture in low-level 405 nm light. Methicillin-sensitive *Staphylococcus aureus* (MSSA) was inactivated following exposure to 60 mW/cm^2 405 nm light after overnight culture in low-level 405 nm light (0.15, 0.5 and 1 mW/cm^2). The inactivation kinetics of dark-cultured MSSA have been included for reference. Each data point is a mean value ± SD (n ≥ 6). * Indicates 405 nm light-cultured samples that were significantly different to those which had been dark-cultured, using one way ANOVA with Dunnett's post-hoc test ($P < 0.05$). No significant changes were observed in the final control populations ($P \geq 0.05$)

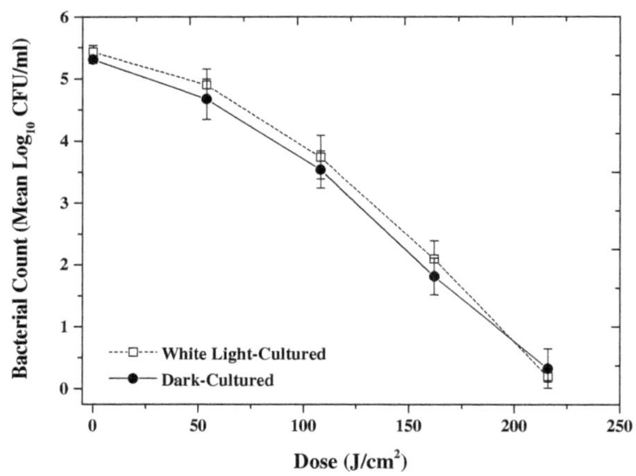

Fig. 3 Inactivation of MSSA following culture in white light or complete darkness. Methicillin-sensitive *Staphylococcus aureus* (MSSA) was inactivated following exposure to 60 mW/cm^2 405 nm light after culture in fluorescent laboratory lighting (white light) or complete darkness. Each data point is a mean value ± SD ($n \geq 6$). No significant differences were found between the susceptibility of the light and dark cultured MSSA, using two-sample t-Test ($P \geq 0.05$). No significant changes were observed in the final control populations ($P \geq 0.05$)

Investigating the minimum inhibitory concentration of H_2O_2

Table 1 shows that the average MIC of H_2O_2 is significantly higher for MSSA cultured in 1 mW/cm^2 405 nm light (P = 0.011) compared to when cultured in white light (P = 0.044) or complete darkness (P = 0.024).

Table 1 Minimum Inhibitory Concentration of H_2O_2 and carotenoid content of *Staphylococcus aureus* following different culture conditions

Growth Conditions	Average Minimum Inhibitory Concentration of H_2O_2 (%) ± SD	Average Carotenoid Absorbance at 465 nm ± SD
Complete Darkness	0.00293 ± 0.00000	0.90 ± 0.22
White Lighting	0.00513 ± 0.00146	0.82 ± 0.24
Low irradiance (1 mW/cm^2) 405 nm Light	0.01831 ± 0.01025*	0.17 ± 0.12*

Differences in the minimum inhibitory concentration (MIC) of hydrogen peroxide (H_2O_2) and carotenoid content of methicillin-sensitive *Staphylococcus aureus* when cultivated in different lighting conditions. Data points represent the mean count (n = 3) ± SD

*represents a significant change ($P < 0.05$)

Carotenoid (Staphyloxanthin) extraction

Results shown in Table 1 demonstrate that the presence of the carotenoid staphyloxanthin is significantly lower in MSSA cultured in 1 mW/cm^2 405 nm light (P = 0.009) compared to that grown in white light (P = 0.015) or complete darkness (P = 0.008).

Bacterial inactivation kinetics following multiple cultures

MSSA was grown in 1 mW/cm^2 405 nm light, sub-cultured onto NA plates, then re-cultured in (a) complete darkness once or (b) 1 mW/cm^2 a further two more times. As can be seen in Fig. 5a, when cultivated in 1 mW/cm^2 followed by cultivation in complete darkness, the level of inactivation returns to that of cultivation in darkness alone, with no significant difference in the level of inactivation (P = 0.395), and similarly the level of inactivation was significantly greater than that of MSSA grown in 1 mW/cm^2 405 nm light (P = 0.043). No significant change was seen in the equivalent non-exposed controls (P = 0.505). Figure 5b also demonstrates that triplicate cultivation in 1 mW/cm^2 does not select for more tolerant cultures. The sensitivity of MSSA to high-intensity 405 nm light returns to a similar level of that when cultivated in complete darkness alone, with an average 0.7 × 10^1 CFU/ml population surviving following a dose of 216 J/cm^2, which is not significantly different to the average 0.3 × 10^1 CFU/ml surviving population which had been grown in darkness (P = 0.230). No significant change was seen in the equivalent non-exposed controls (P = 0.338).

Determining potential for tolerance development following repeated sub-lethal exposure to high-intensity 405 nm light

Repeated sub-lethal exposure

The next stage of this study was to investigate the likelihood of tolerance development when non-proliferating *Staphylococcus aureus* was repeatedly exposed to a sub-lethal dose of high-intensity 405 nm light A dose of 108 J/cm^2 was selected for use, as this had been shown to cause approximately 98% (1.6–1.8 $\log_{10}$) inactivation of the organism (Figs. 3 and 4). As can be seen from Fig. 6a, after repeated sub-lethal exposure there were fluctuations in MSSA inactivation, with the maximum inactivation seen after 7 sub-lethal exposures (1.5 $\log_{10}$ reduction) and minimum after 4 sub-lethal exposures (1.1 $\log_{10}$ reduction). However there was no significant difference (P = 0.242) in MSSA inactivation, compared to equivalent non-exposed controls, after 1 sub-lethal exposure compared to those after 15 sub-lethal exposures, with 1.3 $\log_{10}$ and 1.2 $\log_{10}$ inactivation achieved respectively. Additionally, one-way ANOVA and Dunnett's post-hoc analysis, using Run 1 as the control group, indicated that there was no significant difference in the bactericidal efficiency of 405 nm light ($\log_{10} N_0/N$) between the sub-lethal exposures. No significant change was seen in the equivalent non-exposed controls (P = 0.198).

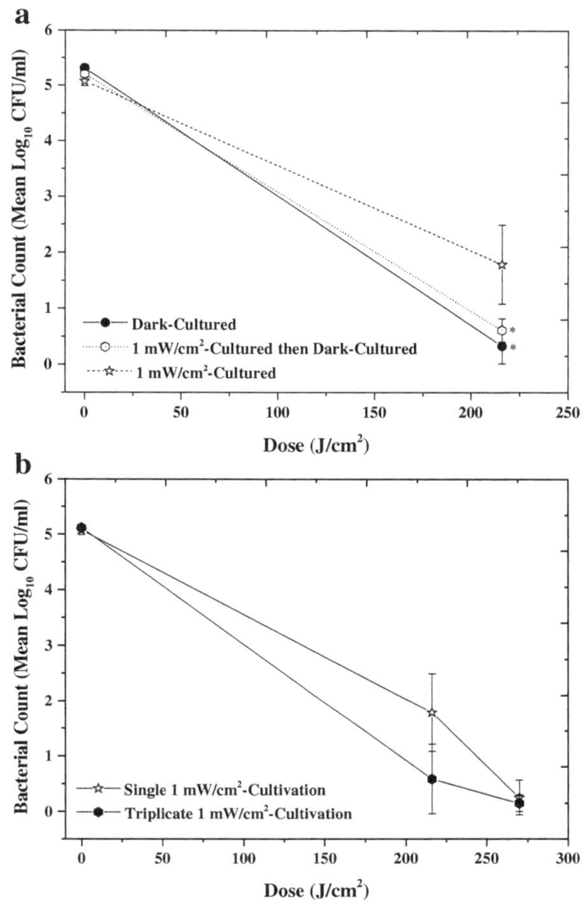

Fig. 5 Comparison of MSSA susceptibility to high-intensity 405 nm light after cultivation in different lighting conditions. **a** Methicillin-sensitive *Staphylococcus aureus* (MSSA) was cultivated in low-intensity (1 mW/cm^2) 405 nm light followed by cultivation in complete darkness, and **b** MSSA was subjected to repeated (three times) cultivation in low-intensity (1 mW/cm^2) 405 nm light. Each cultivation was at 37 °C for 18 h. Following these cultivation conditions, bacteria were exposed to increasing doses of high-intensity 60 mW/cm^2 light to establish the inactivation kinetics. Inactivation kinetics of bacteria which had been pre-cultured once in darkness or low-intensity 405 nm light are given as a comparison. * Indicates cultured samples that were significantly different to those which had been cultured once in 1 mW/cm^2 405 nm light, using one way ANOVA with Dunnett's post-hoc test (P < 0.05). Each data point is a mean value ± SD (n ≥ 6). No significant changes were observed in the final control populations (P ≥ 0.05)

As a comparison a clinical isolate of MRSA was also repeatedly exposed to sub-lethal levels of 405 nm light. Figure 6b demonstrates that similarly to MSSA, there were fluctuations in inactivation of MRSA, with a maximum inactivation after 14 sub-lethal exposures (1.8 $\log_{10}$ reduction) and minimum after 10 sub-lethal exposures (1.1 $\log_{10}$ reduction). Furthermore there was also no significant difference (P = 0.943) between the 1.3 $\log_{10}$ and 1.4 $\log_{10}$

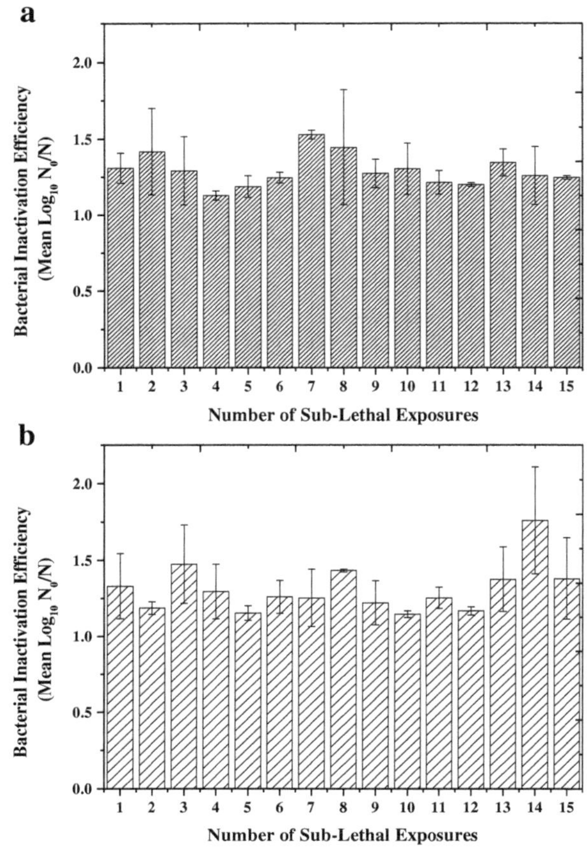

Fig. 6 Average 405 nm light inactivation efficiency following repeated sub-lethal exposure of MSSA and MRSA. 405 nm light inactivation efficiency of 15 sub-lethal exposure cycles of (**a**) methicillin-sensitive *Staphylococcus aureus* (MSSA) and (**b**) methicillin-resistant *Staphylococcus aureus* (MRSA), to a dose of 108 J/cm^2 405 nm light at an irradiance of 60 mW/cm^2. Repeated sub-lethal exposure results are reported as bacterial inactivation efficiency ($\log_{10}$ N_0/N), with N representing the light-exposed population, and N_0 the equivalent non-exposed control population. Each data point is a mean value ± SD (n ≥ 6). No significant changes were observed in the test or final control populations, using one way ANOVA with Dunnett's post-hoc test ($P \geq 0.05$)

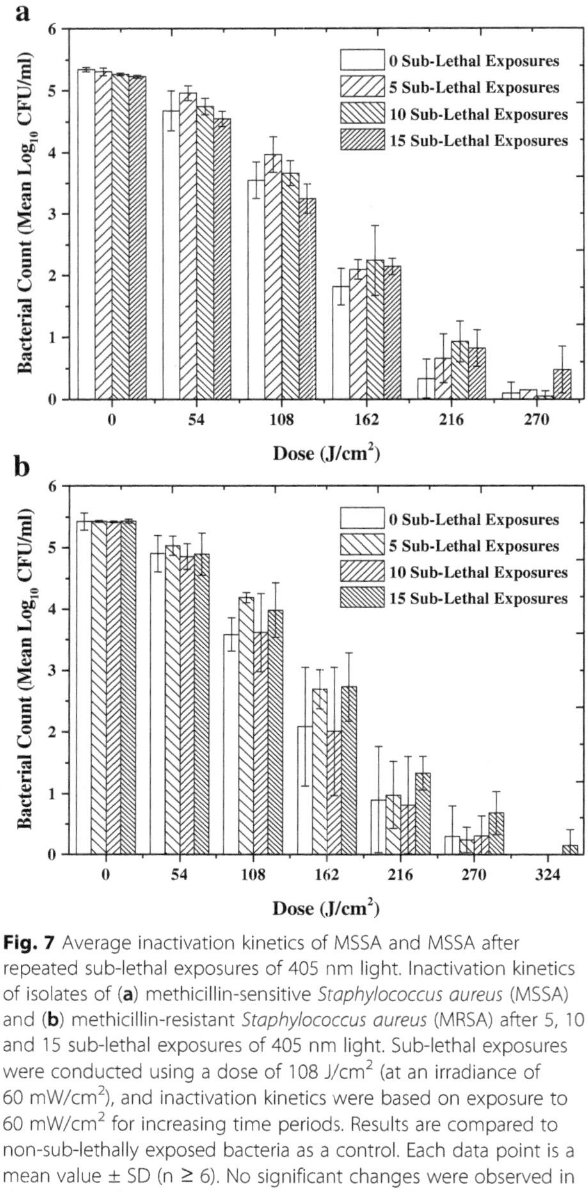

Fig. 7 Average inactivation kinetics of MSSA and MSSA after repeated sub-lethal exposures of 405 nm light. Inactivation kinetics of isolates of (**a**) methicillin-sensitive *Staphylococcus aureus* (MSSA) and (**b**) methicillin-resistant *Staphylococcus aureus* (MRSA) after 5, 10 and 15 sub-lethal exposures of 405 nm light. Sub-lethal exposures were conducted using a dose of 108 J/cm^2 (at an irradiance of 60 mW/cm^2), and inactivation kinetics were based on exposure to 60 mW/cm^2 for increasing time periods. Results are compared to non-sub-lethally exposed bacteria as a control. Each data point is a mean value ± SD (n ≥ 6). No significant changes were observed in the test populations, using one way ANOVA with Dunnett's post-hoc test ($P \geq 0.05$)

reduction after 1 and 15 sub-lethal exposures respectively. Similarly to MSSA, one-way ANOVA and Dunnett's post-hoc analysis, using Run 1 as the control group, indicated that there was no significant difference in the bactericidal efficiency of 405 nm light (log_{10} N_0/N) between the sub-lethal exposures. No significant change was seen in the equivalent non-exposed controls ($P = 0.116$).

Inactivation kinetics of survivors following sub-lethal exposure

The inactivation kinetics of surviving MSSA and MRSA isolates after 5, 10 and 15 sub-lethal exposures to 60 mW/cm^2 light were also determined. Figure 7a shows that after a dose of 270 J/cm^2 (75 mins) there was no significant difference in the level of MSSA inactivation after 5, 10 and 15 sub-lethal exposures, with 5.2 ($P = 0.895$), 5.2 ($P = 0.795$) and 4.8 ($P = 0.583$) $\log_{10}$ reduction achieved, compared to non-sub-lethally exposed MSSA. Similarly, MRSA showed no significant difference in inactivation after a dose of 324 J/cm^2 (90 mins) with 5.4 ($P = 0.193$), 5.4 ($P = 0.259$) and 5.3 ($P = 0.081$) $\log_{10}$ reductions of MRSA after 5, 10 and 15 sub-lethal exposures, respectively.

Antibiotic susceptibility testing

Although little change was seen in bacterial susceptibility to high-intensity 405 nm light after repeated sub-lethal exposure, antibiotic susceptibility was also investigated.

Table 2 shows that there was little variation in the diameter of the zones of inhibition for MSSA after 5, 10 and 15 sub-lethal exposures compared to the initial non sub-lethally exposed populations. There were no significant decreases in the diameter of the zone of inhibition between the initial non sub-lethally exposed MSSA and survivors of 15 sub-lethal exposures ($P > 0.05$). There was a slight decrease in the average diameter of the zone of inhibition caused by mupirocin after 5 sub-lethal exposures, however after 10 and 15 sub-lethal exposures inhibition was comparable to non-stressed cultures ($P > 0.05$).

With regards to the antibiotic susceptibility of MRSA isolates after sub-lethal exposure, there were no significant decreases between the initial non-sub-lethally exposed populations and those after 15 sub-lethal exposures.

Interestingly there were significant increases in the diameter of the zone of inhibition for fusidic acid after 10 sub-lethal exposures and rifampicin after 15 sub-lethal exposures for MSSA and with gentamicin after 15 sub-lethal exposures for MRSA, compared to initial non sub-lethally exposed populations.

Discussion

This study has addressed the question of the potential for *S. aureus* to become tolerant to antimicrobial 405 nm violet-blue light and has provided new information under carefully controlled experimental test conditions.

The results from the first stage of the study, demonstrated that MSSA cultured in 1 mW/cm^2 405 nm light appeared to exhibit a degree of tolerance to high-intensity 405 nm light, compared to when dark-cultured. This suggests that exposure to low-intensity 405 nm light during culture may have acted as a low-level stressor during growth, which could have increased the up-regulation of bacterial oxidative stress responses. Bacteria have developed several mechanisms to overcome oxidative stress, including enzymes to detoxify reactive oxygen species such as catalase, peroxidase and superoxide dismutase [30]. To detect changes in the ability of MSSA to tolerate oxidative stress after culture in the presence of 1 mW/cm^2 405 nm light, compared to white light or complete darkness, a MIC assay using H_2O_2 was carried out, and carotenoid content was measured. Results determined that the average MIC of H_2O_2 was significantly higher for the organism when cultured in low-level (1 mW/cm^2) 405 nm light compared to white light or complete darkness. This demonstrates that during growth in low-irradiance 405 nm light there is likely an increase in the expression of protective enzymes e.g. an increase in catalase enzymes which would act as hydrogen peroxide scavengers. An increase in catalase enzyme, KatA, following photodynamic inactivation of *S. aureus* (using blue light and exogenous porphyrins) was also demonstrated by Doselli et al. [31], which further suggest this enzyme is up-regulated to try to help protect the bacteria against oxidative stress.

The presence of the carotenoid staphyloxanthin was also found to be significantly lower in MSSA cultured in low-level (1 mW/cm^2) 405 nm light compared to when grown in white light or darkness. As carotenoid pigments have anti-oxidative properties, in particular for protecting bacteria against $^1O_2$ stress [32], you would expect MSSA cultivated in 1 mW/cm^2 405 nm light to be more sensitive to subsequent high-intensity 405 nm light exposure, due to the lower levels of staphyloxanthin present. However, as tolerance is increased upon exposure to high-intensity 405 nm light, it is likely there is an up-regulation of other oxidative stress responses within

Table 2 Antibiotic susceptibility of MSSA and MRSA following sub-lethal exposure to 405 nm light

Antibiotic	Conc (μg)	Mean Diameter of Zone of Inhibition of MSSA (mm)				Mean Diameter of Zone of Inhibition of MRSA (mm)			
		0	5	10	15	0	5	10	15
Chloramphenicol	25[a]	21 ± 1.5	21 ± 0.8	21 ± 1.2	21 ± 0.8	24 ± 1.0	24 ± 1.1	23 ± 1.4	23 ± 1.1
Ciprofloxacin	5	22 ± 1.2	21 ± 0.5	22 ± 0.7	22 ± 1.3	26 ± 0.6	26 ± 0.4	26 ± 1.0	26 ± 1.1
Erythromycin	5[a]	21 ± 0.6	21 ± 0.6	22 ± 0.8	21 ± 0.4	23 ± 1.0	22 ± 0.8	23 ± 1.0	23 ± 1.2
Fusidic Acid	10	30 ± 0.0	30 ± 0.8	32 ± 1.0*	31 ± 1.8	31 ± 0.6	30 ± 0.5	30 ± 0.7	30 ± 0.9
Gentamicin	10	21 ± 0.6	21 ± 0.5	21 ± 0.5	20 ± 0.5	21 ± 0.6	21 ± 0.5	22 ± 1.3	23 ± 0.6*
Mupirocin	5[a]	28 ± 0.6	26 ± 0.5*	28 ± 1.4	28 ± 1.1	26 ± 0.6	27 ± 1.1	26 ± 1.2	26 ± 1.3
Oxacillin	5[b]	30 ± 0.0	29 ± 0.9	30 ± 0.6	30 ± 0.9	0 ± 0.0	0 ± 0.0	0 ± 0.0	0 ± 0.0
Rifampicin	5	32 ± 1.0	32 ± 0.7	33 ± 1.8	34 ± 0.6*	31 ± 0.6	30 ± 0.7	31 ± 1.0	31 ± 0.9
Tetracycline	25[a]	28 ± 1.2	28 ± 1.0	28 ± 1.4	29 ± 1.3	27 ± 1.0	27 ± 0.7	27 ± 1.0	26 ± 0.9
Vancomycin	5[b]	15 ± 0.0	14 ± 0.7	15 ± 0.7	15 ± 0.5	14 ± 0.6	15 ± 0.6	15 ± 0.5	14 ± 0.5

Antibiotic susceptibility of methicillin-sensitive *Staphylococcus aureus* (MSSA) and methicillin-resistant *Staphylococcus aureus* (MRSA) after 5, 10 and 15 sub-lethal exposures compared to equivalent non-sub-lethally exposed controls (0). Susceptibility was measured using Disc Diffusion Method

*indicates diameters of zones of inhibition that was significantly different to the equivalent non-sub-lethally exposed control ($P \leq 0.05$). Each data point is a mean value ± SD ($n \geq 3$)

[a]Disc concentration is lower than that recommended by EUCAST

[b]No disc concentration recommended by EUCAST

the bacteria and that the carotenoid pigment provided protection against ROS during growth in low-intensity 405 nm light. Further experiments investigating superoxide dismutase, catalase activity could help to confirm this.

Although the inactivation achieved at 216 J/cm^2 (Fig. 4) was less when the bacteria had been pre-cultured in low-irradiance (1 mW/cm^2) 405 nm light, it is important to note that when exposed to a higher dose of 270 J/cm^2 complete 5 $\log_{10}$ inactivation was still able to be achieved (Fig. 5b). It is likely that complete inactivation is still able to occur due the level of ROS produced being greater than the level that the basal bacterial oxidative stress defence systems are able to scavenge [30].

It is important to consider the possibility that bacteria may become less sensitive to high-irradiance 405 nm light after pre-culture in low-intensity, sub-lethal stress levels of 405 nm light, as this could have implications when violet-blue light is used to inactivate bacteria in nutritious environments where the bacteria are able to replicate, for example within wounds or surgical sites. In these cases it would be important to ensure a bactericidal dose was administered: if the dose administered or irradiance used is too low, the bacteria may not be completely inactivated and cause pathogenic organisms to potentially become more tolerant to subsequent applications of violet-blue light. Additionally, if the dose delivered is too low there may actually be an increase in population concentration, as it is thought visible light can encourage proliferation of microorganisms when used on nutrient rich areas such as wounds [28].

Further investigations were carried out to investigate if growth in low-intensity 405 nm light was selective for MSSA which was able to adapt to a greater level of oxidative stress. Results demonstrated that this was not the case, with the sensitivity of MSSA returning to a similar level of that when cultivated in complete darkness alone. These results additionally suggest that the increased tolerance to high-intensity 405 nm light is caused by an up-regulation in bacterial stress response rather than selection for violet-blue light tolerant colonies due to growth conditions.

Further work should be carried out to investigate the oxidative stress response following growth in low-intensity 405 nm light fully, such as the levels of superoxide dismutase, which has been previously shown to be up-regulated in *S. aureus* sensitive to PDI [33]. Additionally it is known that there is a heat shock protein cascade after PDI [30] and a study by St Denis et al. [34] demonstrated that *E. coli* exposed to external stress, before PDI showed a 2 $\log_{10}$ less reduction in bacterial inactivation compared to normal PDI inactivation levels. Therefore it would be interesting to investigate if there was a heat shock protein cascade during growth in 1 mW/cm^2 violet-blue light, and if this up-regulation of proteins before high-intensity exposure may contribute to the stress tolerance seen. Additionally, investigations should explore why the increased level of tolerance is not seen after repeated growth in the low-level stress conditions. However as the bacteria can still be completely inactivated, and as results indicated repeated growth in low-irradiance light is unlikely to be a selective process, MSSA should continue to be susceptible to high-irradiance 405 nm light after growth in the presence of a low-level stressor.

It is also important to note that the changes in susceptibility observed here are in response to the organisms being pre-cultured in low-level 405 nm light. This is unlikely to occur in non-proliferating bacteria, such as is the case with environmental contamination [17], as these organisms are stressed and not actively growing, thus up-regulation of stress responses is unlikely to occur, and actually when in a stationary stressed state, bacteria should become more susceptible to 405 nm light inactivation [35].

The next stage of this study was to investigate the likelihood of tolerance development when non-proliferating bacteria were repeatedly exposed to a sub-lethal dose of high-intensity 405 nm light. MSSA and MRSA were subjected to 15 exposure-subculture-exposure cycles to 60 mW/cm^2 405 nm light, resulting in a dose of 108 J/cm^2 per sub-lethal exposure. Results demonstrated no significant change in the level of inactivation achieved, with 1.2 $\log_{10}$ and 1.4 $\log_{10}$ inactivation achieved for MSSA and MRSA after 15 sub-lethal exposures respectively, compared to an initial 1.3 $\log_{10}$ inactivation achieved for both.

The dose of 108 J/cm^2 was selected for exposure as it was shown to cause approximately 98% (1.6–1.8 $\log_{10}$) inactivation of the organism used in this study (Figs. 3 and 4). When compared to doses used in other studies to achieve similar levels of inactivation, this dose is somewhat greater [6, 7], however, the dose dependency will vary between studies, as it is specific to the light sources, the irradiances and the organisms used. LED arrays have variations in spectral output in terms of exact peak wavelength and bandwidth, and therefore this will affect the efficiency of bacterial inactivation. In addition, the overall doses used will vary depending on the output irradiance of the light source: the higher power the light source, the higher the irradiance, however, given that there will be a finite number of porphyrins per bacterial cell capable of photon absorption, there is likely to be a point at which the absorption of more photons would have little effect on the inactivation mechanism already in progress, therefore although more energy is being delivered, it may not translate into more effective kill.

Little other evidence has been documented regarding bacterial tolerance to 405 nm light. A short study by

Guffey et al. [26] demonstrated that there was potential for *S. aureus* to become tolerant to a dose of 9 J/cm^2 405 nm light, as following 5 repeated exposures there was a decrease in the kill rate seen. The study demonstrated an initial increase in kill rate from 32.92 to 59.49% after the 1st to 4th sub-lethal exposures, however kill rate subsequently declined, with only 18.04% kill after the 7th repeated sub-lethal exposure, attributed to the development of resistance. These results are conflicting with those in this study, as our results indicate little change in bacterial response to 405 nm light inactivation following 15 sub-lethal exposures. In the present study, which used more than double the number of sub-lethal exposures and higher bacterial populations, natural variation in the level of inactivation occurred after repeated sub-lethal exposure, and this variation would be particularly apparent when using low population densities, as was the case in the study by Guffey et al. [26], so potentially further repeated sub-lethal exposures may have shown a subsequent increase in kill rate.

Additionally, in the present study *S. aureus* was repeatedly sub-lethally exposed whilst suspended in PBS. This allowed investigation of the sole effect that repeated antimicrobial violet-blue light exposure would have on bacterial cultures in a stationary, non-proliferating, state, representative of how bacteria would be found in the clinical environment. In the study by Guffey et al. [26], *S. aureus* was exposed to 405 nm light whilst seeded onto mannitol salt agar plates. Not only is mannitol known to be a ROS scavenger [36], in this scenario the bacteria were likely to be in a metabolic state, tolerating the high salt conditions (7.5% NaCl) and fermenting mannitol, and therefore these processes may have affected the subsequent bacterial stress response to violet-blue light. Consequently the increased tolerance seen may be more relative to results in the earlier phase of this study, where low-level exposure to 405 nm light in nutritious conditions resulted in higher dose requirements for complete inactivation.

Conversely, two studies which exposed *Acinetobacter baumannii* and *P. aeruginosa* to 415 nm light, under exposure conditions similar to this study, demonstrated no evidence of tolerance formation [20, 27]. Results are in keeping with study, with no tolerance to 415 nm light inactivation seen in 10^8 CFU/ml populations of *P. aeruginosa* and *A. baumannii* after 10 repeated sub-lethal exposures to a dose of 36 J/cm^2 and 70.2 J/cm^2 respectively [20, 27]. These previous studies, along with the results in the present study, support the hypothesis that due to the unspecific mechanism of action and broad spectrum of intracellular targets, tolerance is not likely to occur.

Interestingly in the study by Zhang et al. [27] a significant increase in the sensitivity of *A. baumannii* was seen between the 1st exposure (4.52 $\log_{10}$ reduction) and the 10th exposure (6.28 $\log_{10}$ reduction) and inactivation curves revealed an increase in inactivation between 1, 6 and 9 sub-lethal exposures. These results were thought to indicate that a favourable mutation had occurred, increasing bacterial susceptibly to violet-blue light inactivation [27]. To investigate if this phenomenon would also occur in *Staphylococcus aureus*, the inactivation kinetics of surviving isolates after 5, 10 and 15 sub-lethal exposures were determined and all followed similar trends. Although these results do not indicate an increase in sensitivity of MSSA and MRSA to 405 nm light after repeated sub-lethal exposure, they do demonstrate consistent *Staphylococcal* sensitivity to high-irradiance 405 nm light and further supports the hypothesis that tolerance to 405 nm light inactivation in unlikely. However, the potential for tolerance should be evaluated in other microorganisms normally susceptible to 405 nm light inactivation, including multidrug resistant organisms which are currently a great problem in healthcare settings [37, 38].

Antibiotic susceptibility was also analysed to ensure that repeated 405 nm light exposure did not give rise to 'stress hardening', whereby as a result of continued exposure to this sub-lethal stress the bacteria would be able to adapt and develop protection mechanisms against other applied stresses [39, 40]. Little significant variation was seen with the antibiotic susceptibility for both *S. aureus* strains. Although a slight decrease in susceptibility of MSSA to mupirocin was noted after 5 sub-lethal exposures (an observation which was not observed following increased sub-lethal exposures to 10 or 15 cycles), it is worth noting that although the concentration of mupirocin antibiotic disc (5 µg) was below the recommended concentration used by EUCAST (200 µg), the zone of inhibition measured was still far greater (26 mm) than the EUCAST breakpoints for resistance (18 mm). Therefore, indicating that although significantly different to the initial non sub-lethally exposed MSSA, after 5 sub-lethal exposures MSSA is bacteria is still sensitive to mupirocin.

Furthermore, to the best of our knowledge these are the first results comparing repeated sub-lethal 405 nm light exposure and antibiotic susceptibility, and they indicate that sub-lethal exposure is unlikely to result in the development of antibiotic resistance. These findings are further supported by those of Pedigo et al. [23], who demonstrated no antibiotic resistance occurred in MSSA after 25 repeat exposures to PDI, using a methylene blue photosensitizer and 670 nm light, compared to antibiotic resistance in MSSA after only 11 exposures to a 1 µg/ml oxacillin disk. Similarly, Grinholc et al. [41] found no change in antibiotic susceptibility in MRSA before and after exposure to PDI (using protoporphyrin diarginate and 624 nm light) with the 26 different antibiotics tested.

Future studies should involve a greater range of commonly used antibiotics and broth microdilution studies should be carried out to enable the quantification of the MIC of each antibiotic before and after sub-lethal exposure. However, overall these results indicate repeated sub-lethal exposure to 405 nm light is unlikely to affect *S. aureus* susceptibility to antibiotics, and supports the practical application of 405 nm light for decontamination applications within in the clinical environment [42].

This study was designed to generate fundamental microbiological information with regards to the potential for the development of bacterial tolerance to 405 nm light. To investigate this, *S. aureus* was exposed to high-irradiance light whilst in suspension, following either growth in low-level blue light stress conditions or previous sub-lethal exposures to 405 nm light. As discussed earlier, the 405 nm light levels used in the present study permitted establishment of the fundamental responses of the light-exposed bacteria. There is however, interest in utilising this antimicrobial technology for practical decontamination applications and it will therefore be important for future studies to progress investigations towards more clinically-relevant scenarios. This could include repeated exposure of bacteria on inert surfaces with low-irradiance 405 nm light more representative of levels which would be used for environmental decontamination (<1 mW/cm^2) [15–18], or repeated exposure of organisms on tissue models using higher irradiance light, more suited for representation of wound treatments [12]. It would also be important to investigate if there are any differences when bacteria are dried onto clinical surfaces compared to when suspended in biological fluids such as blood and secretions. A previous study by Murdoch et al. [43], also demonstrated that bacteria can be more susceptible to inactivation when exposed whilst dried onto surfaces and in a desiccated state, and it is reasonable to consider that this increased susceptibility when on surfaces is likely to reduce the likelihood of persistent survival and tolerance/resistance. In addition, if the bacteria are present in biological fluids or embedded in a biological matrix then the inactivation effect could be enhanced by the excitation of photosensitive components present in the biological fluids or matrix (which accelerates the production of ROS) [10, 11]. Conversely it must also be considered that inactivation efficacy of the 405 nm light could be hindered by the opaque transmission properties of the suspending fluid/matrix. Clearly much more research is required to understand not only the tolerance response of bacteria to 405 nm light but also the complex interplay between physico-chemical and environmental factors that can impact on the efficacy of the light induced inactivation in real clinical settings.

Finally, it would also be important to establish the influence of strain variance on the potential for tolerance. Although comparisons were made between methicillin sensitive and resistant strains of *S. aureus* other studies have demonstrated that photodynamic inactivation and violet-light exposure can vary between exposed strains of the same organisms [28, 44].

Conclusions

In conclusion, the results in this study provide novel fundamental information surrounding the potential for tolerance development in proliferating *S. aureus* cultivated in low-level 405 nm light. Additionally no evidence of tolerance was generated in non-proliferating antibiotic sensitive and resistant organisms, following repeated sub-lethal exposure. Repeated sub-lethal exposure was also shown to have little effect on inactivation kinetics or antibiotic susceptibility. Whilst previous studies have established that violet-blue light can be safely used for continuous decontamination in occupied environments [15, 16, 18], wound decontamination in mouse models [13, 20, 27, 45], and that it can inactivate a wide range of microorganisms [5–11], our current findings indicate that in fundamental studies using high-intensity light irradiances, bacterial tolerance is unlikely to occur even after repeated use.

These proof-of-principle results offer additional evidence towards the effective use of antimicrobial 405 nm light for decontamination applications within the clinical setting, however further work is needed to translate these findings to use lower, more clinically-relevant irradiance levels and/or longer duration exposures, relevant for applications such as environmental and wound decontamination.

Abbreviations

$^1O_2$: Singlet oxygen; CFU: Colony forming units; EMRSA – 15/MRSA: Epidemic methicillin-sensitive *Staphylococcus aureus*-15; FHWM: Full width at half maximum; H_2O_2: Hydrogen peroxide; LED: Light emitting diode; MH: Mueller-hinton; MIC: Minimum inhibitory concentration; MSSA: Methicillin-sensitive *Staphylococcus aureus*; NA: Nutrient agar; NB: Nutrient broth; PBS: Phosphate buffered saline; PDI: Photodynamic inactivation; ROS: Reactive oxygen species; SD: Standard deviation; UV: Ultraviolet

Acknowledgements

The authors wish to thank the Scottish Reference Laboratory, Glasgow (SMiRL) who supplied a clinical isolate of EMRSA-15. The authors also wish to thank Mr. Daniel Irving for providing assistance with graphic design and The Robertson Trust for their support.

Funding

RMT would like to thank the Scottish Infection Research Network and Chief Scientist Office for their funding support through a Doctoral Fellowship Award, CSO Reference: SIRN/DTF/13/02. The funders had no role in study design, data collection, analysis and interpretation or in the writing of the manuscript.

Authors' contributions

RMT collected, analysed and interpreted the data regarding bacterial tolerance and was the main author of the manuscript. MM also analysed and interpreted the data and contributed to the writing of the manuscript. All authors helped to design the study, and read and approve the final manuscript.

Consent for publication

N/A.

Competing interests

The authors declare that they have no competing interests.

Author details

[1]The Robertson Trust Laboratory for Electronic Sterilisation Technologies (ROLEST), Department of Electronic & Electrical Engineering, University of Strathclyde, Glasgow, UK. [2]Department of Biomedical Engineering, University of Strathclyde, Glasgow, UK. [3]Department of Clinical Microbiology, Glasgow Royal Infirmary, Glasgow, UK.

References

1. Cosgrove SE. The relationship between antimicrobial resistance and patient outcomes: mortality, length of hospital stay, and health care costs. Clin Infect Dis. 2006;42:S82–9.
2. Hamblin MR, Hasan T. Photodynamic therapy: a new antimicrobial approach to infectious disease? Photochem Photobiol Sci. 2004;3:436–50.
3. Maclean M, MacGregor SJ, Anderson JG, Woolsey G. High-intensity narrow-spectrum light inactivation and wavelength sensitivity of *Staphylococcus aureus*. FEMS Microbiol Lett. 2008;285:227–32.
4. Maclean M, MacGregor SJ, Anderson JG, Woolsey GA. The role of oxygen in the visible-light inactivation of *Staphylococcus aureus*. J Photochem Photobiol B. 2008;92:180–4.
5. Guffey JS, Wilborn J. In vitro bactericidal effects of 405-nm and 470-nm blue light. Photomed Laser Surg. 2006;24:684–8
6. Maclean M, MacGregor SJ, Anderson JG, Woolsey G. Inactivation of bacterial pathogens following exposure to light from a 405-nanometer light-emitting diode array. Appl Environ Microbiol. 2009;75:1932–7.
7. Maclean M, Murdoch LE, MacGregor SJ, Anderson JG. Sporicidal effects of high-intensity 405 nm visible light on endospore-forming bacteria. Photochem Photobiol. 2013;89:120–6.
8. McKenzie K, Maclean M, Timoshkin IV, Endarko E, MacGregor SJ, Anderson JG. Photoinactivation of bacteria attached to glass and acrylic surfaces by 405 nm light: potential application for biofilm decontamination. Photochem Photobiol. 2013;89:927–35.
9. Murdoch LE, McKenzie K, Maclean M, MacGregor SJ, Anderson JG. Lethal effects of high intensity violet 405-nm light on *Saccharomyces cerevisiae, Candida albicans* and on dormant and germinating spores of *Aspergillus niger*. Fungal Biol. 2013;117:519–27.
10. Tomb RM, Maclean M, Herron PR, Hoskisson PA, MacGregor SJ, Anderson JG. Inactivation of *Streptomyces* phage ϕC31 by 405 nm light: requirement for exogenous photosensitizers? Bacteriophage. 2014;4:e32129.
11. Tomb RM, Maclean M, Coia JE, Graham E, McDonald M, Atreya CD, MacGregor SJ, Anderson JG. New proof-of-concept in viral inactivation: virucidal efficacy of 405 nm light against feline calicivirus as a model for norovirus decontamination. Food Environ Virol. 2017;9: 159–67.
12. McDonald R, MacGregor SJ, Anderson JG, Maclean M, Grant MH. Effect of 405-nm high-intensity narrow-spectrum light on fibroblast-populated collagen lattices: an *in vitro* model of wound healing. J Biomed Optic. 2011;16:048003.
13. Dai T, Gupta A, Huang YY, Yin R, Murray CK, Vrahas MS, Sherwood ME, Tegos GP, Hamblin MR. Blue light rescues mice from potentially fatal *Pseudomonas aeruginosa* burn infection: efficacy, safety, and mechanism of action. Antimicrob Agents Chemother. 2013;57:1238–45.
14. Ramakrishnan P, Maclean M, MacGregor SJ, Anderson JG, Grant MH. Cytotoxic responses to 405nm light exposure in mammalian and bacterial cells: involvement of reactive oxygen species. Toxicol in Vitro. 2016;33:54–62.
15. Maclean M, Macgregor SJ, Anderson JG, Woolsey GA, Coia JE, Hamilton K, Taggart I, Watson SB, Thakker B, Gettinby G. Environmental decontamination of a hospital isolation room using high-intensity narrow-spectrum light. J Hosp Infect. 2010;76:247–51.
16. Maclean M, Booth MG, Anderson JG, MacGregor SJ, Woolsey GA, Coia JE, Hamilton K, Gettinby G. Continuous decontamination of an intensive care isolation room during patient occupancy using 405 nm light technology. J Infect Prevent. 2013;14:176–81.
17. Maclean M, McKenzie K, Anderson JG, Gettinby G, MacGregor SJ. 405 nm light technology for the inactivation of pathogens and its potential role for environmental disinfection and infection control. J Hosp Infect. 2014;88:1–11.
18. Bache SE, Maclean M, MacGregor SJ, Anderson JG, Gettinby G, Coia JE, Taggart I. Clinical studies of the high-intensity narrow-spectrum light environmental decontamination system [HINS-light EDS], for continuous disinfection in the burn unit inpatient and outpatient settings. Burns. 2012;38:69–76.
19. Moorhead S, Maclean M, Coia JE, MacGregor SJ, Anderson JG. Synergystic efficacy of 405 nm light and chlorinated disinfectants for enhanced decontamination of *Clostridium difficile* spores. Anaerobe. 2016;37:72–7.
20. Amin RM, Bhayana B, Hamblin MR, Dai T. Antimicrobial blue light inactivation of *Pseudomonas aeruginosa* by photo-excitation of endogenous porphyrins: *In vitro* and *in vivo* studies. Lasers Surg Med. 2016; https://doi.org/10.1002/lsm.22474.
21. Tavares A, Carvalho C, Faustino MA, Neves MG, Tomé JP, Tomé AC, Cavaleiro JAS, Cunha Â, Gomes NCM, Alves E, Almeida A. Antimicrobial photodynamic therapy: study of bacterial recovery viability and potential development of resistance after treatment. Mar Drugs. 2010;8:91–105.
22. Lauro FM, Pretto P, Covolo L, Jori G, Bertoloni G. Photoinactivation of bacterial strains involved in periodontal diseases sensitized by porphycene-polylysine conjugates. Photochem Photobiol Sci. 2002;1:468–70.
23. Pedigo LA, Gibbs AJ, Scott RJ, Street CN. Absence of bacterial resistance following repeat exposure to photodynamic therapy. Proc SPIE. 2009;7380:73803H–1.
24. Giuliani F, Martinelli M, Cocchi A, Arbia D, Fantetti L, Roncucci G. In vitro resistance selection studies of RLP068/Cl, a new Zn[II] phthalocyanine suitable for antimicrobial photodynamic therapy. Antimicrob Agents Chemother. 2010;54:637–42.
25. Bartolomeu M, Rocha S, Cunha Â, Neves MGPMS, Faustino MA, Almeida A. Effect of photodynamic therapy on the virulence factors of *Staphylococcus aureus*. Front Microbiol. 2016;7:267.
26. Guffey JS, Payne W, Jones T, Martin K. Evidence of resistance development by *Staphylococcus aureus* to an in vitro, multiple stage application of 405 nm light from a supraluminous diode array. Photomed Laser Surg. 2013;31:179–82.
27. Zhang Y, Zhu Y, Gupta A, Huang Y, Murray CK, Vrahas MS, Sherwood ME, Baer DG, Hamblin MR, Dai T. Antimicrobial blue light therapy for multidrug-resistant *Acinetobacter baumannii* infection in a mouse burn model: implications for prophylaxis and treatment of combat-related wound infections. J Infect Dis. 2014;209:1963–71.
28. Lipovsky A, Nitzan Y, Friedmann H, Lubart R. Sensitivity of *Staphylococcus aureus* strains to broadband visible light. Photochem Photobiol. 2009;85:255–60.
29. Matuschek E, Brown DFJ, Kahlmeter G. Development of the EUCAST disk diffusion antimicrobial susceptibility testing method and its implementation in routine microbiology laboratories. Clin Microbiol Infect. 2014;20:O255–66.
30. Maisch T. Resistance in antimicrobial photodynamic inactivation of bacteria. Photochem Photobiol Sci. 2015;14:1518–26.
31. Dosselli R, Millioni R, Puricelli L, Tessari P, Arrigoni G, Franchin C, Segalla A, Teardo E, Reddi E. Molecular targets of antimicrobial photodynamic therapy identified by a proteomic approach. J Proteome. 2012;77:329–43.
32. Liu GY, Essex A, Buchanan JT, Datta V, Hoffman HM, Bastian JF, Fierer J, Nizet V. *Staphylococcus aureus* golden pigment impairs neutrophil killing and promotes virulence through its antioxidant activity. J Exp Med. 2005;202:209–15.
33. Nakonieczna J, Michta E, Rybicka M, Grinholc M, Gwizdek-Wiśniewska A, Bielawski KP. Superoxide dismutase is upregulated in *Staphylococcus aureus* following protoporphyrin-mediated photodynamic inactivation and does not directly influence the response to photodynamic treatment. BMC Microbiol. 2010;10:323.
34. St Denis TG, Huang L, Dai T, Hamblin MR. Analysis of the bacterial heat shock response to photodynamic therapy-mediated oxidative stress. Photochem Photobiol. 2011;87:707–13.
35. McKenzie K, Maclean M, Timoshkin IV, MacGregor SJ, Anderson JG. Bactericidal effect of 405nm light on *Escherichia coli* and *Listeria monocytogenes* in the presence of sub-lethal stress. Int J Food Microbiol. 2014;170:91–8.
36. Santos AL, Gomes NCM, Henriques I, Almeida A, Correia A, Cunha Â. Contribution of reactive oxygen species to UV-B-induced damage in bacteria. J Photochem Photobiol B Biol. 2012;117:40–6.

37. Pendleton JN, Gorman SP, Gilmore BF. Clinical relevance of the ESKAPE pathogens. Expert Rev Anti-Infect Ther. 2013;11:297–308.
38. Vasoo S, Barreto JN, Tosh PK. Emerging issues in gram-negative bacterial resistance: an update for the practicing clinician. Mayo Clin Proc. 2015;90:395–403.
39. Koutsoumanis KP, Kendall PA, Sofos JN. Effect of food processing related stresses on acid tolerance of *Listeria monocytogenes*. Appl Environ Microbiol. 2003;69:514–7516.
40. McMahon MA, Xu J, Moore JE, Blair IS, McDowell DA. Environmental stress and antibiotic resistance in food-related pathogens. Appl Environ Microbiol. 2007;73:211–7.
41. Grinholc M, Szramka B, Olender K, Graczyk A. Bactericidal effect of photodynamic therapy against methicillin-resistant *Staphylococcus aureus* strain with the use of various porphyrin photosensitizers. Acta Biochim Pol. 2007;54:665–70.
42. Boyce JM. Modern technologies for improving cleaning and disinfection of environmental surfaces in hospitals. Antimicrob Res Infect Cont. 2016;5:10.
43. Murdoch LE, Maclean M, Endarko E, MacGregor SJ, Anderson JG. Bactericidal effects of 405 nm light exposure demonstrated by inactivation of *Escherichia*, *Salmonella*, *Shigella*, *Listeria*, and *Mycobacterium* species in liquid suspensions and on exposed surfaces. Sci World J. 2012;2012:137805.
44. Halstead FD, Thwaite JE, Burt R, Laws TR, Raguse M, Moeller R, Webber MA, Oppenheim BA. Antibacterial activity of blue light against nosocomial wound pathogens growing planktonically and as mature biofilms. Appl Environ Microbiol. 2016;82:4006–16.
45. Dai T, Gupta A, Huang YY, Sherwood ME, Murray CK, Vrahas MS, Kielian T, Hamblin MR. Blue light eliminates community-acquired methicillin-resistant *Staphylococcus aureus* in infected mouse skin abrasions. Photomed Laser Surg. 2013;11:531–8.

14

High burden of antimicrobial resistance among gram negative bacteria causing healthcare associated infections in a critical care unit of Nepal

Narayan Prasad Parajuli[1,2*], Subhash Prasad Acharya[3], Shyam Kumar Mishra[1], Keshab Parajuli[1], Basista Prasad Rijal[1] and Bharat Mani Pokhrel[1]

Abstract

Background: Healthcare associated infections (HCAI) and antimicrobial resistance are principal threats to the patients of intensive care units and are the major determining factors for patient outcome. They are associated with increased morbidity, mortality, excess hospitalization and financial costs. The present study is an attempt to investigate the spectrum and antimicrobial resistance of bacterial isolates involved in healthcare associated infections (HCAI) in the patients of a critical care unit at a tertiary care university hospital in Kathmandu, Nepal.

Methods: A laboratory based study was conducted over the period of 15 months (January 2014 to March 2015) among the patients of intensive care unit of Tribhuvan University Teaching Hospital, Kathmandu, Nepal. Clinical specimens from patients with suspected healthcare-associated infection were processed and bacterial isolates were identified with standard microbiological methods. Antimicrobial susceptibilities of the isolated strains were determined according to the CLSI guidelines and β-lactamases (ESBL, AmpC, MBL and KPC) were detected by various phenotypic tests.

Results: One hundred and forty nine clinical specimens received from 135 patients suspected of HCAI (out of 491 patients) were found with significant bacterial growth. Specimens were from patients suspected of hospital-acquired pneumonia (16%, 79/491), bloodstream infections (5.7%, 28/491), surgical site infections (4.7%, 23/491), and urinary tract infections (3.9%, 19/491). *Acinetobacter* spp., *Klebsiella* spp., *Escherichia coli* and *Burkholderia cepacia* were the leading bacterial pathogens. Extremely high level of drug resistance (95.8%) along with the production of β-lactamases (ESBL; 43.7%, AmpC; 27.5%), MBL; 50.2% and KPC; 4.2%) was observed among Gram negative bacterial isolates.

Conclusion: Healthcare associated infections are very common in our ICU. Gram negative bacterial pathogens are major culprits associated with these infections and there is alarming state of drug resistance among these isolates. Continuous surveillance and establishment of preventive and control measures of healthcare associated infections are urgently needed in our setting.

Keywords: Healthcare associated infections, ICU, MDR bacteria, β-lactamases, Nepal

* Correspondence: narayan.parajuli@iom.edu.np
[1]Department of Clinical Microbiology, Institute of Medicine, Tribhuvan University Teaching Hospital, Kathmandu, Nepal
[2]Department of Laboratory Medicine, Manmohan Memorial Institute of Health Sciences, Khola Pravesh Marg, Soalteemode, P.O. Box No. 15201, Kathmandu, Nepal
Full list of author information is available at the end of the article

Background

Infection is the most common presentation among hospitalized patients of intensive care unit (ICU), and in many instances, is a determining factor for patient outcomes [1, 2]. Healthcare associated infections (HCAIs), in particular, are the major risks associated with critically ill patients of ICU, due to the reduced host defenses, frequent use of invasive medical devices, administration of multiple drugs, cross transmission of pathogens among patients and staffs, and inadequate infection control procedures [3, 4]. Hence, intensive care units (ICUs) are now often recognised as the epicenter of infections in the hospital [5]. Pneumonia, surgical-site infections, catheter-related bloodstream infections and urinary tract infections are currently the most common cause of death in ICU due to healthcare associated infections [6]. According to a large surveillance study, more than 70% of critically ill patients receive an antimicrobial drug during their ICU stay either for prophylaxis or for therapy [1]. Nevertheless, in the recent years, therapeutic drugs are being progressively ineffective against bacterial infections, threatning the success of routine treatment [7]. The major consequences of this problem are increased patient morbidity, mortality, health care related expenses and treatment failure [8, 9].

β-lactam antibiotics are the major bulk of prescribed antibiotics in ICUs across the globe because of their efficacy, broad spectra and low toxicity [10]. However, irrational use of these antibiotics has resulted in the development and spread of drug resistant bacterial pathogens especially in the developing countries [11]. Of the particular concern, increased occurrence of Gram negative bacteria, including multidrug resistant nonfermenters (*Acinetobacter baumannii and Pseudomonas* species) and Enterobacteriaceae producing extended-spectrum beta-lactamase(ESBL) and carbapenemases in severe healthcare-associated infections has evolved as a significant clinical threat for medical fraternity in the recent decades [12, 13]. The broad substrate profile of these enzymes may affect entire beta lactam agents, and also the organisms with these enzymes are additionally found resistant to aminoglycosides and fluoroquinolones, further compromising the therapeutic choices for severe infections in ICU [14, 15].

In Nepal, international guidelines on initial antibiotic selection are generally applied in ICUs and empiric choices are made for serious ICU related infections. Thorough knowledge of epidemiology, spectrum and nature of infections along with susceptibilities of causative organisms are extremely valuable for empirical treatment of severe infections in intensive care hospital settings. Therefore, it would be an effective measure for policy formulation of judicious antimicrobial therapy for critically ill patients in the intensive care units of various hospitals in our country. In this perspective, we aimed to determine the incidence of multidrug resistant bacteria, their susceptibilities and common mechanisms of drug resistance involved in healthcare associated infections in the critically ill patients of an intensive care unit at a tertiary care teaching hospital in Kathmandu, Nepal.

Methods

A laboratory based study was conducted at the department of clinical microbiology of the Tribhuvan University Teaching Hospital in Kathmandu, Nepal from January 2014 to March 2015 (over a period of 15 months). All clinical specimens from the patients suspected of healthcare associated infections (after 48 h of admission to the ICU) representing various body systems viz. blood, urine, endotracheal aspirate (ETA), bronchoalveolar lavage fluid (BAL), pleural fluid, pus, peritoneal fluid, cerebrospinal fluid (CSF), CSF shunt, central venous catheter (CVC) etc. were included in the study. The specimens were collected appropriately by trained ICU nurses and transported to the clinical microbiology laboratory with minimal time delay. Specimens that strictly met the criteria recommended by the American Society for Microbiology (ASM) [16] were selected for further processing and analysis. However, specimens not fulfilling the ASM criteria and duplicate specimens from the same patient were excluded.

Inoculation of the specimen and identification of the isolates

The clinical specimens were inoculated onto suitable culture medium according to their specific requirements. Respiratory specimens and CSF samples were cultured on Chocolate agar (CHA), 5% Sheep Blood Agar (BA) and MacConkey Agar (MA) (HiMedia, Mumbai, India) plates. Blood specimens were first enriched with Brain Heart Infusion broth (BHI) and then subcultured on to the 5% Sheep Blood Agar (BA) and MacConkey Agar (MA) (HiMedia, Mumbai, India) plates. The vascular catheter tips (CVC tips) were inoculated onto 5% Sheep blood Agar (BA), MacConkey agar (MA) (HiMedia Mumbai, India) according to Maki's roll plate method [17] by semiquantitative technique. Similarly, surgical specimens, wound swab, pus and urine specimens were plated onto 5% Sheep Blood Agar (BA) and MacConkey Agar (MA) (HiMedia, Mumbai, India) plates. The CHA plates were incubated in a CO_2 incubator (10% CO_2) at 37 °C for 24 h. The BA and MA plates were incubated at 37 °C for 24 h in an aerobic atmosphere. Identification of significant isolates that are associated with healthcare associated infections was performed following standard microbiological techniques which involved morphological appearance of the colonies; Gram's staining, catalase test, coagulase test, oxidase test with other biochemical parameters [16]. Assurance of pure culture inoculum was done by setting purity plate along with the biochemical tests.

Antibiotic susceptibility testing
The susceptibility of bacterial isolates against different antibiotics was determined by the disk diffusion method [modified Kirby-Bauer method] on Mueller Hinton agar (Hi-Media, India) following standard procedures recommended by the Clinical and Laboratory Standards Institute (CLSI), Wayne, USA [18]. For this purpose following antibiotics with specified concentrations were used; ampicillin (10 μg), ampicillin-sulbactam (10/10 μg), ceftazidime (30 μg), ceftriaxone (30 μg), cefepime (30 μg), cefoxitin (30 μg), piperacillin-tazobactam (100/10 μg, aztreonam (30 μg), imipenem (10 μg), meropenem (10 μg), gentamycin (10 μg), amikacin (30 μg), ciprofloxacin (5 μg), ofloxacin (5 μg), levofloxacin (5 μg), trimethoprim-sulphamethoxazole/co-trimoxazole (25 μg), polymixin B (300unit), colistin sulphate (10 μg)] and tigecycline (30 μg) from HiMedia Laboratories, India. Interpretations of antibiotic susceptibility results were made according to the guidelines of interpretative zone diameters of CLSI [18]. *Escherichia coli* ATCC 25922 and *Pseudomonas aeruginosa* ATCC 27853 were used as the control organisms for antibiotic sensitivity.

Identification of Multidrug Resistant (MDR), Extensively Drug Resistant (XDR) and Pan Drug Resistance (PDR) isolates
Multidrug resistant (MDR) bacterial isolates were identified according to the criteria recommended by international expert committee of the European Centre for Disease Prevention and Control (ECDC) and the Centers for Disease Control and Prevention (CDC) [19]. In this study, the isolate resistant to at least one antimicrobial from three different group of first line drugs tested was regarded as multidrug resistant (MDR). Extensively drug resistant (XDR) isolates were identified when the isolates were resistant to at least one agent in all but two or fewer antimicrobial categories (i.e. bacterial isolates remain susceptible to only one or two categories). Pan drug resistant (PDR) was defined as non-susceptibility to all agents in all antimicrobial categories (i.e. no agents tested were susceptible for that organism) [19].

Detection of ESBL, MBL, AmpC and KPC β-lactamases
Testing of extended spectrum β-lactamase (ESBL) producers
The initial screening test for the ESBL production was performed by using one of three antibiotics; ceftriaxone (CRO 30 μg), ceftazidime (CAZ 30 μg) or cefotaxime (CTX 30 μg) disks (HiMedia, Mumbai, India). If the zone of inhibition (ZOI) was ≤25 mm for CRO,≤22 mm for CAZ and/or ≤ 27 mm for CTX, the isolate was considered a potential ESBL producer as recommended by CLSI [18]. Isolates that were suspected as ESBL-producer by screen test were tested further by combination disk test (CDT). In this test, Ceftazidime (30 μg) disks alone and in combination with clavulanic acid (ceftazidime + clavulanic Acid, 30/10 μg) disks, were applied onto a plate of Mueller Hinton Agar (MHA) which was inoculated with the test strain and then incubated in ambient air for 16-18 h of incubation at 35 ± 2 °C. Isolate that showed increase of ≥5 mm in the zone of inhibition of the combination discs in comparison to that of the ceftazidime disk alone was considered an ESBL producer [18].

Testing of metallo β-lactamase (MBL) producers
Isolates that were found non-susceptible to third generation cephalosporins (ceftazidime), imipenem or meropenem in Kirby Bauer disk diffusion method were presumptively considered MBL producers and were confirmed by the imipenem disk with ethylene diamine tetra acetic acid (EDTA) method. Briefly, the test inoculums (comparable to 0.5 McFarland standards) were prepared and transferred on to Mueller Hinton agar plates. In the combination disk test for MBL, two imipenem (IPM) disks (10 μg), a plain imipenem disk and another containing 10 μl of 0.1 M (292 μg) anhydrous EDTA (Sigma Chemicals, St. Louis, MO), were placed 20 mm apart. An increase in the zone size of more than or equal to 7 mm for imipenem-EDTA disk compared to imipenem disk alone indicated MBL producer strain as described by Yong et al. [20].

Testing of AmpC β-lactamase producers
Screening of AmpC β-lactamase production was carried out by cefoxitin disk. Isolates that yielded a zone diameter less than 18 mm (screen positive) were further subjected to confirmatory testing. Cefoxitin (30 μg) disk alone and cefoxitin (30 μg) disk containing 10 μl of 300 μg/ml PBA (Phenyl Boronic Acid) were placed at 20 mm distance. An increase in zone of inhibition by at least 5 mm around Cefoxitin disk containing Boronic acid after overnight incubation at 37 °C were considered as positive for AmpC production by the isolates [21].

Testing of *Klebsiella pneumoniae* carbapenemase (KPC) producers
The isolates that tested for MBL detection were also subjected to KPC production. Phenotypic test for KPC detection was performed by combination disk method. In this test, meropenem (MEM) (10 μg) disk alone and a meropenem disk containing 10 μl (300 μg/ml) 3-AminoPhenyl Boronic Acid (3-APBA) (Tokyo Chemical Co. Ltd., Japan) were placed 20 mm apart centre to centre. An increase in zone diameter of more than 5 mm around the MEM- PBA disk compared to that of

the MEM disk alone was considered positive for KPC. To exclude the AmpC overproduction in the same isolate, four disk test for differentiation of carbapenemeses described by Tsakris et al. was used [22].

Ethical consideration

Written approval (Ref No: 129(6-11-E)/2070/71) was obtained from Institutional Review Board (IRB) of Institute of Medicine after submitting and presenting research proposal. In addition, written consent was taken from every patient or their guardian for participation into this study before enrollment.

Data processing and analysis

Data regarding patient demographics, HCAI types, bacterial isolates, antimicrobial susceptibilities and resistance determinants were entered in to a computer program. Data were analyzed using SPSS 20.0 version and interpreted according to frequency distribution, percentage.

Results

Patient demographics

During the study period, a total of 568 patients were admitted to the intensive care unit of our hospital. Forty six patients were transferred to another unit, 17 died and 14 patients left against medical advice within 48 h of their admission. Among 491 patients stayed more than 48 h in the ICU, male patients (280/491, 57%) were more than their female counterparts (211/491, 43%). The median age of patient was 41.4 years (IQR; 35-60) and maximum numbers of patients were from the age group 46-55 years.

Distribution of specimens by suspected HCAI

After clinico-bacteriological analysis, 149 clinical specimens received from 135 patients (out of 491 patients admitted to the ICU) suspected of HCAI were found to be associated with significant bacterial growth. Among specimens with significant growth, majority were from suspected hospital acquired pneumonia [(53.0%, 79/149), (overall; 16.0%, 79/491)] followed by bloodstream infections [(18.8%, 28/149), (overall; 5.7%, 28/491)], surgical site infections [(15.4%, 23/149), overall (4.7%, 23/491)] and urinary tract infections (12.8%,19/149), overall (3.9%, 19/491)] (Table 1).

Table 1 Distribution of specimens by suspected Healthcare Associated Infections (HCAI)

Type of Infections	No.	%	Overall incidence %
Hospital acquired pneumonia	79	53.0	16.0
Bloodstream infections	28	18.8	5.7
Surgical site infections	23	15.4	4.7
Urinary tract infections	19	12.8	3.9
Total	149	100.0	27.4

Distribution of bacterial isolates

Diverse bacterial etiology was noted among HCAIs (Table 2). *Acinetobacter* spp. (51, 34.9%) was the leading organism followed by *Klebsiella* spp. (37, 25.3%), *Escherichia coli* (31, 21.2%), and *Pseudomonas* spp. (24, 16.4%). Hospital acquired pneumonia were predominantly associated with *Acinetobacter* spp. (38.1%) and *Klebsiella* spp. (21.6%) while bloodstream infections were caused by *Burkholderia cepacia* (47.3%), surgical site infections caused by *Pseudomonas* spp. (31.0%) and urinary tract infections caused by *Klebsiella* spp. (42.8%). Among total 28 bloodstream infections, 19 were associated with Gram negative bacteria and remaining 9 were Gram positive bacteria (data not presented).

Antimicrobial susceptibility pattern of isolates

Antibiogram of nonfermenters

Gram negative nonfermenters were variably resistant to tested antimicrobials (Table 3). Entire isolates of *Acinetobacter* and *Burkholderia* spp. were resistant to cephalosporins, while almost 92% of *Pseudomonas* spp. were cephalosporin resistant. Resistant to fluoroquinolones was observed higher (upto100%) in *Burkholderia* spp. when compared to that in *Acinetobacter* spp. (94.2%) and *Pseudomonas* spp. (95.8%). Carbapenems, the preferred regimens in ICU, were highly resistant in *Acinetobacter* spp. (upto86.4%) and *Pseudomonas* spp. (62.5%) but were effective against *Burkholderia* spp. (20% resistance).

Antibiogram of Enterobacterial isolates

In this study, entire isolates of enterobacteriaceae were resistant to third generation cephalosporins. *Klebsiella* spp. were resistant to ciprofloxacin (86.4%), gentamycin (83.7%), piperacillin tazobactam (81.0%) and imipenem (48.6%). Almost similar rates of resistance were observed in *Escherichia coli,* except for carbapenems (19.3% resistance). Although, the number of *Citrobacter* spp. was small, majority of them were resistant to cephalosporins, fluoroquinolones and aminoglycosides (Table 4).

MDR, XDR and β-lactamase producing bacterial isolates

Nearly 96% of the Gram negative bacterial isolates causing nosocomial infections were found multidrug resistant and 43.3% isolates were extensively drug resistant (XDR). In this study, rates of beta lactamase producing bacterial isolates was extremely high (ESBL; 43.7%, AmpC; 27.5%), MBL; 50.2% and KPC; 4.2%). *Escherichia coli* was major ESBL producer (70.9%) followed by *Citrobacter* spp. (62.5%) and *Klebsiella* spp. (59.4%). Major MBL enzyme producers were *Acinetobacter* spp. (78.8%),

Table 2 Distribution of Bacterial isolates

Bacterial isolates	Total number (%)			
	HAP(*n* = 79)	BSI(*n* = 28)	SSI (*n* = 23)	UTI (*n* = 19)
Acinetobacter spp. (*n* = 51)	37(38.1)	3(15.7)	7(24.1)	4(19.0)
Klebsiella spp. (*n* = 37)	21(21.6)	1(5.2)	6(20.6)	9(42.8)
Escherichia coli (*n* = 31)	19(19.5)	5(26.3)	2(6.9)	5(23.9)
Pseudomonas spp.(*n* = 24)	12(12.4)	0(0.0)	9(31.0)	3(14.3)
Burkholderia cepacia (*n* = 14)	6(6.2)	9(47.3)	0(0.0)	0(0.0)
Citrobacter spp. (*n* = 8)	2(2.0)	1(5.2)	5(17.2)	0(0.0)
Total isolates (*n* = 165)	97(100.0)	19(100.0)	29(100.0)	21(100.0)

Pseudomonas spp. (62.5%) and *Klebsiella* spp. (48.6%). Small proportion of *Klebsiella* (10.8%) and *Acinetobacter* spp. (5.7%) were KPC producers (Table 5).

Discussion

Increased consumption of antimicrobial regimens, higher prevalence and dissemination of drug resistance among nosocomial pathogens and poor infection control strategies for prevention of healthcare associated infections are the rising problems in Nepalese hospitals [23]. The problem is several-folds high in the intensive care units where collection of severely ill patients from all over the hospital units with varieties of pathological profile and etiological agents exists. Therefore, identification of the underlying pattern of drug resistance among microorganisms in every hospital is the key to success in the appropriate treatment of patients. This issue is of interest especially in Nepalese ICUs where the highest prevalence of patients on antibiotic treatment is frequently reported.

The rate of healthcare associated infections varies globally and higher rates have been reported from developing countries [24]. Moreover, the type of hospital setting (ward or intensive care unit), patient population and the precise definition and surveillance techniques used to identify the healthcare associated infections are responsible for variable incidences [25]. Healthcare associated infections are frequent in our study as previously described by Sah et al. from same hospital [26], although they have included the patients from all sections of hospital, providing heterogeneity of the cases. However, extremely high incidences have been documented in recent reports from India (11.9-17.7%) [27, 28]. In the well

Table 3 Antibiogram of Nonfermenters (*n* = 90)

Antibiotics	% Resistance among bacterial isolates		
	Acinetobacter spp. (*n* = 51)	*P. aeruginosa* (*n* = 24)	*Burkholderia* spp. (*n* = 15)
Cotrimoxazole	100	-	0
Ceftazidime	100	91.6	100
Cefepime	100	91.6	100
Ciprofloxacin	94.2	95.8	100
Levofloxacin	76.5	87.5	93.3
Gentamycin	92.2	62.5	86.6
Amikacin	84.4	37.5	67
Piperacillin Tazobactam	92.2	67	60
Ampicillin Sulbactam	92.2	-	-
Cefoperazone Sulbactam	90.2	67	86.6
Imipenem	86.4	62.5	20
Meropenem	84.4	62.5	20
Polymixin B	0	0	–
Colistin Sulphate	0	0	–
Tigecycline	0	–	–

Table 4 Antibiogram of Enterobacterial isolates (*n* = 76)

Antibiotics	% Resistance among bacterial isolates		
	Escherichia coli (*n* = 31)	*Klebsiella* spp. (*n* = 37)	*Citrobacter* spp. (*n* = 8)
Ampicillin	100	–	–
Cotrimoxazole	64.5	100	100
Cefotaxime	100	100	100
Cefepime	100	100	100
Ciprofloxacin	90.3	86.4	100
Levofloxacin	77.4	72.9	100
Gentamycin	64.5	83.7	100
Amikacin	45.1	83.7	100
Piperacillin Tazobactam	48.3	81.0	87.5
Cefoperazone Sulbactam	48.3	83.7	87.5
Imipenem	19.3	48.6	25
Meropenem	19.3	48.6	25
Polymixin B	0	0	0
Colistin Sulphate	0	0	0
Tigecycline	0	0	0

Table 5 MDR,XDR and β-lactamse producing bacterial isolates

Bacterial isolates	% MDR	% XDR	β- lactamases producers			
			% ESBL	% MBL	% AmpC	% KPC
Escherichia coli	100	19.3	70.9	16.1	38.7	0
Klebsiella spp.	100	48.6	59.4	48.6	32.4	10.8
Acinetobacter spp.	94.2	84.4	15.4	78.8	42.3	5.7
Pseudomonas spp.	83.3	62.5	33.4	62.5	–	0
Burkholderia spp.	100	20	53.4	20	–	0
Citrobacter spp.	100	25	62.5	25	–	0
Total	95.8	43.3	43.7	50.2	27.5	4.2

known EPIC II study by Vincent et al., 51% of the patients in ICU were found infected [1]. Another multicentre cohort study yielded the rate of infections in ICU patients around the globe to be ranging from 2.3 to 49.3% [29]. However, the higher rates in multicentre studies are due to the heterogeneous patients, study parameters, voluntary participation and reporting, as well as the variation in surveillance techniques [30].

We observed hospital acquired pneumonia (53%) to be the most common healthcare associated infection in this study, followed by bloodstream infections (18.8%), surgical site infections (15.4%) and urinary tract infections (12.8%) which are comparable to the findings of large EPIC II study [1]. Similar findings were also been reported from epidemiological study of infections in ICU population by Cosic et al. from Brazil [31] and Dasgupta et al. from India [28]. However, in a recent report, Mythri and Kashinath pointed UTI as the most common infection, followed by pneumonia and surgical site infections [27]. The site distribution of infections in various studies might be attributable to the type of ICUs and patient population. Our report broadly corroborates to the findings of earlier studies mentioned above.

Non fermentative Gram negative bacteria including enterobacteriaceae are increasingly reported as the cause of healthcare associated infections worldwide [32]. *Acinetobacter* species, major pathogenic organism in health-care-associated infections, was found to be the most common organisms in our ICU. Majority of the infections associated with *Acinetobacter* were pneumonia and surgical site infections. Similar spectrum of bacterial pathogens in healthcare associated infections in ICU has been documented by other studies too [26, 33]. However, *Burkholderia cepacia* was the most common bacteria isolated from bloodstream infections in our ICU. Increased use of pharmaceutical derivatives and accumulation of sicker patients with variable infections might be the reason for our shifting etiology.

Antimicrobial resistance is a recognized problem in South Asian region with high levels of resistance among Gram negative organisms reported frequently [34]. It is well known fact that resistance is due to extreme antimicrobial consumption [11], and overuse of antibiotics can be surmised as one of the factors contributing to the high rates of antimicrobial resistance in Nepal. In this study, many microorganisms found as resistant to different antimicrobial agents and in some cases to nearly all agents representing an alarming scenario in our intensive care setting. Nearly 96% of the Gram negative bacterial isolates causing nosocomial infections were found multidrug resistant, which is highest ever rate of MDR bacteria reported from our country. Earlier reports from Nepal have reported upto 95% of the nosocomial isolates as drug resistant [35, 36]. Further in this study, not only the isolates were multidrug resistant, a significant proportion (43.3%) of our isolates was extensively drug resistant (XDR). The high level of drug resistance in Gram negative isolates have been described as a result of the production of different -lactamases, multiple efflux pumps, decreased drug uptake, and other drug modifying enzymes [37].

Gram negative non-fermenters were more resistant to antimicrobial drugs in this study. *Acinetobacter* isolates were found highly resistant to carbapenem (86.4%), aminoglycosides (93%) and cephalosporins (100%) groups of antibiotics which is nearly twofold high than that reported by Mishra et al. from same hospital (nearly 89% resistance in cephalosporins and 50% in carbapenem) [35]. However, the resistance rate of Gram negative nonfermenters in our study is comparable to the study of Xia et al. from China [38] and Fatima et al. from Pakistan [39]. Moreover, a SENTRY study also reported that Gram negative bacterial resistance to imipenem changed from 34.5% in 2006 to 59.8% in 2009 across the world [40]. In addition to this, the increasing emergence of highly aminoglycosides-resistant strains is also cause of major concern. Our result on amikacin resistance (up to 85%) is higher than that (54%) of previous study from same hospital [35]. Although none of the *Acinetobacter* strains in our study was tigecycline and colistin resistant, it has been indicated as an emerging therapeutic problem which may severely compromise the treatment of MDR *Acinetobacter* spp. infections [41]. This high prevalence of multi drug resistance in *Acinetobacter spp.* may be due to high chance of acquisition of resistance gene and their ability to persist and multiply in hospital environment [42]. On the other hand, *Pseudomonas aeruginosa* and *Burkholderia cepacia* are intrinsically resistant to several antibiotics because of the low permeability of their outer-membrane, the constitutive expression of various efflux pumps, and the production of antibiotic-inactivating enzymes (e.g., cephalosporinases) [43].

Enterobacteriaceae, including *Escherichia coli, Klebsiella* spp. and *Citrobacter* spp. were also found resistant to multiple antibiotics. Resistance of enterobacterial strains towards cephalosporins (100%), fluoroquinolones (86.4 to 100%), aminoglycosides (45.1 to 100%) and carbapenems (19.3 to 48.6%) was considerably high when compared to the reported rates from previous studies [36, 44]. However, tigecycline and polymixins showed excellent effect against MDR Gram-negative enterobacterial isolates. High antibiotic resistance rate against commonly used antibiotics is a disadvantage for health care system in countries like Nepal as it can greatly affect patient management especially in critical care units.

Beta lactamases are the hydrolytic enzymes thwarting the functional part of β-lactam antibiotics used for the treatment of most bacterial infections. The menacing state of resistance in Gram negative isolates towards the cephalosporins, carbapenems and other antibiotics could be attributed to ESBL, AmpC β-lactamase, carbapenamase producers and some other relevant underlying mechanisms [45]. In this study, the rates of beta lactamase production, including ESBL, AmpC, MBL, and KPC were alarmingly high. *Escherichia coli, Klebsiella* spp., *Citrobacter* spp., *Pseudomonas* spp. and *Burkholderia* spp. were major ESBL producers. Previously, Shrestha et al. in 2011 have also reported 28.57% of *Escherichia coli*, 8.33% of *Klebsiella spp.* and 2.38% of *Pseudomonas aeruginosa* were ESBL producers [46]. However, in an Indian study, the rate of ESBL production among nosocomial isolates was 50% in *Escherichia coli* and 67% in *Klebsiella pneumoniae* respectively [41]. Variations in ESBL rates may be ascribed to antibiotic prescribing habits and endemicity of pathogens harboring the genes for ESBL production. Furthermore, we detect 27.5% AmpC producing isolates, including *Acinetobacter spp.* (42.3%) followed by *Escherichia coli* (38.7%) and *Klebsiella pneumoniae* (32.4%) which is comparative to the previous reports of Baral et al. [47] and Khanal et al. [36] from nearby hospital. However, in an Indian study lower rate (14.2%) of AmpC producing isolates were documented [48].

High resistance of carbapenems in our study has been supported by the detection of carbapenemase enzyme in the bacterial isolates. Major bacterial isolates producing MBL were *Acinetobacter* spp., *Pseudomonas* spp., *Klebsiella* spp. and *Burkholderia* spp. Although, till date, there is no single article regarding detection of KPC from Nepal, this study attempted to find out the KPC producing bacterial isolates in ICU population. In Nepal, carbapenamase producing bacteria are poorly reported. Mishra et al. documented the rate of MBL producers to be 1.3% including *Acinetobacter* (4.3%), *Pseudomonas* (3.3%) [49], but in a study by Shrestha et al. the rate of MBL was 17.43% among nosocomial isolates including *Acinetobacter* (47.22%), *Pseudomonas* (2.38%) and of *Klebsiella* spp. (4.17%) [46]. The emergence of carbapenamase in Gram negative bacilli is becoming a therapeutic challenge as these enzymes possess high hydrolytic activity that leads to degradation of higher generation cephalosporins and carbapenems. Furthermore, these plasmid mediated genes have the ability spread rapidly to other species of Gram negative bacilli [50]. Therefore rapid detection of these resistance determinants is necessary to modify therapy and to initiate effective infection control to prevent their dissemination.

Limitations

We could not evaluate the risk factors and outcomes of nosocomial infections associated with drug resistant bacteria. Due to the unavailability of sufficient data from the patients without healthcare associated infections, statistical comparison between the patients with and without healthcare associated infections could not been made. Further, it was limited to a mixed adult ICU of a teaching hospital leaving other surgical and pediatric ICU patients. Furthermore, molecular characterization of the resistant phenotypes and their epidemiology would be more significant in public health perspective.

Conclusion

From this study, it becomes clear that healthcare associated infections caused by drug resistant bacteria are major problems in our ICU. Menacing state of drug resistance among Gram negative pathogens associated with these infections is particularly worrisome. It is very important to control this situation before it takes a deadly shape. Established recommendations including adequately identifying the pathogen, choosing correct antibiotics, limiting their excess use, improving resistance surveillance systems will help controlling this situation.

Abbreviations

ASM: American Society for Microbiology; BSI: Bloodstream infection; CLSI: Clinical and Laboratory Standards Institute; ESBL: Extended spectrum β-lactamases; HAP: Hospital acquired pneumonia; HCAI: Healthcare associated infection; ICU: Intensive care unit; KPC: Klebsiella pneumoniae carbapenamase; MBL: Metallo β-lactamases; MDR: Multidrug resistant; SSI: Surgical site infection; UTI: Urinary tract infection; XDR: Extensively drug resistant

Funding

No monetary benefit was received for this study.

Authors' contributions

NPP and BMP- conceived the design of study, reviewed the literature performed necessary interventions including laboratory investigations. NPP, SPA, SKM, KP and BPR- case identification, entry and data analysis. NPP-prepared the manuscript with the help of SPA, SKM, KP, BPR and BMP. All authors read the final version of manuscript and approved for publication.

Competing interests

The authors declare that they have no competing interests.

Consent for publication
Informed consent for relevant investigations and publication of the findings were taken from every patient and co-authors.

Author details
[1]Department of Clinical Microbiology, Institute of Medicine, Tribhuvan University Teaching Hospital, Kathmandu, Nepal. [2]Department of Laboratory Medicine, Manmohan Memorial Institute of Health Sciences, Khola Pravesh Marg, Soalteemode, P.O. Box No. 15201, Kathmandu, Nepal. [3]Department of Anesthesiology and Critical Care, Institute of Medicine, Tribhuvan University Teaching Hospital, Kathmandu, Nepal.

References
1. Vincent JL, Rello J, Marshall J, Silva E, Anzueto A, Martin CD, et al. International study of the prevalence and outcomes of infection in intensive care units. JAMA. 2009;302(21):2323–9.
2. Vincent JL, Bihari DJ, Suter PM, Bruining HA, White J, Nicolas-Chanoin MH, et al. The prevalence of nosocomial infection in intensive care units in Europe. Results of the European Prevalence of Infection in Intensive Care (EPIC) Study. EPIC International Advisory Committee. JAMA. 1995; 274(8):639–44.
3. Trilla A. Epidemiology of nosocomial infections in adult intensive care units. Intensive Care Med. 1994;20(Suppl 3):S1–4.
4. Majumdar SS, Padiglione AA. Nosocomial infections in the intensive care unit. Anaesth Intens Care Med. 13(5):204–8.
5. Brusselaers N, Vogelaers D, Blot S. The rising problem of antimicrobial resistance in the intensive care unit. Ann Intensive Care. 2011;1:47.
6. Meric M, Baykara N, Aksoy S, Kol IO, Yilmaz G, Beyazit N, et al. Epidemiology and risk factors of intensive care unit-acquired infections: a prospective multicentre cohort study in a middle-income country. Singap Med J. 2012;53(4):260–3.
7. Laxminarayan R, Duse A, Wattal C, Zaidi AKM, Wertheim HFL, Sumpradit N, Vlieghe E, Hara GL, Gould IM, Goossens H, Greko C, So AD, Bigdeli M, Tomson G, Woodhouse W, Ombaka E, Peralta AQ, Qamar FN, Mir F, Kariuki S, Bhutta ZA, Coates A, Bergstrom R, Wright GD, Brown ED, Cars O. Antibiotic resistance the need for global solutions. The Lancet Infectious Diseases. 2013;13(12):1057–98
8. Vasudevan A, Memon BI, Mukhopadhyay A, Li J, Tambyah PA. The costs of nosocomial resistant gram negative intensive care unit infections among patients with the systemic inflammatory response syndrome- a propensity matched case control study. Antimicrob Resist Infect Control. 2015;4(1):1–8.
9. Horcajada JP, Belvis F, Castells X, Grau S, Riu M, Morales E, et al. Hospital costs of nosocomial multi-drug resistant Pseudomonas aeruginosa acquisition. BMC Health Serv Res. 2012;12
10. Kollef MH. Optimizing antibiotic therapy in the intensive care unit setting. Crit Care. 2001;5(4):189–95.
11. Byarugaba DK. Antimicrobial resistance in developing countries and responsible risk factors. Int J Antimicrob Agents. 24(2):105–10.
12. Fraimow HS, Tsigrelis C. Antimicrobial resistance in the intensive care unit: mechanisms, epidemiology, and management of specific resistant pathogens. Crit Care Clin. 27(1):163–205.
13. Rahal JJ. Antimicrobial resistance among and therapeutic options against gram-negative pathogens. Clin Infect Dis. 2009;49(Suppl 1):S4–s10.
14. Yamamoto M, Pop-Vicas AE. Treatment for infections with carbapenem-resistant Enterobacteriaceae: what options do we still have? Crit Care. 2014;18(3):1–8.
15. Ruppé É, Woerther P-L, Barbier F. Mechanisms of antimicrobial resistance in Gram-negative bacilli. Ann Intensive Care. 2015;5:21.
16. Isenberg HD. Clinical Microbiology procedure handbook, vol. 1. 2nd ed. Washington DC: American Society for Microbiology; ASM press; 2004.
17. Maki DG, Weise CE, Sarafin HW. A semiquantitative culture method for identifying intravenous-catheter-related infection. N Engl J Med. 1977; 296(23):1305–9.
18. CLSI. Performance standards for antimicrobial disk susceptibility tests, vol. M02-A11. Wayne: Clinical and Laboratory Standards Institute; 2012.
19. Magiorakos AP, Srinivasan A, Carey RB, Carmeli Y, Falagas ME, Giske CG, et al. Multidrug-resistant, extensively drug-resistant and pandrug-resistant bacteria: an international expert proposal for interim standard definitions for acquired resistance. Clin Microbiol Infect. 2012;18(3):268–81.
20. Yong D, Lee K, Yum JH, Shin HB, Rossolini GM, Chong Y. Imipenem-EDTA disk method for differentiation of metallo-beta-lactamase-producing clinical isolates of pseudomonas spp. and acinetobacter spp. J Clin Microbiol. 2002; 40(10):3798–801.
21. Coudron PE. Inhibitor-based methods for detection of plasmid mediated AmpC β-lactamases in Klebsiella spp., Escherichia coli, and Proteus mirabilis. J Clin Microbiol. 2005;43:5.
22. Tsakris A, Poulou A, Pournaras S, Voulgari E, Vrioni G, Themeli-Digalaki K, et al. A simple phenotypic method for the differentiation of metallo-beta-lactamases and class A KPC carbapenemases in Enterobacteriaceae clinical isolates. J Antimicrob Chemother. 2010;65(8):1664–71.
23. Shrestha S, Tada T, Miyoshi-Akiyama T, Ohara H, Shimada K, Satou K, et al. Molecular epidemiology of multidrug-resistant Acinetobacter baumannii isolates in a university hospital in Nepal reveals the emergence of a novel epidemic clonal lineage. Int J Antimicrob Agents. 2015;46(5):526–31.
24. Allegranzi B, Bagheri Nejad S, Combescure C, Graafmans W, Attar H, Donaldson L, et al. Burden of endemic health-care-associated infection in developing countries: systematic review and meta-analysis. Lancet (London, England). 2011;377(9761):228–41.
25. Gastmeier P, Sohr D, Just HM, Nassauer A, Daschner F, Ruden H. How to survey nosocomial infections. Infect Control Hosp Epidemiol. 2000;21(6):366–70.
26. Sah M, Mishra S, Ohora H, Kirikae T, Sherchan J, Rijal B. Nosocomial bacterial infection and antimicrobial resistant pattern in a tertiary care hospital in Nepal. J Inst Med. 2015:38(1).
27. Mythri H, Kashinath K. Nosocomial infections in patients admitted in intensive care unit of a tertiary health center, India. Ann Med Health Sci Res. 2014;4(5):738–41.
28. Dasgupta S, Das S, Chawan NS, Hazra A. Nosocomial infections in the intensive care unit: Incidence, risk factors, outcome and associated pathogens in a public tertiary teaching hospital of Eastern India. Indian J Crit Care Med. 2015;19(1):14–20.
29. Alberti C, Brun-Buisson C, Burchardi H, Martin C, Goodman S, Artigas A, et al. Epidemiology of sepsis and infection in ICU patients from an international multicentre cohort study. Intensive Care Med. 2002;28(2):108–21.
30. Toufen C Jr, Hovnanian AL, Franca SA, Carvalho CR. Prevalence rates of infection in intensive care units of a tertiary teaching hospital. Rev Hosp Clin Fac Med Sao Paulo. 2003;58(5):254–9.
31. Ćosić Gorana ĐJ, Smiljana R, Ristić M, Ikonić N. nosocomial infections and microbiological agents in an intensive care unit. Arch Biol Sci Belgrade. 2012;64(4):6.
32. Mehrad B, Clark NM, Zhanel GG, Lynch JP 3rd. Antimicrobial resistance in hospital-acquired gram-negative bacterial infections. Chest. 2015;147(5):1413–21.
33. Habibi S, Wig N, Agarwal S, Sharma SK, Lodha R, Pandey RM, et al. Epidemiology of nosocomial infections in medicine intensive care unit at a tertiary care hospital in northern India. Trop Dr. 2008;38(4):233–5.
34. Bhatia R, Narain JP. The growing challenge of antimicrobial resistance in the South-East Asia Region - Are we losing the battle? Indian J Med Res. 2010; 132(5):482–6.
35. Mishra SK, Rijal BP, Pokhrel BM. Emerging threat of multidrug resistant bugs–Acinetobacter calcoaceticus baumannii complex and methicillin resistant Staphylococcus aureus. BMC Res Notes. 2013;6:98.
36. Khanal S, Joshi DR, Bhatta DR, Devkota U, Pokhrel BM. beta -lactamase-producing multidrug-resistant bacterial pathogens from tracheal aspirates of intensive care unit patients at national institute of neurological and allied sciences, Nepal. ISRN Microbiol. 2013;2013:847569.
37. Tenover FC. Mechanisms of antimicrobial resistance in bacteria. Am J Med. 2006;119(6 Suppl 1):S3–10. discussion S62-70
38. Xie DS, Xiong W, Lai RP, Liu L, Gan XM, Wang XH, et al. Ventilator-associated pneumonia in intensive care units in Hubei Province, China: a multicentre prospective cohort survey. J Hospital Infect. 2011;78(4):284–8.
39. Fatima A, Naqvi SB, Khaliq SA, Perveen S, Jabeen S. Antimicrobial susceptibility pattern of clinical isolates of Pseudomonas aeruginosa isolated from patients of lower respiratory tract infections. SpringerPlus. 2012;1(1):70.
40. Gales AC, Jones RN, Sader HS. Contemporary activity of colistin and polymyxin B against a worldwide collection of Gram-negative pathogens: results from the SENTRY Antimicrobial Surveillance Program (2006-09). J Antimicrob Chemother. 2011;66(9):2070–4.
41. Joseph NM, Sistla S, Dutta TK, Badhe AS, Rasitha D, Parija SC. Ventilator-associated pneumonia in a tertiary care hospital in India: role of multi-drug resistant pathogens. J Infect Dev Ctries. 2010;4(4):218–25.
42. Peleg AY, Seifert H, Paterson DL. Acinetobacter baumannii: emergence of a successful pathogen. Clin Microbiol Rev. 2008;21(3):538–82.

43. Hancock RE. Resistance mechanisms in Pseudomonas aeruginosa and other nonfermentative gram-negative bacteria. Clin Infect Dis. 1998;27(Suppl 1):S93–9.
44. Mishra SK, Awal BK, Kattel HP, Acharya J, Gyawali P, Bhatt CP, et al. Drug resistant bacteria are growing menace in a University Hospital in Nepal. Am J Epidemiol Infect Dis. 2014;2(1):19–23.
45. Livermore DM. Current epidemiology and growing resistance of gram-negative pathogens. Korean J Intern Med. 2012;27(2):128–42.
46. Shrestha S, Kattel HP, Mishra SK, Dahal RK, Ohara H, Pokhrel BM. Prevalence of nosocomial lower respiratory tract infections caused by Multidrug resistance pathologens. J Inst Med. 2011;33:8.
47. Baral P, Neupane S, Shrestha B, Ghimire KR, Marasini BP, Lekhak B. Clinical and microbiological observational study on AmpC beta-lactamase-producing Enterobacteriaceae in a hospital of Nepal. Braz J Infect Dis. 2013; 17(2):256–9.
48. Grover N, Sahni AK, Bhattacharya S. Therapeutic challenges of ESBLS and AmpC beta-lactamase producers in a tertiary care center. Med J Armed Forces India. 2013;69(1):4–10.
49. Mishra SK, Acharya J, Kattel HP, Koirala J, Rijal BP, Pokhrel BM. Metallo-beta-lactamase producing gram-negative bacterial isolates. J Nepal Health Res Counc. 2012;10(22):208–13.
50. Walsh TR, Weeks J, Livermore DM, Toleman MA. Dissemination of NDM-1 positive bacteria in the New Delhi environment and its implications for human health: an environmental point prevalence study. Lancet Infect Dis. 2011;11(5):355–62.

Vancomycin-resistant *Enterococcus faecium* sequence type 796 - rapid international dissemination of a new epidemic clone

Andrew A. Mahony[1,2*†], Andrew H. Buultjens[3†], Susan A. Ballard[1,4], Elizabeth A. Grabsch[5], Shirley Xie[5], Torsten Seemann[6], Rhonda L. Stuart[7], Despina Kotsanas[7], Allen Cheng[8], Helen Heffernan[9], Sally A. Roberts[10], Geoffrey W. Coombs[11,12], Narin Bak[13], John K. Ferguson[14], Glen C. Carter[4], Benjamin P. Howden[3,4], Timothy P. Stinear[3] and Paul D. R. Johnson[1,2,3*]

Abstract

Background: Vancomycin-resistant *Enterococcus faecium* (VRE) is a leading cause of hospital-acquired infections. New, presumably better-adapted strains of VRE appear unpredictably; it is uncertain how they spread despite improved infection control. We aimed to investigate the relatedness of a novel sequence type (ST) of *vanB E. faecium* - ST796 - very near its time of origin from hospitals in three Australian states and New Zealand.

Methods: Following near-simultaneous outbreaks of ST796 in multiple institutions, we gathered then tested colonization and bloodstream infection isolates' antimicrobial resistance (AMR) phenotypes, and phylogenomic relationships using whole genome sequencing (WGS). Patient meta-data was explored to trace the spread of ST796.

Results: A novel clone of *vanB E. faecium* (ST796) was first detected at one Australian hospital in late 2011, then in two New Zealand hospitals linked by inter-hospital transfers from separate Melbourne hospitals. ST796 also appeared in hospitals in South Australia and New South Wales and was responsible for at least one major colonization outbreak in a Neonatal Intensive Care Unit without identifiable links between centers. No exceptional AMR was detected in the isolates. While WGS analysis showed very limited diversity at the core genome, consistent with recent emergence of the clone, clustering by institution was observed.

Conclusions: Evolution of new *E. faecium* clones, followed by recognized or unrecognized movement of colonized individuals then rapid intra-institutional cross-transmission best explain the multi-center, multistate and international outbreak we observed.

Keywords: VRE, Whole genome sequencing, Molecular epidemiology, Outbreak, Infection control

Background

Enterococcus faecium has become a major cause of healthcare-associated bloodstream infections (BSI) worldwide [1, 2]. It is often postulated that antibiotic resistance mechanisms in *E. faecium* explain this success in hospitals. However, molecular typing has now defined clear lineages of hospital-associated *E. faecium* strains, nearly all of which belong to clade A1 (also defined as multi-locus sequence type [MLST] clonal complex 17), that are distinct from animal and non-hospitalized human commensal *E. faecium* [3–6]. Some researchers argue that hospital-adapted *E. faecium* is sufficiently different to qualify as a separate species [7].

Vancomycin-resistant enterococcus (VRE) was first detected in Australasia in 1994, as *vanA E. faecium* in a clinical specimen from a liver transplant patient at Austin

* Correspondence:
andrew.mahony@austin.org.au; paul.johnson@austin.org.au
†Equal contributors
[1]Department of Infectious Diseases, Austin Health, 145 Studley Rd, Heidelberg, VIC 3084, Australia
Full list of author information is available at the end of the article

Health in Melbourne [8]. For the next 10 years, VRE colonization and infection remained uncommon in Australia and New Zealand. From 2005, several geographically separate hospitals in Australia noted increasing numbers of VRE colonized patients and VRE BSI caused by *E. faecium*. In contrast to the United States and Europe, these VRE have predominantly been *vanB E. faecium*, a phenomenon that may relate to *vanB* carriage within bowel anaerobes in the healthy population [9–11]. It was assumed that the sudden increase in detection was due to failures in infection control and cross transmission of existing endemic VRE clones. However, a detailed outbreak investigation at Austin Health documented the arrival in 2005 of a new sequence type of *E. faecium*, ST203 [12], initially as vancomycin-susceptible *E. faecium* (VSE), with subsequent acquisition of *vanB* determinants on multiple separate occasions in several distinct clones of ST203 VSE [13]. Results from national surveys demonstrated a similar sequence of events in other hospitals so that by 2011, ST203 VSE and VRE had become the most common cause of *E. faecium* BSI in hospitals across all Australian states [14]. Notably, in New Zealand VRE colonization and infection remained very uncommon.

Improved cleaning protocols were introduced at Austin Health following the ST203 VRE outbreak, which reduced the incidence of VRE BSI between 2009 and 2011 [15]. However despite ongoing enhanced cleaning, we once again observed an abrupt increase in *vanB* VRE *E. faecium* BSI from 2012 onwards that was caused by a novel ST – we lodged the alleles with the MLST Database (https://pubmlst.org/efaecium) and received the designation ST796 in September 2012 [16]. Although unknown prior to 2011, by 2013 *vanB* ST796 *E. faecium* had caused a large outbreak of colonization in a Melbourne Neonatal Intensive Care Unit (NICU) [17], and by 2014 was responsible for 66% of *E. faecium* VRE BSI in five separate Melbourne hospitals, largely replacing its ST203 predecessor [18].

To investigate the emergence of ST796 we established a multi-institutional working group to study the early history of ST796 *E. faecium* by whole genome sequencing (WGS). Our principal research question was whether this near-simultaneous multi-institution outbreak was best explained by repeated introductions from unrecognised VSE followed by independent acquisition of *vanB*, VRE community colonization, or by VRE cross-transmission in and between affected hospitals. We now describe the clinical impact, antibiotic resistance and phylogenetic relatedness of this newly emerged *E. faecium*.

Methods

Working group participants from eastern Australia and northern New Zealand contributed ST796 *E. faecium* isolates from their local outbreaks – Fig. 1 shows the geographic distribution and number of isolates per institution. Initial identification of *E. faecium* was performed by the source hospital microbiology laboratory. Most isolates were originally classified as likely ST796 by Single Nucleotide Polymorphism High Resolution Melt (SNP HRM – in short, a rapid typing system based on the melt curves of common SNPs with variable G + C content) after referral to Austin Health [19]. Subsequently, speciation was re-confirmed by MALDI-TOF mass spectrometry or Vitek® 2 and the vancomycin resistance genotype determined by PCR as previously described [20]. A summary of the isolates with their epidemiological and meta-data is provided in Additional file 1: Table S1 and described in outline below.

Rates of *Enterococcus faecium* bacteremia at Austin health

Using discharge data collected by Austin Health's information management system, rates of VRE *E. faecium* bacteremia by ST over 6-month periods per 1000 discharged patients were calculated from 2011 to 2014. These were compared with previously published rates from 1998 to 2010 [12].

Antibiotic susceptibility testing

Antibiotic susceptibility testing was performed on all Austin Health, Alfred Health and John Hunter Hospital ST796 *E. faecium* blood culture isolates using the Vitek® 2 and Gram Positive Susceptibility card, AST-P612, according to the manufacturer's instructions (bioMérieux). Austin Health isolates were further assessed by Etest® according to the manufacturer's instructions (bioMérieux) for susceptibility to streptomycin, daptomycin, tigecycline, quinupristin-dalfopristin and chloramphenicol. Minimum Inhibitory Concentrations (MICs) were interpreted according to the Clinical and Laboratory Standards Institute (CLSI) guidelines where applicable.

Provenance of 131 *Enterococcus faecium* isolates that underwent WGS

Alfred Health

Alfred Health, a university teaching hospital in Melbourne with solid organ and allogeneic bone marrow transplantation units, experienced a marked increase in VRE BSI in 2014; 17 consecutive VRE BSI isolates (all *E. faecium*) were investigated as the STs and relatedness of isolates were unknown. Sixteen isolates were found to be ST796 (the other was ST203). One BSI isolate from 2013 identified retrospectively via SNP HRM typing as likely to be ST796 was included in the analysis [21].

Auckland City Hospital

Thirteen isolates were referred from Auckland City Hospital, New Zealand, during a VRE colonization

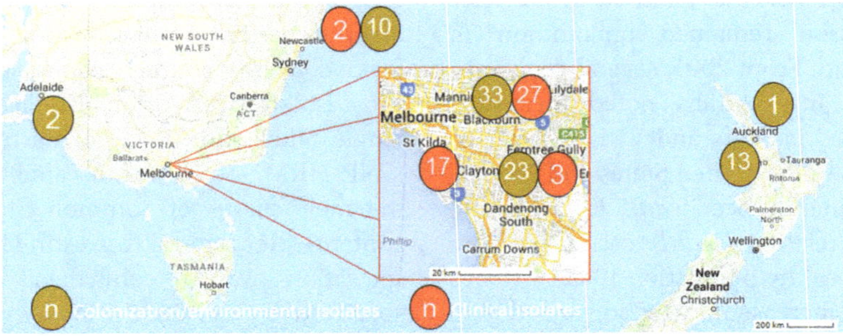

Fig. 1 Source of 131 ST796 *E. faecium* isolates from seven hospitals across Australia and New Zealand

outbreak that affected more than 50 hospitalized patients in 2012. The outbreak appeared to be clonal by pulsed field gel electrophoresis (PFGE, data not shown) performed at the national reference laboratory (ESR, Wellington, New Zealand), and followed the repatriation in 2012 from Monash Health in Melbourne of a patient who had been hospitalized while travelling in Australia and acquired VRE prior to transfer. This patient was found to have two PFGE pulsotypes of colonizing VRE *E. faecium*, detected serendipitously on antibiotic susceptibility testing, with a double zone of inhibition observed around a streptomycin disc; one matched the outbreak ST796 by MLST, whereas the other pulsotype was ST203. The patient's earlier rectal colonization and liver abscess VRE *E. faecium* isolates from Monash Health were identified as ST203.

A single colonizing isolate from a patient in another Auckland hospital, with no known links to Auckland City Hospital, also typed as ST796 by MLST so was included in WGS; this patient had similarly been transferred from a Melbourne hospital in 2012.

Austin Health

To capture the first appearance of ST796 in Austin BSI cases and to monitor its incidence compared to other STs over time, 79 consecutive *E. faecium* isolates obtained from all episodes of BSI at Austin Health from 1st January 2011 to 31st December 2014 were assessed. Thirty-nine were *vanB* VRE, and 24 of these ST796. Three additional isolates from early 2015 were subsequently identified as ST796, so were included in phenotypic and phlyogenomic analyses. Additionally, 32 colonizing isolates of *E. faecium* over the same period obtained from high-risk patients who are routinely screened for VRE rectal colonization, and one environmental isolate detected on surveillance, with matching SNP HRM genotype to the first ST796 BSI isolate, were included – one VSE, 30 *vanB*, one *vanA* and one with both *vanA* and *vanB*.

John Hunter Hospital

One hundred nine *E. faecium* blood culture and selected screening isolates from John Hunter Hospital in New South Wales (NSW) obtained between 2007 and 2015 were available for WGS. Of these we identified 12 ST796 isolates, all from 2015. These comprised one VSE and one VRE from adults with positive blood cultures, and ten screening isolates from a NICU colonization outbreak.

Monash Health

A large outbreak of VRE colonization in the NICU and special care nurseries at Monash Health in Melbourne was recognized in October 2013, with VRE never previously detected in these wards [17]. WGS was performed on 26 isolates (two environmental swab isolates, one urine culture, one eye swab, one blood culture and 21 screening samples from more than 40 colonized neonates).

Royal Adelaide Hospital

Two of five patient isolates from a VRE colonization outbreak in September 2013 at the Royal Adelaide Hospital in South Australia matched the SNP HRM type of ST796 so were included in WGS analysis.

WGS and bioinformatic analyses

Short read sequencing libraries were generated from genomic DNA using the Illumina Nextera XT DNA sample preparation kit. Libraries were sequenced on the Illumina platform using either the MiSeq with 250-cycle paired end chemistry or the NextSeq 500 with 150-cycle paired end chemistry according to the manufacturer's instructions.

Snippy v3.2 (https://github.com/tseemann/snippy) was used to map sequence reads against the fully assembled Ef_aus0233 genome (GenBank accession no. PRJEB14733), a representative of the ST796 lineage [22]. Single nucleotide polymorphisms (SNPs) in core genome positions were used to construct a Maximum Likelihood tree with

FastTree v2.1.8 [23]. The tree was used as a guide for ClonalFrame v1.7 to infer regions of recombination [24]. As previously described, a robust and recombination-free tree was generated [22]. Tree branches with less than 70% bootstrap support (500 replicates) were collapsed. Pairwise core non-recombinogenic SNP differences between isolates were tabulated and visualized using a custom R-script (https://github.com/MDU-PHL/pairwise_snp_differences).

Ethics approval

VRE isolates were collected and compared, along with rates of BSI, using non-identifying data as part of standard infection control procedures under appropriately constituted infection control committees at each institution.

Results

Bacteremia at Austin Health

To better understand the changing epidemiology of *E. faecium* BSI at Austin Health, we plotted the rates at six-month intervals between 1998 and 2014 of VRE *E. faecium* BSI by ST (Fig. 2). This analysis showed the dominance of ST203 in 2009, then ST796 emerging in mid-2011 and becoming dominant by mid-2012. Of the 40 VSE (51% of all *E. faecium* BSI), nine were ampicillin-susceptible with all of these being community-associated infections, and none were ST796. Although ST796 and ST203 *E. faecium* caused BSI in roughly equal measure during 2012, the next 16 consecutive cases of VRE BSI over 15 months were all *vanB* ST796, almost completely replacing ST203.

Phenotypic antibiotic resistance

Forty-six ST796 blood culture isolates underwent antimicrobial susceptibility testing (27 from Austin Health, 17 from Alfred Health, and two from John Hunter Hospital). All were ampicillin-resistant and all except one harboured *vanB*. Thirty-nine of 45 *vanB* isolates (87%) tested vancomycin-resistant, but two tested susceptible (MIC ≤4 mg/L) and four intermediate (MIC 8-16 mg/L). Thirty isolates (65%) had high-level gentamicin resistance. Two (4%) had intermediate susceptibility to linezolid (with none of the known 23S rRNA mutations or *optrA* genes; data not shown). All were susceptible to teicoplanin.

Additional testing of the Austin Health isolates revealed one with high-level streptomycin resistance, but no resistance to tigecycline, quinupristin-dalfopristin or chloramphenicol. All isolates were susceptible to daptomycin (although most had MICs of 3-4 mg/L). The ST796 isolates did not have additional antibiotic resistance or higher MICs than the ST203 clones they replaced (data not shown).

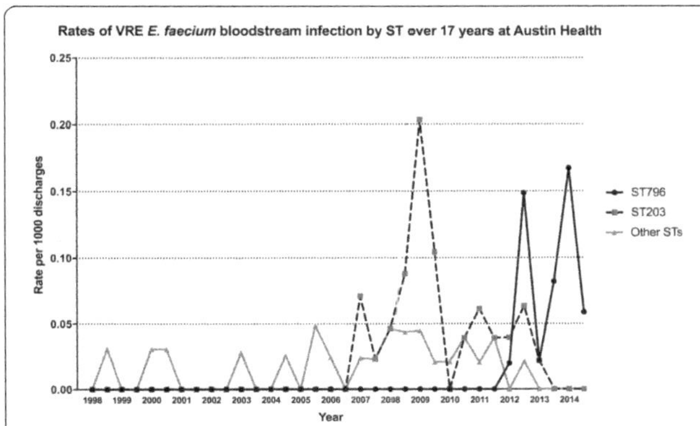

Fig. 2 Rates of VRE *E. faecium* bacteremia by ST over 17 years at Austin Health, Melbourne. We have observed two recent outbreaks of VRE bacteremia, the first with ST203 which has now been almost completely replaced by ST796. *One isolate from 2010 was not typed

Phylogenomics

The core genomes of 131 ST796 isolates were compared. SNPs were identified between these genomes and used to create a maximum likelihood phylogenomic tree (Fig. 3). To focus on the clonal heritage of the isolates, SNPs within regions of recombination (411 and 1895 clonal and recombinogenic core SNPs, respectively) were omitted from the sequence alignment that was used for tree building (Fig. 3).

The 128 *vanB* isolates formed a cohesive and monophyletic phylogroup (9.5 mean core SNPs) while the single *vanA* and two VSE ST796 isolates formed distinct phylogroups (20 core SNPs between the VSE isolates). The VSE phylogroup was furthest from the ST796 Most Recent Common Ancestor (MRCA) and was separated from the *vanA* and *vanB* phylogroups by 89 and 123 mean core SNPs, respectively. The single *vanA* isolate was separated from the VSE and *vanB* phylogroups by 89 and 61 mean core SNPs, respectively and was phylogenomically further from the ST796 MRCA than that of the *vanB* phylogroup.

The basal position of the *vanB* to that of the VSE isolates suggests that these isolates may have lost *vanB*. This feature of ST796 population structure was also observed in an accompanying study that focused on the genomic evolution of this emerging clone [22]. Similarly, this would also imply that the *vanA* isolate may have evolved from an ST796 progenitor that was originally *vanB*. One ST796 isolate with both *vanA* and *vanB* genotypes was identified; interestingly, this isolate clustered tightly within the *vanB* phylogroup, suggesting that it was originally harbouring *vanB* then horizontally acquired the *vanA* plasmid.

Despite the limited core SNP diversity observed among the *vanB* isolates, the existence of signature SNPs was linked to an isolate's institution of origin. For some *vanB* isolates from a common institution there was

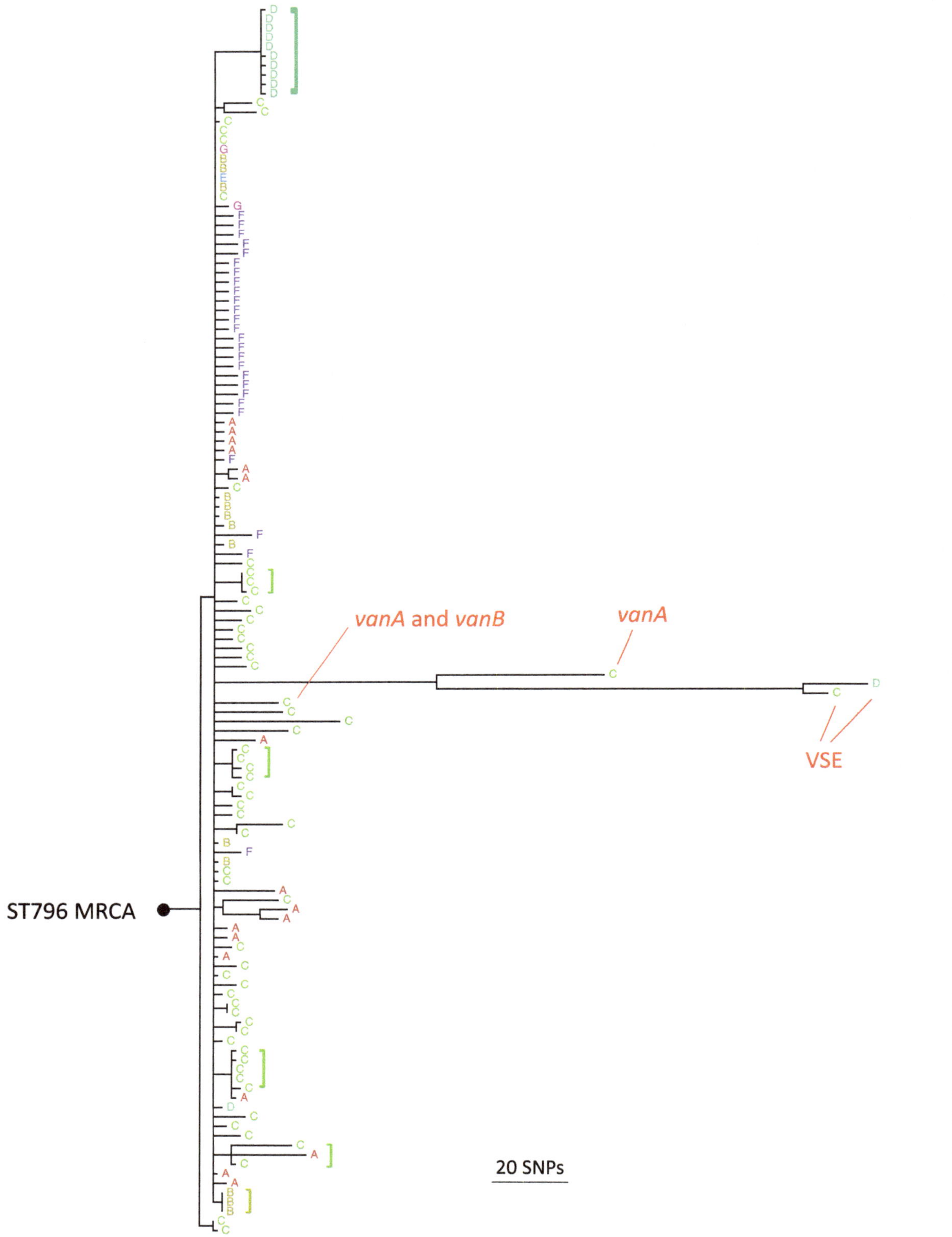

Fig. 3 (See legend on next page.)

(See figure on previous page.)
Fig. 3 Maximum likelihood phylogenomic tree of 131 ST796 isolates. The tree was constructed from non-recombinogenic core SNPs and branches with less than 70% bootstrap support (500 replicates) were collapsed. The VSE, *vanA* and *vanB* isolates formed distinct and robust phylogroups. The single *vanA* + *vanB* isolate clustered within the *vanB* phylogroup. Branch lengths are proportional to core SNP differences with the scale as indicated. The inferred occurrences of intra-hospital evolution among the *vanB* isolates are labelled (brackets). The phylogenomic position of the ST796 most recent common ancestor (MRCA) in the ST796 tree was identified by using *Enterococcus hirae* (hirae_ATCC_9790, GenBank accession no. CP003504) as an outgroup. A = Alfred Health, Melbourne; B = Auckland City Hospital; C = Austin Health, Melbourne; D = John Hunter Hospital, Newcastle; E = other Auckland hospital; F = Monash Health, Melbourne; G = Royal Adelaide Hospital

sufficient core SNP identity to group them on a single node. The existence of isolates with identical core SNPs is indicative of sustained intra-institution circulation, where the founding bacteria have undergone a population bottleneck and consequently developed conserved alleles that are institution-specific. Despite such groupings, other *vanB* isolates formed singleton branches that radiate outward from the *vanB* MRCA. The singleton branches likely represent rapid evolutionary radiations from the *vanB* MRCA – a hallmark of a recently emerged and rapidly disseminated clone.

To examine the relationship between the number of core SNP differences and the originating institutions, a pairwise core SNP comparison was undertaken (Fig. 4). The expectation for a clonal population is low intra-group diversity and higher inter-group diversity. Here, discrepancies between the intra-group and inter-group comparisons for all institutions were very modest and in some cases non-existent, indicating they do not contain single ST796 genotypes but rather multiple genotypes. Such substantial intra-institution diversity is consistent with a scenario of multiple inter-hospital transmission events.

Discussion

E. faecium ST796 was first recognised at Austin Health at the beginning of 2012 and by 2014 had completely replaced the predecessor ST203 as a cause of BSI at that institution. This was not due to additional antibiotic resistance so the apparent enhanced fitness of ST796 is likely due to an alternative survival advantage. ST796 appeared almost simultaneously in two hospitals in Auckland New Zealand in 2012, and by 2015 had reached Newcastle, NSW. Using WGS to investigate this outbreak

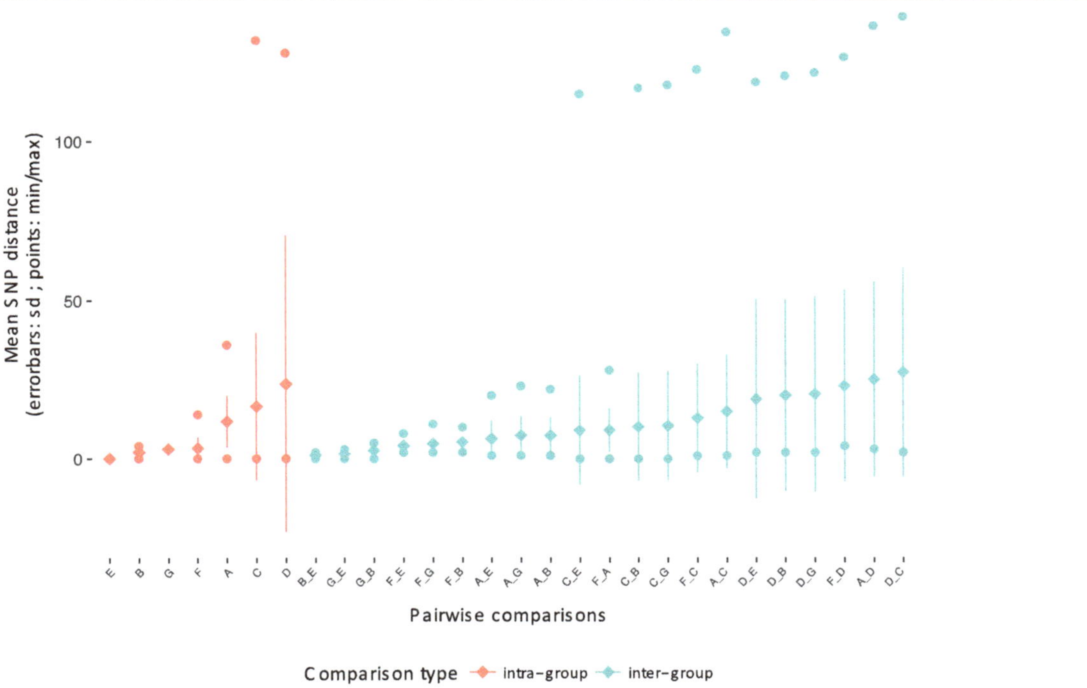

Fig. 4 Pairwise comparisons of non-recombinogenic core SNP differences according to institution of origin. Overall, intra-hospital diversity is equal to or greater than inter-hospital diversity, indicating that there is substantial ST genomic admixture within each hospital. Comparisons are ordered according to increasing means. A = Alfred Health, Melbourne; B = Auckland City Hospital; C = Austin Health, Melbourne; D = John Hunter Hospital, Newcastle; E = other Auckland hospital; F = Monash Health, Melbourne; G = Royal Adelaide Hospital

we observed genomic signals that were indicative of both rapid inter-hospital transmission and in some cases, sustained secondary intra-institution circulation. Our observation of a surge in BSI at Austin Health due to the appearance of ST796 is supported by results from Australian national surveys of *E. faecium* BSI from the Australian Group on Antimicrobial Resistance (AGAR). In the 2010 survey, ST796 was not detected, however in 2014, ST796 was responsible for 66% of BSI isolates in Victorian hospitals, 14% in Tasmania and 4% in South Australia [18, 25, 26]. Notably ST796 was not detected in other Australian states, even though we now know it had reached John Hunter Hospital in NSW as a colonizing and infecting strain. This very rapid spread within Victoria indicates high transmissibility of ST796, but may also reflect different infection control procedures at the time of inter-hospital transfer or greater mixing of patients between institutions compared with other states. Similarly, a recent Victorian outbreak of carbapenem-resistant *Enterobacteriaceae* is now understood to be linked to admission or transfer from a single center [27].

In addition to BSI, ST796 *E. faecium* also caused rapid, clinically silent outbreaks of colonization in several locations: two hospitals in New Zealand, NICUs at Monash Health, and John Hunter Hospital, more than 800 km away. It is likely that undetected transfer of VRE between patients preceded the sharp rise in BSI in Victoria. In New Zealand, ST796 colonization was shown to be linked to international transfer of patients from hospitals in Victoria. We did not identify epidemiological links between other Melbourne hospitals and those where ST796 was identified in South Australia or NSW. However it seems likely that ST796 was disseminated in a similar manner, carried by undetected colonized patients.

All *vanB* ST796 isolates we assessed are very closely related at the core genome level, irrespective of the location or date of isolation over three years. In contrast, significant differences in relationship were observed between the two ST796 VSE isolates and the ST796 *vanA* isolate when compared to their ST796 *vanB* counterparts (including the single *vanA* and *vanB* ST796 isolate). These differences are not explained by the presence or absence of different vancomycin resistance elements as these are excluded when determining core genome. Furthermore, all but one of the ST796 *E. faecium* isolated from blood cultures were vancomycin-resistant. This contrasts markedly with the previous ST203 outbreak at Austin Health and other mainland Australian states in which ST203 isolates were frequently clonally diverse and included VSE and VRE isolates [19], and with the complexity and diversity of hospital outbreak strains in a single center from Sydney [28].

This report has a number of limitations. Firstly, it is an observational study, with VRE screening not standardized across the institutions. Secondly, WGS was not performed on all new rectal colonization VRE isolates from the study sites due to cost, so we cannot assess the distribution of colonizing *E. faecium* STs, nor calculate the "attack rate" of ST796 from colonization to BSI. Thirdly, we cannot explain why the population structure of ST796 VRE has remained so clonal compared with the much greater diversity found within the previous ST203 outbreak strain. This suggests a survival advantage in hospitals of ST796 VRE over its predecessors but what exactly this is remains to be determined.

Cost, lack of single rooms and isolation fatigue make VRE control for those hospitals with endemic colonization a major challenge [21, 29]. Where VRE is not endemic, swift recognition and enhanced infection control may still be effective [17, 30]. Our data suggest that if we wish to control VRE colonization and infection in hospitals that are not yet endemic then more attention must be paid to movements of patients and possibly staff who have had contact with VRE-endemic hospitals.

Conclusion

In conclusion, we have tracked a novel clone of ST796 *E. faecium* close to the start of its existence in Victoria Australia, where it has largely displaced ST203 as the leading cause of VRE BSI. In contrast ST796 has not caused significant invasive disease despite extensive colonization in a Melbourne NICU, John Hunter Hospital in NSW or in hospitals in Auckland – possibly due to differences in patients' underlying medical conditions. WGS has demonstrated an essentially clonal population structure of ST796, but unlike the multi-drug-resistant gram-negatives, emerging healthcare-associated strains of *E. faecium* do not appear to depend for their success on enhanced antibiotic resistance. This suggests that other determinants of clonal success drive the rapid appearance and dissemination of new successful clones. One possibility is resistance to biocides rather than antibiotics per se; we are now actively investigating this possibility [31].

Acknowledgements
Not applicable.

Funding
This work was supported by the National Human Medical Research Council of Australia [grant number 1027874, and NHMRC Fellowships to TPS. and BPH.]; and the University of Melbourne [Australian Postgraduate Award to AAM.]. These funding bodies had no role in the design of the study, collection, analysis, and interpretation of data or in writing the manuscript.

Authors' contributions
AM coordinated the study, performed additional phenotypic antibiotic susceptibility testing of isolates, calculated rates of bacteremia over time, and

prepared the manuscript. AB contributed phylogenomic analyses, with whole genome sequencing data from SB and bioinformatics from TS. EG and SX performed additional microbiologic analyses of isolates. RS, DK, AC, HH, SR, GWC, NB, JF and GCC contributed site-specific isolate and epidemiologic data. BH, TS and PJ oversaw all aspects of the study. All authors read and approved the final manuscript.

Consent for publication
Not applicable.

Competing interests
The authors declare that they have no competing interests.

Author details
[1]Department of Infectious Diseases, Austin Health, 145 Studley Rd, Heidelberg, VIC 3084, Australia. [2]Department of Medicine, The University of Melbourne, Heidelberg, VIC 3084, Australia. [3]Department of Microbiology and Immunology, The University of Melbourne at The Peter Doherty Institute for Infection and Immunity, Melbourne, VIC 3000, Australia. [4]Microbiological Diagnostic Unit Public Health Laboratory, The University of Melbourne at The Peter Doherty Institute for Infection and Immunity, Melbourne, VIC 3000, Australia. [5]Department of Microbiology, Austin Health, Heidelberg, VIC 3084, Australia. [6]Melbourne Bioinformatics, The University of Melbourne, Parkville, VIC 3010, Australia. [7]Monash Infectious Diseases, Monash Health, Clayton, VIC 3168, Australia. [8]Department of Infectious Diseases, Alfred Health, School of Public Health and Preventive Medicine, Monash University, Prahran, VIC 3181, Australia. [9]Antimicrobial Reference Laboratory, Institute of Environmental Science and Research (ESR), Wellington 5022, New Zealand. [10]Department of Clinical Microbiology, Auckland District Health Board, Auckland 1051, New Zealand. [11]School of Veterinary and Life Sciences, Murdoch University, Murdoch, WA 6150, Australia. [12]Microbiology Department, PathWest Laboratory Medicine – WA, Fiona Stanley Hospital, Murdoch, WA 6150, Australia. [13]Department of Infectious Diseases, Royal Adelaide Hospital, Adelaide, South Australia 5000, Australia. [14]Division of Microbiology, Health Pathology, NSW Department of Immunology and Infectious Diseases, John Hunter Hospital, University of Newcastle, Newcastle, NSW 2305, Australia.

References
1. Pinholt M, Ostergaard C, Arpi M, et al. Incidence, clinical characteristics and 30-day mortality of enterococcal bacteraemia in Denmark 2006-2009: a population-based cohort study. Clin Microbiol Infect. 2014;20:145–51.
2. Tedim AP, Ruiz-Garbajosa P, Rodriguez MC, et al. Long-term clonal dynamics of Entercoccus faecium strains causing bloodstream infections (1995-2015) in Spain. J Antimicrob Chemother. 2017;71:48–55.
3. Homan WL, Tribe D, Poznanski S, et al. Multilocus sequence typing scheme for enterococcus faecium. J Clin Microbiol. 2002;40:1963–71.
4. Willems RJ, Top J, van Schaik W, et al. Restricted gene flow among hospital subpopulations of enterococcus faecium. MBio. 2012;3:e00151–12.
5. Galloway-Pena J, Roh JH, Latorre M, Qin X, Murray BE. Genomic and SNP analyses demonstrate a distant separation of the hospital and community-associated clades of enterococcus faecium. PLoS One. 2012;7:e30187.
6. Tedim AP, Ruiz-Garbajosa P, Corander J, et al. Population biology of intestinal enterococcus isolates from hospitalized and nonhospitalized individuals in different age groups. Appl Environ Microbiol. 2015;81:1820–31.
7. Lebreton F, van Schaik W, McGuire AM, et al. Emergence of epidemic multidrug-resistant *Enterococcus faecium* from animal and commensal strains. MBio. 2013;4:e00534–13.
8. Kamarulzaman A, Tosolini FA, Boquest AL, Geddes JE, Richards MJ. Vancomycin-resistant enterococcus faecium in a liver transplant patient [abstract]. Australia New Zealand. J Med. 1995;25:260.
9. Stinear TP, Olden DC, Johnson PD, Davies JK, Grayson ML. Enterococcal vanB resistance locus in anaerobic bacteria in human faeces. Lancet. 2001;357:855–6.
10. Graham M, Ballard SA, Grabsch EA, Johnson PD, Grayson ML. High rates of fecal carriage of nonenterococcal vanB in both children and adults. Antimicrob Agents Chemother. 2008;52:1195–7.
11. Ballard SA, Pertile KK, Lim M, Johnson PD, Grayson ML. Molecular characterization of vanB elements in naturally occurring gut anaerobes. Antimicrob Agents Chemother. 2005;49:1688–94.
12. Johnson PD, Ballard SA, Grabsch EA, et al. A sustained hospital outbreak of vancomycin-resistant enterococcus faecium bacteremia due to emergence of vanB E. Faecium sequence type 203. J Infect Dis. 2010;202:1278–86.
13. Howden BP, Holt KE, Lam MM, et al. Genomic insights to control the emergence of vancomycin-resistant enterococci. MBio. 2013;4:e00412–3.
14. Coombs GW, Pearson JC, Daley DA, et al. Molecular epidemiology of enterococcal bacteremia in Australia. J Clin Microbiol. 2014;52:897–905.
15. Grabsch EA, Mahony AA, Cameron DR, et al. Significant reductionin vancomycin-resistant enterococcus colonization and bacteraemia after introduction of a bleach-based cleaning-disinfection programme. J Hosp Infect. 2012;82:234–42.
16. Mahony AA, Grabsch EA, Ballard SA, et al. Vancomycin-resistant enterococcus faecium sequence type 796, the new trans-Tasman epidemic clone [abstract 41]. In: Program and abstracts of the Australian Society for Antimicrobials - antimicrobials 2014 (Melbourne). Australian Society for Antimocrobials; 2014.
17. Lister DM, Kotsanas D, Ballard SA, et al. Outbreak of vanB vancomycin-resistant *Enterococcus faecium* colonization in a neonatal service. Am J Infect Control. 2015;43:1061–5.
18. Coombs GW, Daley DA, Thin Lee Y, et al. Australian group on antimicrobial resistance Australian Enterococcal Sepsis outcome Programme annual report, 2014. Comun Dis Intell Q Rep. 2016;40:E236–43.
19. Tong SY, Xie S, Richardson LJ, et al. High-resolution melting genotyping of enterococcus faecium based on multilocus sequence typing derviced single nucleotide polymorphisms. PLoS One. 2011;6:e29189.
20. Grabsch EA, Chua K, Xie S, et al. Improved detection of vanB2-containing enterococcus faecium with vancomycin susceptibility by Etest using oxgall supplementation. J Clin Microbiol. 2008;46:1961–4.
21. Karki S, Land G, Aitchison S, et al. Long-term carriage of vancomycin-resistant enterococci in patients discharged from hospitals: a 12-year retrospective cohort study. J Clin Microbiol. 2013;51:3374–9.
22. Buultjens AH, Lam MM, Ballard S, et al. Evolutionary origins of the emergent ST796 clone of vancomycin resistant enterococcus faecium. PeerJ. 2017;5:e2916.
23. Price MN, Dehal PS, Arkin AP. FastTree 2 - approximately maximum-likelihood trees for large alignments. PLoS One. 2010;5:e9490.
24. Didelot X, Wilson DJ. ClonalFrameML: efficient inference of recombination in whole bacterial genomes. PLoS Comput Biol. 2015;11:e1004041.
25. Coombs GW, Pearson JC, Le T, et al. Australian Enterococcal Sepsis outcome Progamme, 2011. Commun Dis Intell Q Rep. 2014;38:E247–52.
26. Coombs GW, Pearson JC, Daley DA, et al. Australian enterococcal sepsis outcome programme annual report, 2013. Commun Dis Intell Q Rep. 2014;38:E320–6.
27. Chang LW, Buising KL, Jeremiah CJ, et al. Managing a nosocomial outbreak of carbapenem-resistant Klebsiella pneumoniae: an early Australian hospital experience. Intern Med J. 2015;45:1037–43.
28. van Hal SJ, Ip CLC, Ansari MA, et al. Evolutionary dynamics of enterococcus faecium reveals complex genomic relationships between isolates with independent emergence of vancomycin resistance. Microbial Genomics. 2016;2:e000048.
29. Karki S, Leder K, Cheng AC. Should we continue to isolate patients with vancomycin-resistant enterococci in hospitals? Med J Aust. 2015;202:234–6.
30. Cheng VC, Tai JW, Ng ML, et al. Extensive contact tracing and screening to control the spread of vancomycin-resistant enterococcus faecium ST414 in Hong Kong. Chin Med J. 2012;125:3450–7.
31. Stinear TP, Pidot SJ, Lam MC, et al. Increasing tolerance of hospital Enterococcus faecium to hand-rub alcohols. bioRxiv. 2016; https://doi.org/10.1101/053728.

16

Antibiotic resistance, ability to form biofilm and susceptibility to copper alloys of selected staphylococcal strains isolated from touch surfaces in Polish hospital wards

Anna Różańska[1*], Agnieszka Chmielarczyk[1], Dorota Romaniszyn[1], Małgorzata Bulanda[1], Monika Walkowicz[2], Piotr Osuch[2] and Tadeusz Knych[2]

Abstract

Background: Despite the employment of sanitary regimes, contact transmission of the aetiological agents of hospital infections is still exceedingly common. The issue of microbe transmission becomes particularly important when facing multidrug-resistant microorganisms such as methicillin-resistant staphylococci. In the case of deficiencies in cleaning and disinfection procedures, hospital equipment made of copper alloys can play an important role, complementing traditional hospital hygiene procedures.

The objective of this study was to characterize staphylococcal strains isolated from touch surfaces in Polish hospital wards in terms of their drug resistance, ability to form biofilm and susceptibility to antimicrobial activity of copper alloys.

Methods: The materials for the study were 95 staphylococcal strains isolated from touch surfaces in 13 different hospital wards from Małopolska province (the south of Poland). Phenotypic and genotypic antibiotic resistance were checked for erythromycin, clindamycin, gentamycin, ciprofloxacin, trimethoprim/sulfamethoxazole and mupirocin. Biofilm formation ability for the tested strains was checked with the use of culture on Congo red agar. Susceptibility to copper, tin bronze, brass and new silver was tested using a modification of the Japanese standard.

Results: Over 67% of the analysed staphylococcal strains were methicillin-resistant (MR). Four strains were resistant to all of the tested antibiotics, and 14 were resistant to all except mupirocin. Strains classified as MR had significantly increased resistance to the remaining antibiotic groups. About one-third of the analysed strains revealed biofilm-forming ability. Among the majority of species, biofilm-forming and non-biofilm-forming strains were distributed evenly; in the case of *S. haemolyticus* only, negative strains accounted for 92.8%. Susceptibility to copper alloys was different between strains and rather lower than in the case of the SA strain selected for comparison.

Conclusions: Coagulase-negative staphylococci, the most commonly isolated in Polish hospital wards, should not be neglected as an infection risk factor due their high antibiotic resistance. Our experiments confirmed that touch surfaces made of copper alloys may play an important role in eliminating bacteria from the hospital environment.

Keywords: Hospital environment contamination, Staphylococci, Antibiotic resistance, Antimicrobial copper, Biofilm-forming staphylococci

* Correspondence: a.rozanska@uj.edu.pl
[1]Jagiellonian University Medical College, Faculty of Medicine, Chair of Microbiology, Czysta str. 18, 31-121 Kraków, Poland
Full list of author information is available at the end of the article

Background

Despite the employment of sanitary regimes, contact transmission of the aetiological agents of hospital infections is still exceedingly common [1]. The issue of microbe transmission becomes particularly important when multidrug-resistant microorganisms, such as methicillin-resistant staphylococci (MRSA, MRCoNS), vancomycin-resistant enterococci (VRE), or non-fermentative bacilli, appear in the hospital environment [2]. The spread of methicillin-resistant *S. aureus* (MRSA) or *S. epidermidis* (MRSE) outside hospital units (hotels, buses) is also described, but it is of greater significance when the drug-resistant bacteria present themselves in hospitals [3–6]. Methicillin-resistant staphylococcal strains are frequently resistant not only to beta-lactam antibiotics but also to the majority of antibiotics used for therapy. Rapidly increasing resistance among both staphylococci and Gram-negative bacilli is a very serious problem in hospitals as it limits effective treatment of infections, especially in patients with severe infections treated in ICUs [7, 8]. The most common vector mediating the transfer of microbes is the hands of the staff and of patients, and the reservoir is represented by surfaces most often touched (door handles, countertops, light switches and others), on which these microorganisms can survive over long periods of time – many days or even months [9]. Cleaning and disinfection of these surfaces is an action obviously applied that has significance in controlling MRSA and MRCoNS [9]. Solutions to this problem are searched for in many directions, and understanding bacterial mechanisms of resistance enables one to seek new drugs tackling this resistance, but there is also a search for new substances that could be used in disinfectants and new materials (e.g., metal alloys) for use in commercial (touch) surfaces.

The objective of the present study was to describe the antibiotic resistance (phenotypes and genotypes), the ability to create biofilm and the susceptibility to selected copper alloys of the most numerous staphylococcal strains (n = 95) isolated from hospital unit touch surfaces.

Methods

The materials for the study were strains cultured from touch surfaces in 13 different units in three hospitals of various sizes and profiles located in Małopolska province (the south of Poland). Swabs for testing were collected from the following surfaces that may be a reservoir for microbes: worktop in sickroom, bedside table top, drip stand, bed frame, soap dispenser, disinfecting fluid dispenser, light switch, ventilator monitor, mobile phone, department landline phone receiver, computer keyboard, dressing (or surgical) trolley worktop, door handle, protective glove container, and tissue package. The detailed methodology and results of environmental screening are described elsewhere [10], but the most numerous isolates were coagulase-negative staphylococci (85.7%), followed by *Staphylococcus aureus* (2.7%), streptococci (including *E. faecalis*) (8.9%), Gram-negative bacilli (1.8%) and others (0.9%). In the most numerous group of coagulase-negative staphylococci, the following species were isolated: *Staphylococcus epidermidis, Staphylococcus haemolyticus, Staphylococcus hominis, Staphylococcus warneri, Staphylococcus capitis, Staphylococcus simulans, Staphylococcus pettenkoferi, Staphylococcus caprae* and coagulase-positive ones - *S. aureus.*

The collected strains were stored in the Department of Microbiology at −70 °C (according to the procedure of Microorganism Preservation System Protect TS/80-MX).

Drug resistance study

All isolates were tested using disk diffusion antimicrobial susceptibility methods on Mueller-Hinton agar plates according to the current guidelines of the European Committee on Antimicrobial Susceptibility Testing (EUCAST Tables v. 6.0; http://www.eucast.org v.6.0 accessed 1.12.2016). Antibiotics used in this study included erythromycin (2 μg), clindamycin (15 μg), gentamycin (10 μg), ciprofloxacin (5 μg), trimethoprim/sulfamethoxazole (1.25/23.75 μg), and mupirocin (200 μg). All disks were obtained from Oxoid (Basingstoke, United Kingdom). The MRSA resistance phenotype was detected using a cefoxitin disc (30 μg) according to the current EUCAST guidelines. The macrolide-lincosamide-streptogramin B (MLSB) resistance phenotype of the isolates was determined by D-test according to a previously published protocol [11].

DNA isolation

DNA was extracted from isolates using the Genomic Mini kit (A&A Biotechnology, Gdynia, Poland) according to the manufacturer's instructions.

Polymerase chain reaction (PCR) screening for selected resistance genes

MRSA phenotype was confirmed by detection of the *mec*A gene in PCR amplification using previously published primers (Table 1) [12]. Erythromycin resistance genes (*erm*A, *erm*B, *erm*C, and *msr*A/B) were detected by multiplex PCR, and amplification of a 456 bp fragment of the *mup* gene (mupirocin resistance gene) was performed by single PCR (Table 1) [13, 14]. As positive controls, *S. aureus* ATCC 33591 and ATCC BAA 1708 were employed.

Biofilm

Isolate biofilm formation was screened using the method described by Arciola et al. [15] with Congo red agar (CRA). CRA plates were prepared by adding 0.8 g of Congo red and 36 g of saccharose (Sigma, Missouri,

Table 1 Sequences of starters used for detection of resistance genes

Gen	Primer sequences 5′-3′	Product of amplification	References
mecA	TAG AAA TGA CTG AAC GTC CG TTG CGA TCA ATG TTA CCG TAG	154 bp	Pereira 2010 [12]
mup	TAT ATT ATG CGA TGG AAG GTT GG AAT AAA ATC AGC TGG AAA GTG TTG	458 bp	Anthony RM 1999 [14]
ermA	TCT AAA AAG CAT GTA AAA GAA CTT CGA TAG TTT ATT AAT ATT AGT	645 bp	Sutcliffe 1996 [13]
ermB	GAA AAG GTA CTC AAC CAA ATA AGT AAC GGT ACT TAA ATT GTT TAC	639 bp	Sutcliffe 1996 [13]
ermC	TCA AAA CAT AAT ATA GAT AAA GCT AAT ATT GTT TAA ATC GTC AAT	642 bp	Sutcliffe 1996 [13]
msrA/B	GCA AAT GGT GTA GGT AAG ACA ACT ATC ATG TGA TGT AAA CAA AAT	399 BP	Sutcliffe 1996 [13]

USA) to 1 L of brain heart infusion agar (Oxoid, Basingstoke, Hampshire, England). The plates were incubated for 24 h at 37 °C and subsequently overnight at room temperature. On CRA, slime-producing strains form black colonies, whereas non-producing strains develop red colonies. For an accurate assessment of all the possible chromatic variations exhibited by the cultured colonies, a six-colour scale was used [15]. The scale ranged from very black (vb), through black (b), and almost black (ab) to bordeaux (brd, red (r) and very red (vr) (Fig. 1). Very black and black colonies were considered normal slime producer strains, while dark, almost black colours were considered indicative of weak slime production activity. Conversely, very red to bordeaux coloured colonies were considered grades of red and classified as strains unable to produce slime.

Chosen copper alloys and their preparation

Metal samples measuring 2.5 cm × 2.5 cm with a thickness of 1–2.5 mm were provided by the Faculty of Non-ferrous Metals, AGH University of Science and Technology, Kraków. Before their delivery for microbiological testing, the samples underwent mechanical polishing, cleaning and degreasing by immersion in acetone. Prior to use for microbiological testing, the samples were sterilized by wiping with 96% alcohol. Studies were conducted on the following copper alloys: brass CuZn37, tin bronze CuSn6, and nickel silver CuNi18Zn20 with ETP copper (99.9% Cu) as a positive control (presumed highest antimicrobial efficacy) and stainless steel as a negative control (assumed lack of antimicrobial properties). The copper alloys selected for this study are the most well known and most frequently used in various industries. The alloys used in the study with data on the concentration percentage of copper are listed in Table 2.

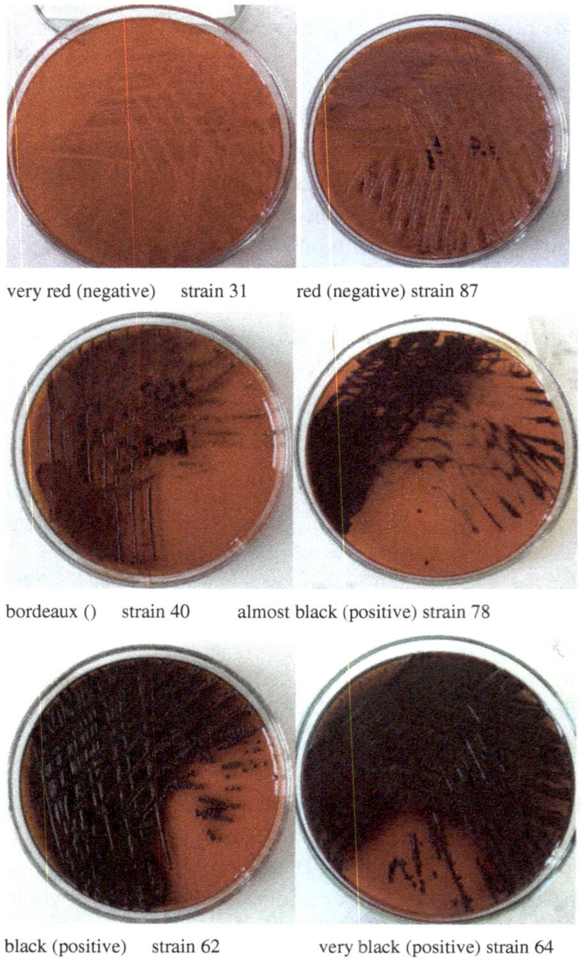

Fig. 1 Examples of strains with and without ability to biofilm formation on plates with Congo *red* agar

Table 2 Compositions (%) of the tested commercial copper alloys

Common name	UNS code	Cu	As	Bi	Cd	Fe	Mn	Al	Ni	P	Pb	Sb	Si	Sn	Zn
Copper Cu-ETP	C11000	99.9	0.0	0.001	0.001	0.002	0.001	0.0	0.0	0.030	0.002	0.000	0.008	0.0	0.0
Yellow Brass CuZn37	C27400	63.2	0.001	0.001	0.001	0.001	0.001	0.001	0.06	0.001	0.004	0.001	0.008	0.0	36.7
Phosphor Bronze CuSn6	C51900	94.1	0.006	0.002	0.0	0.001	0.001	0.016	0.01	0.222	0.038	0.001	0.002	5.5.	0.1
Nickel silver CuNi18Zn20	C75200	63.1	0.001	0.001	0.001	0.027	0.12	0.001	17.9.	0.001	0.001	0.008	0.001	0.001	18.9.
Stainless Steel	S30400	Fe 68.8, C 0.07, Cr 19, Mn 2, N 0.1, Ni 10, P 0.045, S 0.015, Si 1													

UNS (Unified Numbering System), *ETP* Electrolytic Tough Pitch

Quantitative culture method to determine the antimicrobial effectiveness of copper and its alloys

In this study, wet exposure was used (modified methodology of the Japanese Standard [16]) to assess the antimicrobial properties of the selected copper alloys. The testing procedure is described in detail below.

For susceptibility to copper alloys four CNS strains were chosen and, for comparison, one *Staphylococcus aureus* strain (ATCC 12493). The following strains were chosen to examine antimicrobial properties of copper alloys: *S. epidermidis* no. 65 (MSSE), also sensitive to ciprofloxacin and gentamicin, biofilm-forming (category: black); *S. epidermidis* no. 62 (MRSE), resistant to the remaining antibiotics, biofilm-forming (category: black); *S. haemolyticus* no. 93 (MSSH), sensitive to all antibiotics, non-biofilm-forming (category: bordeaux) and *S. haemolyticus* no. 89 (MRSH), resistant to the remaining antibiotics, non-biofilm-forming (category: bordeaux) (Table 3). The strain numbers are internal laboratory numbers in this study.

The tested bacterial strains were stored in glycerol at −70 °C. One day before antimicrobial efficacy testing, a small amount of the suspension was taken from a frozen sample, inoculated onto solid Muller-Hinton agar (MHA, BIOCORP, Warsaw, Poland) (clean culture) and then incubated for 24 h at 37 °C. From the obtained culture, a suspension was prepared in saline at a density of 0.5 McFarland standard (controlled using a densitometer bioSan, Ryga, Latvia). Subsequently, 100 μL of the suspension with a density of 0.5 McFarland standard was transferred to 900 μL of TSB. Each time, a control for the viability of the bacteria obtained in the culture on solid medium and a control for the precise initial concentration (its density expressed in CFU/mL) was performed.

Samples of the metals tested were placed in a sterile container made of PVC with a capacity of 100 mL that was 6 cm in diameter, and then, 100 μL of a test suspension was applied (the composition depended on the variant of the experiment). Next, the container was covered with sterile polypropylene foil measuring 2 cm × 2 cm to provide close contact between the bacterial suspension and the metal surface. The container was covered to prevent contamination of the sample with microbes from the air, but it remained loose enough that aerobic conditions were maintained throughout the course of exposure and when left for a specified period of time (0, 30, 60, 90, 120, 180, 240, and 300 min) at approx. 22 °C (room temperature).

After a certain period of time, 5 mL of TSB solution and approx. 30 sterile glass beads that were 2 mm in diameter were placed into the container and shaken for 2 min in a shaker (shaker-incubator ES-20/60, Ryga, Latvia). Then, 100 μL of the wash was collected, and 4 serial decimal dilutions were prepared, of which 100 μL was inoculated onto solid MHA for each time-point. After a 24-h incubation, individual colonies were counted on the plates when the resulting number was countable.

For each metallic material, each exposure time for all microbes was repeated three times. To count the amount of CFU/mL after exposure of the bacterial suspension to the studied materials, the average of triplicates was used. The formula for the calculation was CFU/mL = (n x f x v1)/(v2 x v3), where n is the average number of colonies/plate in dilution, f is the dilution factor, v1 is the volume of TSB used for washing the bacteria that survived after exposure, v2 is the volume used and applied on metallic coupons, and v3 is the volume of the plated material (v1-3 in mL).

To evaluate the effectiveness of the antimicrobial activity, the criteria used by Souli et al. [17] were adopted, according to which a suspension density reduction ranging from ≤2 to <3 log means the presence of bacteriostatic properties, whereas a reduction of >3 log means bactericidal properties. Ole et al. estimated that the microbiological load of touch surfaces, such as door

Table 3 Characteristic of selected for tests of susceptibility for copper alloys CNS strains

Number of strain/ strain code	Species	Biofilm	Cefoxitin resistance
65/ MSSE 65	*S.epidermidis*	black (+)	S
62/ MRSE 62	*S.epidermidis*	black (+)	R
93/ MSSH 93	*S.haemolyticus*	bordeaux (−)	S
89/MRSH 89	*S.haemolyticus*	bordeaux (−)	R
ATCC 12493	*S. aureus*	very black (+)	R

handles in hospital wards, was 1–6 × 10^3 CFU [18] and therefore, the criteria proposed by Souli et al. can be deemed to be appropriate for testing the antimicrobial efficacy of products made of copper and its alloys. The results are presented in Fig. 2.

Statistical analysis

Test of comparison between fractions was used for analysis of statistical significance of antimicrobial resistance within CoNS species and between strains presenting resistance vs. susceptibility to methicillin – in case of characterization of antimicrobial resistance.

Results of susceptibility tests for the copper alloys tested were shown as charts of CFU/ml values in chosen time periods and were expressed as the mean ± SEM. Two-way Anova with repeated measures analysis of variance was used to evaluate the effects of both time and strain for every tested alloy. *P* values less than 0.05 were considered statistically significant.

Results

Microbes of the genus *Staphylococcus* accounted for the vast majority of the population of bacteria cultured from touch surfaces in the hospital environment. Among staphylococci, of which almost 97% were CoNS *(coagulase-negative staphylococci)*, there were 8 different species, the most frequent of which were *S. epidermidis, S. haemolyticus* and *S. hominis*, accounting for 34%, 30% and 15% of all CNS isolates, respectively.

Drug resistance

More than 67% (n = 64) of the analysed staphylococcal strains were methicillin-resistant, which is equivalent to resistance to all beta-lactam antibiotics. The presence of the *mec*A gene was confirmed in 68.4% of isolates (n = 65). Two *S. haemolyticus* isolates that were resistant to cefoxitin did not have the *mec*A gene, and three *S. epidermidis* isolates had the *mec*A gene and simultaneous susceptibility to cefoxitin (Table 4).

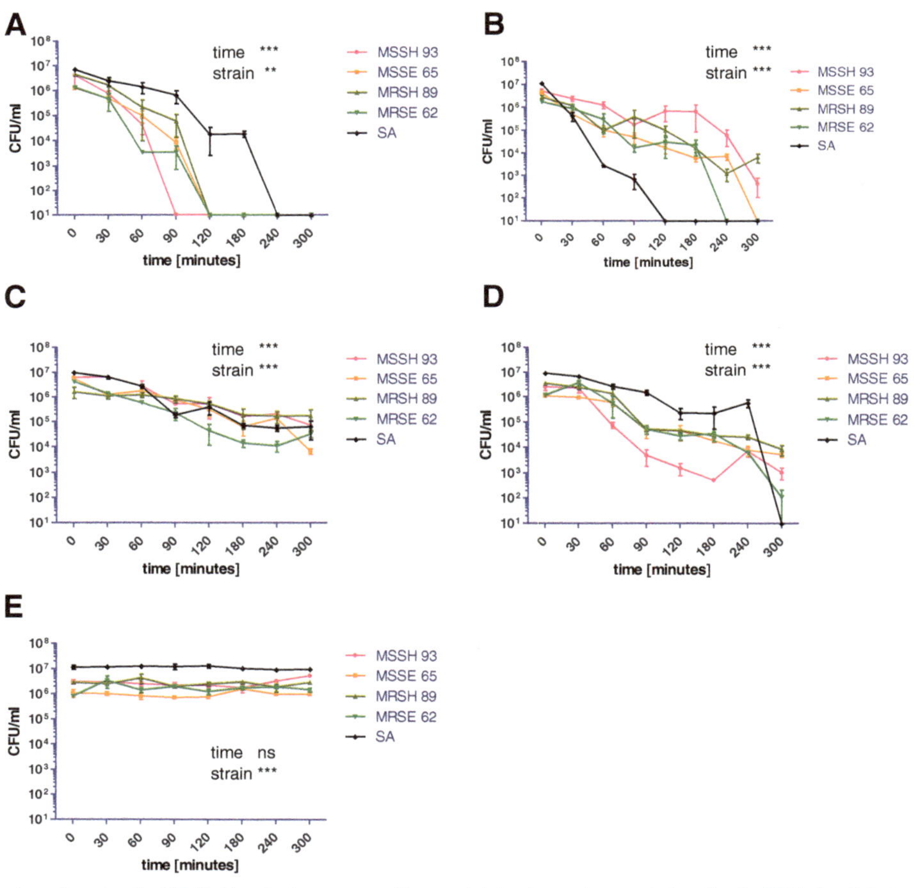

Fig. 2 Tested bacteria inoculum density (CFU/mL) reduction on metallic materials in chosen time periods. **a** for Cu-ETP, **b** for CuSn6, **c** for CuZn37, **d** for CuNi18Zn20, **e** for stainless steel. MSSH 93 - methicillin sensitive *Staphylococcus haemolyticus*, strain no. 93, MSSE 65 - methicillin sensitive *Staphylococcus epidermidis*, strain no. 65, MRSH 89 - methicillin-resistant *Staphylococcus haemolyticus*, strain no. 89, MRSE 62 - methicillin-resistant *Staphylococcus epidermidis* strain no. 62, SA – *Staphylococcus aureus* ATCC 12493. *** - $p < 0.001$, ** - $p < 0.01$, ns – not statistically significant

Table 4 Distribution of phenotypic and genotypic antibiotic resistance among tested staphylococcal strains

Species	n (%)	Methicillin resistance phenotype n (%)	Gen mecA n (%)	Phenotypes of macrolides resistance			erm (A, B, C) genes n (%)	Msr gen n (%)	Mupirocin resistence - phenotype n (%)	Mup gen n (%)
				cMLSB n (%)	iMLSB n (%)	MSB n (%)				
S. epidermidis	32 (33.7)	20 (21.1)	23 (24.2)	9 (9.5)	5 (5.3)	8 (8.4)	1 (1.1)	10 (10.5)	8 (8.4)	7 (7.4)
S. haemolyticus	28 (29.5)	22 (23.2)	20 (21.1)	17 (17.9)	0 (0)	5 (5.3)	0 (0)	15 (15.8)	3 (3.2)	6 (6.3)
S. hominis	14 (14.7)	13 (13.7)	13 (13.7)	3 (3.2)	6 (6.3)	2 (2.1)	0 (0)	0 (0)	2 (2.1)	5 (5.3)
S. capitis	6 (6.3)	4 (4.2)	4 (4.2)	3 (3.2)	0 (0)	0 (0)	0 (0)	1 (1.1)	1 (1.1)	0 (0)
S. warnerii	6 (6.3)	1 (1.1)	1(1.1)	0 (0)	0 (0)	2 (2.1)	0 (0)	2 (2.1)	0 (0)	0 (0)
S. simulans	3 (3.2)	1 (1.1)	1 (1.1)	0 (0)	3 (3.2)	0 (0)	0 (0)	0 (0)	0 (0)	0 (0)
S. aureus	3 (3.2)	1 (1.1)	1 (1.1)	1 (1.1)	0 (0)	0 (0)	0 (0)	0 (0)	0 (0)	0 (0)
S. pettenkoferi	2 (2.1)	2 (2.1)	2 (2.1)	1 (1.1)	1 (1.1)	0 (0)	0 (0)	0 (0)	0 (0)	0 (0)
S. caprae	1 (1.1)	0 (0)	0 (0)	0 (0)	0 (0)	0 (0)	0 (0)	0 (0)	0 (0)	0 (0)
Total	95 (100)	64 (67.4)	65 (68.4)	34 (35.8)	15 (15.8)	17 (17.9)	1 (1.1)	28 (29.5)	14 (14.7)	18 (18.9)

n number

In the group of the remaining antibiotics, the highest level of resistance was to erythromycin (70.5%) and clindamycin (52.6%). Resistance to gentamycin was demonstrated by 43.2% of the isolates. Resistance not exceeding 40% was found to ciprofloxacin, SXT and mupirocin (Table 4). Four strains were resistant to all of the tested antibiotics, and 14 to all except for mupirocin.

Resistance to macrolides and lincosamides can be conditioned by three mechanisms. The first mechanism, consisting of modification of the destination on the ribosome, was detected in 51.6% (n = 49) of the isolates (constitutive resistance phenotype cMLSB and inducible iMLSB). Expression of cMLSB resistance occurred in 34 isolates (35.8%) and that of iMLSB in 15 isolates (15.8%). The gene encoding the ribosomal methylase enzyme (*erm*B) was detected in only one strain from that group, and the *msr*A gene encoding the membrane transporter was detected in 15 isolates from that group.

The second mechanism of resistance is active removal of the antibiotic from the cell (efflux). The phenotype of resistance to erythromycin and preserved susceptibility to clindamycin (MSB) was confirmed in 17 isolates (17.9%), and the *msr*A gene was detected in 12 isolates from this group. One isolate had the *msr*A gene despite a lack of resistance to macrolides and lincosamides. The *msr* gene was thus detected in 28 isolates (29.5%).

Phenotypic resistance to mupirocin was found in 14 strains, and the *mup* gene was shown in 18 strains.

The incidence of MLSB and MSB phenotypes correlated with the incidence of MRCoNS and MRSA phenotypes; 52 (54.8%) isolates had both of these mechanisms at the same time.

Strains classified as MRCoNS had significantly increased resistance to the remaining antibiotic groups (p < 0.00001) (Table 5), but no statistically significant differences were observed in the proportion of methicillin resistance in specific CoNS species (p = 0.297).

Examination of antimicrobial activity of copper alloys on selected CoNS vs. SA strains

The material with greatest bactericidal properties is ETP copper, with which the density of the initial suspension, when in contact with the copper, decreased from 10^6 to 10^7 CFU/mL depending on the strain, and reached zero density in less than 4 h. For three of the tested CoNS strains, a complete reduction was observed after 2 h (Table 6). Three out of four tested coagulase-negative staphylococcal strains underwent complete reduction quicker than the SA strain, whereas the time needed for complete reduction of the MSSH93 strain was the same as for SA (Table 6).

Slightly lower antibacterial efficacy was exhibited by tin bronze (CuSn6). In only one of the strains tested (resistant to all antibiotics investigated) was complete reduction not observed (MRSH89 strain) after 300 min of exposure, and there was even no evidence of bacteriostatic activity – the suspension density decreased over a period of 6 h from 2.68E + 06 to 1.10E + 05 (Table 6). When the tested strains were exposed to CuSn6, the fastest complete reduction in suspension density was demonstrated for SA – after 2 h; and for the studied CoNS strains, the fastest complete reduction was found for strain MRSE62, demonstrating biofilm-forming properties (Table 6).

With respect to all of the studied staphylococcal strains, brass (CuZn37) demonstrated bacteriostatic properties after 300 min; the reduction in suspension density ranged from ≥2 log <3 log (Table 6).

In the case of material made from CuNi18Zn20 (nickel silver), a complete reduction in suspension density was observed for one of the studied MRSE62 strains, resistant to the majority of the examined antibiotics and exhibiting biofilm-forming properties (Table 6). Regarding the MRSH89 strain, resistant to all of the tested antibiotics, the CuNi18Zn20 material displayed neither bactericidal nor bacteriostatic effects; the degree of reduction of the initial bacterial suspension for the

Table 5 Antibiotic resistance of methicilline-resistant vs. sensitive staphylococcal strains isolated from touch surfaces

Antibiotic tested	Resistance for other antibiotics of CoNS (total) (n, %)	Resistance for other antibiotics of MRCoNS strains (n, %)	Resistance for other antibiotics of MSCoNS strains (n, %)
cefoxitin	63 (66.3)	63 (66.3)	29 (30.5)
erythromycin	66 (69.5)	53 (55.8)	13 (13.7)
clindamycin	49 (51.6)	43 (45.3)	6 (6.3)
ciprofloxacin	37 (38.9)	35 (36.8)	2 (2.1)
gentamycin	40 (42.1)	35 (36.8)	5 (5.3)
trimethoprim/sulfamethoxazole	33 (34.7)	31 (32.6)	2 (2.1)
mupirocin	14 (14.7)	12 (12.6)	2 (2.1)

MR methicillin resistant, *MS* methicillin sensitive

Table 6 Tested bacteria inoculum density (CFU/mL) reduction on Cu-ETP, CuSn6, CuZn37, CuNi18Zn20, stainless steel, in chosen time periods

Time [min]	MSSE 65[a]	MRSE 62	MSSH 93	MRSH 89	SA
Cu-ETP					
0	1.25E + 06	1.38E + 06	4.22E + 06	4.52E + 06	7.49E + 06
30	4.83E + 05	4.67E + 05	7.50E + 05	1.68E + 06	2.33E + 06
60	1.00E + 05	3.50E + 03	3.33E + 04	8.60E + 05	7.92E + 05
90	8.50E + 03	4.17E + 03	1.67E + 05	3.73E + 04	3.87E + 05
120	1.00E + 00	1.00E + 00	8.33E + 05	1.00E + 00	4.67E + 04
180	1.00E + 00	1.00E + 00	1.67E + 05	1.00E + 00	1.00E + 04
240	1.00E + 00	1.00E + 00	1.00E + 00	1.00E + 00	1.00E + 00
300	1.00E + 00	1.00E + 00	1.00E + 00	1.00E + 00	1.00E + 00
CuSn6					
Time [min]	MSSE 65	MRSE 62	MSSH 93	MRSH 89	SA
0	4.43E + 06	1.73E + 06	5.05E + 06	2.68E + 06	1.13E + 07
30	5.17E + 05	9.00E + 05	2.35E + 06	1.23E + 06	4.33E + 05
60	1.00E + 05	3.00E + 05	1.23E + 06	1.32E + 05	3.08E + 03
90	4.50E + 04	1.67E + 04	1.72E + 05	3.90E + 05	1.17E + 03
120	1.50E + 04	3.00E + 04	2.48E + 05	9.67E + 04	1.00E + 00
180	5.00E + 03	2.17E + 04	6.37E + 05	1.17E + 04	1.00E + 00
240	1.67E + 03	1.00E + 00	5.83E + 04	1.67E + 03	1.00E + 00
300	1.00E + 00	1.00E + 00	1.00E + 00	1.10E + 05	1.00E + 00
CuZn37					
Time [min]	MSSE 65	MRSE 62	MSSH 93	MRSH 89	SA
0	5.62E + 06	4.17E + 06	6.17E + 06	1.68E + 06	1.01E + 07
30	1.25E + 06	1.43E + 06	6.38E + 06	1.13E + 06	6.55E + 06
60	1.72E + 06	5.83E + 05	2.83E + 06	1.25E + 06	2.78E + 06
90	7.33E + 05	6.67E + 04	3.67E + 05	8.50E + 05	1.47E + 05
120	3.02E + 05	4.00E + 04	5.00E + 05	5.25E + 05	3.97E + 05
180	6.33E + 04	1.67E + 04	1.83E + 05	1.88E + 05	7.10E + 05
240	1.30E + 05	8.33E + 03	1.92E + 05	1.68E + 05	4.70E + 05
300	6.67E + 03	3.33E + 04	3.17E + 04	1.72E + 05	6.50E + 04
CuNi18Zn20					
Time [min]	MSSE 65	MRSE 62	MSSH 93	MRSH 89	SA
0	1.05E + 06	1.17E + 06	2.45E + 06	4.25E + 05	9.20E + 06
30	9.17E + 05	3.68E + 06	2.18E + 06	2.25E + 05	6.77E + 06
60	5.67E + 05	5.67E + 05	1.23E + 05	3.63E + 05	2.70E + 06
90	4.83E + 04	3.67E + 04	5.00E + 03	5.33E + 04	1.50E + 06
120	4.50E + 04	3.00E + 04	1.00E + 00	3.52E + 05	2.38E + 05
180	2.00E + 04	3.67E + 04	1.00E + 00	1.83E + 04	2.12E + 05
240	5.00E + 03	8.33E + 03	1.00E + 00	1.67E + 04	5.77E + 05
300	1.67E + 03	1.00E + 00	1.00E + 00	2.50E + 04	2.83E + 03
SS					
Time [min]	MSSE 65	MRSE 62	MSSH 93	MRSH 89	SA
0	1.05E + 06	8.17E + 06	2.98E + 06	3.33E + 06	1.18E + 07
30	9.83E + 05	3.40E + 06	2.87E + 06	2.20E + 06	1.20E + 07

Table 6 Tested bacteria inoculum density (CFU/mL) reduction on Cu-ETP, CuSn6, CuZn37, CuNi18Zn20, stainless steel, in chosen time periods *(Continued)*

60	8.00E + 05	1.43E + 06	2.45E + 06	4.63E + 06	1.27E + 07
90	7.00E + 05	2.02E + 06	2.22E + 06	1.80E + 06	1.25E + 07
120	7.33E + 05	1.23E + 06	2.12E + 06	2.10E + 06	1.30E + 07
180	1.55E + 06	1.80E + 06	1.73E + 06	3.43E + 06	1.05E + 07
240	9.67E + 05	1.92E + 06	3.20E + 06	1.50E + 06	9.33E + 06
300	9.50E + 05	1.50E + 06	5.15E + 06	3.08E + 06	9.77E + 06

[a]strains codes - see Table 3

remaining CoNS and SA strains was within the limits of bacteriostatic activity.

As for stainless steel, no bacteriostatic or bactericidal properties were found for any of the tested strains (Table 6).

The speed and degree of reduction of bacterial suspensions density for the tested strains on ETP copper, copper alloys and stainless steel, together with the results of statistical significance for strains and time points, are presented in Fig. 2. Only for stainless steel no significant reduction of bacterial density in time was observed. Significant differences were observed between strains for all tested metals (for stainless steel it was the result of difference in bacterial suspension density in time zero between SA and CoNS strains).

Biofilm

The environmental strains subjected to analysis were examined in terms of their biofilm formation capabilities: there were 32 (33.7%) biofilm-forming strains (categories: very black, black and almost black), including very black – 1 strain, black – 11 and almost black – 20, and 63 (66.3%) non-biofilm-forming strains (categories: bordeaux, red and very red), including bordeaux – 54, red – 4, and very red – 5 (Fig. 1).

Among the majority of species, biofilm-forming and non-biofilm-forming strains were distributed evenly; in the case of *S. haemolyticus* only, negative strains accounted for 92.8%.

Discussion

The staphylococcal strains that were found on touch surfaces were primarily CoNS. Fewer than 3% of *S. aureus* species found were coagulase-positive isolates. Staphylococcal strains on touch surfaces can come from both the normal human flora (hand skin) and the environment, especially the air. CoNS are not dangerous to people with a properly functioning immune system but, in hospitals, they may pose a threat especially for patients who are severely ill, older, immunocompromised, hospitalized in the ICU or newborns in the NICU [19, 20]. *S. epidermidis, S. haemolyticus,* and *S. hominis* are the most frequent CoNS found to be responsible for causing skin infections as well as severe invasive infections [21–23]. Additionally, treating infections caused by CoNS can be difficult due to their drug resistance [23, 24].

In our study, among CoNS species, *S. epidermidis* and *S. haemolyticus* were predominant, which differs from studies on air also conducted in the south of Poland where *S. saprophyticus* and *S. warneri* were prevailing [25]. The reason for this difference might be the different places of isolation (touch surfaces, not air) as well as the method applied for species identification. In this work, we employed the state-of-the-art and most recommended method, that is, Matrix Assisted Laser Desorption Ionization Time of Flight (MALDI-TOF). In other studies in which authors employed the MALDI method for environmental research, strains from the species *S. haemolyticus, S. hominis* [4], *S. haemolyticus* and *S. epidermidis* [26] were most common. Additionally, Mkrtchyan et al. showed that results may vary when different identification methods are applied [27].

S. aureus, which is the main cause of hospital-acquired infections, was not isolated in large numbers, which can be surprising but has been confirmed by recent studies in Poland and abroad [4, 25, 28].

Many CoNS strains were methicillin-resistant (as many as 65%), which greatly limits therapeutic options in the case of potential opportunistic infections that they cause, due to inapplicability of the entire group of beta--lactam antibiotics [29]. For the vast majority of isolates, phenotypic resistance was confirmed through the detection of the *mec*A gene. Three *S. epidermidis* strains had the *mec*A gene and retained sensitivity to cefoxitin – similar strains were found for the species *S. aureus* [30].

Surprisingly, many isolates were also resistant to erythromycin (over 2/3) and clindamycin (a 1/2). Additionally, almost 55% of isolates had simultaneous resistance to methicillin and the MLSB mechanism of resistance.

The most frequent phenotypically detected mechanism of resistance to macrolide antibiotics, lincosamides and streptogramins B was the constitutive MLSB mechanism (35.8%), which agrees with the study by Lina [31] (here, it was 36.6%) and is a little less than Castro-Alarcon's results [32] (47%) but different from Lenart-Boroń's findings (where it was present only in 4% of the strains and where the inducible mechanism was predominant) [25]. The phenotype of resistance to erythromycin and retained sensitivity to clindamycin (MSB) was confirmed in 17 isolates (17.9%), and for Lenart-Boroń, it was 28% [25]. The gene associated with resistance to macrolides that was most often detected in our study was the *msr*A gene encoding a pump responsible for active efflux of the antibiotic from the cell (29.5% of the strains); the *erm*B gene, one of the genes encoding a methylase, was present in only 1 strain. Castro-Alarcon had contrasting results in which 32% of strains had the *erm*A gene [32]. The differences between the genes detected and the phenotypic detection of mechanisms of resistance may stem from testing only several selected genes – we did not look, e.g., at different variants of the *msr* gene, *mph* genes (encoding phosphotransferase), or the flax gene (responsible for resistance to lincosamides). We also did not examine the problem of gene expression. Our aim was not only to study the mechanisms of resistance; we also wanted to select strains for research on antibacterial properties of copper alloys.

Sensitivity to mupirocin concerned the greatest number of strains, and the *mup* gene was found in approx. 18% of strains.

One of the significant virulence factors of CoNS strains is their ability to form biofilm. The biofilm testing method applied here is a screening method. However, it allowed us to estimate that approximately 1/3 of the strains are potentially biofilm-forming, fewer than in the study by Szczuka, where 64% of CoNS strains formed biofilm [33].

The copper alloys that we tested have Environmental Protection Agency (USA) certificates, but EPA recommendations are based on tests for such bacterial species as *Staphylococcus aureus*, *Escherichia coli*, *Enterobacter aerogenes* and *Pseudomonas aeruginosa*, which are the bacteria that cause the majority of hospital-acquired infections [34, 35]. Coagulase-negative staphylococci, however, have also been identified as aetiologic agents of infection [12, 15, 19], and their drug resistance and ability to form biofilms, demonstrated in this study and by other researchers [24, 26], justify activity assays of copper alloys for potential use on touch surfaces in hospital departments. Four strains of the most often isolated CoNS species were selected for research on their antimicrobial properties. They differed in their resistance to antibiotics and their ability to form biofilm, and our experiments also revealed differences in susceptibility to the copper alloys.

The tests conducted showed that only for Cu-ETP was similar or higher bactericidal activity found against the studied CoNS strains than against *Staphylococcus aureus* – the maximum bacterial suspension density reduction from the level of approx. 10^7 CFU/mL to 0 was observed in 120 to 240 min, depending on the strain.

Tin bronze demonstrated a faster bactericidal effect against the tested SA strain. Complete reduction in suspension density was observed after 120 min, but in the case of three of the tested CoNS strains, this time was 240 or 300 min, while for the MRSH89 strain (methicillin-resistant, non-biofilm-forming), after 300 min, the reduction in suspension density was lower by 2 log.

A similar course and degree of reduction in initial suspension density was observed for all of the examined CoNS and SA on brass CuZn37 – the boundary criterion for determining bacteriostatic effects. On CuNi18Zn20, two of the tested CoNS strains demonstrated greater susceptibility than SA.

Noyce et al. examined sensitivity to copper and bronze for three different methicillin-resistant *Staphylococcus aureus* strains [36]. The authors observed similar susceptibility of the tested MRSA strains to copper (C19700) – total reduction of the initial suspension density from approx. 1E + 07 to zero in under 90 min – and for two MRSA strains on bronze (C24000), they found total reduction after approximately 4.5 h, while for one of the tested strains, the degree of reduction after 360 min did not meet the qualification criterion for bacteriostatic properties [36].

The study that we conducted shows that coagulase-negative staphylococci, most often isolated from touch surfaces in Polish hospital wards [13], are not only highly drug-resistant but also perhaps less sensitive to copper alloys than *Staphylococcus aureus*. However, most of the CoNS strains tested in this study demonstrated susceptibility to copper alloys, which as a result are useful as a complementary solution for traditional cleaning and disinfection in hospitals.

Additionally, in Poland, there are no official recommendations for testing the antimicrobial effectiveness of materials dedicated for touch surfaces in healthcare settings. In the case of developing such recommendations, perhaps research on antimicrobial properties of materials intended for use as touch surfaces should also include representative coagulase-negative staphylococci because, as was shown in this study, they can be a reservoir of antibiotic-resistance genes. The advantage of copper as a material with antimicrobial properties intended for touch surfaces is its cidal activity, consisting of the destruction of genetic material as shown in other studies [37], and hence the possibility that it can eliminate genes for antibiotic resistance.

Conclusions

1. Coagulase-negative staphylococci, the most commonly isolated in Polish hospital wards, should not be neglected as infection risk factors due to their high antibiotic resistance.

2. About one-third of the tested environmental staphylococcal strains revealed biofilm-forming ability, and this may be a reason for the common contamination of hospital environments by these bacteria.
3. In the case of tin bronze, we observed lower antimicrobial activity against tested CoNS strains compared to an SA strain (longer times of bacterial density reduction). Despite this, our experiments confirmed that touch surfaces made of copper alloys may play an important role in eliminating bacteria from the hospital environment.

Abbreviations

ATCC: American Type Culture Collection; CFU: Colony forming units; cMLSB: Constitutive macrolide-lincosamide-streptogramin B; CoNS: Coagulase-negative staphylococci; CRA: Congo red agar; EPA: Environmental Protection Agency; ETP: Electrolytic Tough Pitch; EUCAST: The European Committee on Antimicrobial Susceptibility Testing; iMLSB: Inducible macrolide-lincosamide-streptogramin B; MRCoNS: Methicillin-resistant coagulase negative staphylococci; MRSA: Methicillin-resistant *Staphylococcus aureus*; MRSE: Methicillin-resistant *Staphylococcus epidermidis*; MRSH: Methicillin-resistant *Staphylococcus haemolyticus*; MSB: Macrolide-streptogramin B; MSCoNS: Methicillin sensitive coagulase-negative staphylococci; MSSE: Methicillin sensitive *Staphylococcus epidermidis*; MSSH: Methicillin sensitive *Staphylococcus haemolyticus*; PCR: Polymerase chain reaction; R: Resistant; S: Sensitive; SA: *Staphylococcus aureus*; TSB: Tryptic soy broth; VRE: Vancomycin-resistant enterococci

Acknowledgements

Not applicable

Funding

This project was financially supported by The Polish National Center for Research and Development and awarded on the basis of decision PBS3/A9/32/2015.

Authors' contributions

AR planned the experiments, performed laboratory microbiological tests, analysed and interpreted the data and was a major contributor in writing the manuscript; ACH and DR performed laboratory microbiological tests and drafted the manuscript; MW and PO prepared the metallic samples for the study, planned the experiments, and drafted the manuscript; MB and TK coordinated the project and drafted the manuscript. All authors read and approved the final manuscript.

Consent for publication

Not applicable

Competing interests

The authors declare that they have no competing interests.

Author details

[1]Jagiellonian University Medical College, Faculty of Medicine, Chair of Microbiology, Czysta str. 18, 31-121 Kraków, Poland. [2]Faculty of Non-Ferrous Metals, Department of Metal Working and Physical Metallurgy of Non-Ferrous Metals, AGH University of Science and Technology, al. Mickiewicza 30, 30-059 Kraków, Poland.

References

1. Rampling A, Wiseman S, Davis L, Hyett AP, Walbridge AN, Payne GC, et al. Evidence that hospital hygiene is important in the control of methicillin-resistant *Staphylococcus aureus*. J Hosp Infect. 2001;49(2):109–16.
2. Dancer SJ. Controlling hospital-acquired infection: focus on the role of the environment and new technologies for decontamination. Clin Microbiol Rev. 2014;27(4):665–90.
3. Siegel JD, Rhinehart E, Jackson M, Chiarello L, Healthcare Infection Control Practices Advisory Committee. Management of multidrug-resistant organisms in health care settings, 2006. Am J Infect Control. 2007;35(10 Suppl 2):S165–93.
4. Xu Z, Mkrtchyan HV, Cutler RR. Antibiotic resistance and mecA characterization of coagulase-negative staphylococci isolated from three hotels in London, UK. Front Microbiol. 2015;6:947.
5. Roberts MC, Soge OO, No D, Helgeson SE, Meschke JS. Characterization of Methicillin-resistant Staphylococcus aureus isolated from public surfaces on a university campus, student homes and local community. J Appl Microbiol. 2011;110(6):1531–7.
6. Simões RR, Aires-de-Sousa M, Conceição T, Antunes F, da Costa PM, de Lencastre H. High prevalence of EMRSA-15 in Portuguese public buses: a worrisome finding. PLoS One. 2011;6(3):e17630.
7. Shurland S, Zhan M, Bradham DD, Roghmann MC. Comparison of mortality risk associated with bacteremia due to methicillin-resistant and methicillin-susceptible Staphylococcus aureus. Infect Control Hosp Epidemiol. 2007;28(3):273–9.
8. Chmielarczyk A, Pomorska-Wesołowska M, Szczypta A, Romaniszyn D, Pobiega M, Wójkowska-Mach J. Molecular analysis of meticillin-resistant *Staphylococcus aureus* strains isolated from different types of infections from patients hospitalized in 12 regional, non-teaching hospitals in southern Poland. J Hosp Infect. 2017;95(3):259–67.
9. Dancer SJ, White LF, Lamb J, Girvan EK, Robertson C. Measuring the effect of enhanced cleaning in a UK hospital: a prospective cross-over study. BMC Med. 2009;7:28. doi:10.1186/1741-7015-7-28.
10. Różańska A, Romaniszyn D, Chmielarczyk A, Bulanda M. Contamination with bacteria of otuch surfaces inPolish hospital wards. Med Pr. 2017;68(4):459–67. doi:10.13075/mp.5893.00575.
11. Leclercq R. Mechanisms of resistance to macrolides and lincosamides: nature of the resistance elements and their clinical implications. Clin Infect Dis. 2002;34(4):482–92.
12. Pereira EM, Schuenck RP, Malvar KL, Iorio NL, Matos PD, Olendzki AN, et al. Staphylococcus aureus, Staphylococcus epidermidis and Staphylococcus haemolyticus: methicillin-resistant isolates are detected directly in blood cultures by multiplex PCR. Microbiol Res. 2010;165(3):243–9.
13. Sutcliffe J, Grebe T, Tait-Kamradt A, Wondrack L. Detection of erythromycin resistant determinants by PCR. Antimicrob Agents Chemother. 1996;40(11):2562–6.
14. Anthony RM, Connor AM, Power EG, French GL. Use of the polymerase chain reaction for rapid detection of high-level mupirocin resistance In staphylococci. Eur J Clin Microbiol Infect Dis. 1999;18:30–4.
15. Arciola CR, Campoccia D, Gamberini S, Cervellati M, Donati E, Montanaro L. Detection of slime production by means of an optimised Congo red agar plate test based on a colourimetric scale in *Staphylococcus epidermidis* clinical isolates genotyped for ica locus. Biomaterials. 2002;23(21):4233–9.
16. Japanese Industrial Standard JIS Z 2801 "Antimicrobial products – Test for antibacterial activity and efficacy". https://law.resource.org/pub/jp/ibr/jis.z.2801.e.2010.pdf. Accessed 21 Apr 2017.
17. Souli M, Galani I, Plachouras D, Panagea T, Armaganidis A, Petrikkos G, et al. Antimicrobial activity of copper surfaces against carbapenemase-producing contemporarty Gram-negative clinical isolates. J Antimicrob Chemother. 2012. doi: 10.1093/jac/dks473
18. Ojell M, Jermann C, Holah J, Denyer SP, Maillard J-Y. Evaluation of new in vitro efficacy test for antimicrobial surface activity reflecting UK hospital conditions. J Hosp Infect. 2013;85:274–81.
19. Bouchami O, Achour W, Mekni MA, Rolo J, BenHassen A. Antibiotic resistance and molecular characterization of clinical isolates of methicillin-resistant coagulase-negative staphylococci solated from bacteremic patients in oncohematology. Folia Microbiol (Praha). 2011;56:122–30. doi:10.1007/s12223-011-0017-1.
20. Klingenberg C, Rønnestad A, Anderson AS, Abrahamsen TG, Zorman J, Villaruz A, et al. Persistent strains of coagulase-negative staphylococci in a neonatal intensive care unit: virulence factors and invasiveness. Clin Microbiol Infect. 2007;13(11):1100–11.
21. Huebner J, Goldmann DA. Coagulase-negativestaphylococci:role aspathogens. Annu Rev Med. 1999;50:223–36. doi:10.1146/annurev.med.50.1.223.

22. Basaglia G, Moras L, Bearz A, Scalone S, Paoli PD. *Staphylococcus cohnii* septicaemia in a patient with colon cancer. J Med Microbiol. 2003;52:101–2. doi:10.1099/jmm.0.05002-0.
23. Becker K, Heilmann C, Peters G. Coagulase-negative staphylococci. Clin Microbiol Rev. 2014;27(4):870–926.
24. Monsen T, Karlsson C, Wiström J. Spread of clones of multidrug-resistant, coagulase-negative staphylococci within a university hospital. Infect Control Hosp Epidemiol. 2005;26(1):76–80.
25. Lenart-Boroń A, Wolny-Koładka K, Stec J, Kasprowic A. Phenotypic and molecular antibiotic resistance determination of airborne coagulase negative Staphylococcus spp. strains from healthcare facilities in Southern Poland. Microb Drug Resist. 2016;22(7):515–22.
26. Singh S, Dhawan B, Kapil A, Kabra SK, Suri A, Sreenivas V, et al. Coagulase-negative staphylococci causing blood stream infection at an Indian tertiary care hospital: prevalence, antimicrobial resistance and molecular characterisation. Indian J Med Microbiol. 2016;34(4):500–5.
27. Mkrtchyan HV, Russell CA, Wang N, Cutler RR. Could public restrooms be an environment for bacterial resistomes? PLoS One. 2013;8(1):e54223.
28. Augustowska M, Dutkiewicz J. Variability of airborne microflora in a hospital ward within a period of one year. Ann Agric Environ Med. 2006;13(1):99–106.
29. Talebi M, Shafiee M, Sadeghi J, Moghadam NA, Saifi M, Pourshafie MR. Genotypic diversity of methicillin-resistant coagulase-negative staphylococci isolated from inpatients and outpatients. Microb Drug Resist. 2016;22(2): 147–54. doi:10.1089/mdr.2014.0195.
30. Andrade-Figueiredo M, Leal-Balbino TC. Clonal diversity and epidemiological characteristics of Staphylococcus aureus: high prevalence of oxacillin-susceptible mecA-positive Staphylococcus aureus (OS-MRSA) associated with clinical isolates in Brazil. BMC Microbiol. 2016;16(1):115.
31. Lina G, Quaglia A, Reverdy ME, Leclercq R, Vandenesch F, Etienne J. Distribution of genes encoding resistance to macrolides, lincosamides, and streptogramins among staphylococci. Antimicrob Agents Chemother. 1999;43(5):1062–6.
32. Castro-Alarcón N, Ribas-Aparicio RM, Silva-Sánchez J, Calderón-Navarro A, Sánchez-Pérez A, Parra-Rojas I, et al. Molecular typing and characterization of macrolide, lincosamide and streptogramin resistance in Staphylococcus epidermidis strains isolated in a Mexican hospital. J Med Microbiol. 2011;60(Pt 6):730–6.
33. Szczuka E, Jabłońska L, Kaznowski A. Coagulase-negative staphylococci: pathogenesis, occurrence of antibiotic resistance genes and in vitro effects of antimicrobial agents on biofilm-growing bacteria. J Med Microbiol. 2016; 65(12):1405–13.
34. Kock R, Becker K, Cookson B, van Gemert-Pijnen JE, Harbath S, Kluytmans J, et al. Systemic literature analysis and review of targeted preventive measures to limit healthcare-associated infections by meticillin-resistant *Staphylococcus aureus*. Eur Secur. 2014;19(29).23–49.
35. European Centre for Disease Prevention and Control. Antimicrobial resistance surveillance in Europe 2013. Annual Report of the European Antimicrobial Resistance Surveillance Netwoerk (EARS-Net). Stockholm: ECDC; 2014.
36. Noyce JO, Michels H, Keevil CW. Potential use of copper surfaces to reduce survival of epidemic meticillin-resistant *Stapnylococcus aureus* in the healthcare environment. J Hosp Infect. 2006;63:289–97.
37. Weaver L, Michels HT, Keevil CW. Survival of Clostridium difficile on copper and steel: futuristic options for hospital hygiene. J Hosp Infect. 2008;68(2):145–51.

17

Outbreak report: a nosocomial outbreak of vancomycin resistant *enterococci* in a solid organ transplant unit

Peter Kreidl[1], Astrid Mayr[1*], Guido Hinterberger[1], Michael Berktold[1], Ludwig Knabl[1], Stefan Fuchs[1], Wilfried Posch[1], Stephan Eschertzhuber[2], Alois Obwegeser[3], Cornelia Lass-Flörl[1] and Dorothea Orth-Höller[1]

Abstract

Background: Vancomycin resistant *enterococci* (VRE) are an emerging problem in health care settings. The purpose of the investigation was to assess the extent of the outbreak including environmental contamination and to limit further transmission.

Methods: We used retrospective patient and laboratory data including pulse field gel electrophoresis (PFGE) typing and virulence and resistance gene analysis. For comparison of medians the Mann-Whitney and for comparison of proportions the Fisher exact tests were used.

Results: PFGE typing of VRE strains of an outbreak of 15 VRE cases in a solid transplant unit revealed that nine of the cases belonged to one identical pattern (A), which was only found twice in the environment. Eleven further positive environmental samples showed a different, but identical PFGE pattern E. Only one patient was infected with this environmental strain.
Two of nine (22.2%) PFGE A, but nine of eleven (81.2%) PFGE E samples were positive for gelatinase E ($p = 0.01$), which is described as enhancing biofilm production, suggesting a survival benefit for this strain on inanimate surfaces.

Conclusion: Routine disinfection was not able to stop the cluster, but after repeated enforcement of the infection prevention and control (IPC) bundle such as training, strict adherence to hand hygiene and surface disinfection no further cases were observed. We conclude that certain VRE strains predominate in the environment whereas others predominate in humans. Enforcement of the IPC bundle is essential for controlling VRE outbreaks and reducing further transmission.

Keywords: Solid organ transplant unit, Vancomycin resistant *enterococci*, Outbreak, Survival benefit, Infection control

Background

Vancomycin resistant *enterococci* (VRE) are important causes of morbidity and mortality especially in health care settings where they easily disseminate [1]. Effective treatment is limited and thus VRE remain a major challenge for infection control.

Vancomycin resistance of invasive *Enterococcus faecium* isolates ranges between 0 and 46.3% in countries of the European Union and European Economic Area (EU/EEA). The proportion of VRE in Austria (4.3% in 2016) was below the EU population weighted mean of 11.8% (95% confidence interval (CI) 11–13%) [2]. Monoclonal and polyclonal outbreaks of VRE were described worldwide; the largest reported outbreaks comprised up to 72 cases [3].

The most important transmission-routes of VRE are still not fully understood, but cross contamination via the hands of health care workers' (HCW) is believed to play a major role. HCW act as a vector between colonized or infected patients, inanimate surfaces and previously unaffected patients [4]. The reservoir for VRE is believed to be the human intestine [5].

* Correspondence: astrid.mayr@i-med.ac.at
[1]Department of Hygiene, Microbiology and Social Medicine, Division of Hygiene and Medical Microbiology, Medical University of Innsbruck, Innsbruck, Schoepfstr. 41, 6020 Innsbruck, Austria
Full list of author information is available at the end of the article

Known risk factors for acquisition of VRE include previous use of antibiotics, prolonged hospital stay, underlying diseases, admission to high risk departments such as oncology, hematology, transplant or intensive care units (ICU), the nurse to patient ratio, and occupancy to a room where previously a patient harboring VRE was admitted [6]. The transmission in high risk wards via contaminated inanimate surfaces is believed to be important but it remains a challenge to quantify the attributable risk [6] of environmental contamination.

We describe an outbreak which was identified on 7th January 2017 after detection of five cases within 2 months following the Orion statement [7].

The objective of this investigation was to assess the extent of the outbreak including the environmental contamination, to limit further transmission and to evaluate the effectiveness of implemented control measures. Further important objectives were to foster infection prevention and control (IPC) education by the infection control team (ICT) of the University Hospital Innsbruck (LKI).

Methods

Study design

We used retrospective data analysis including PFGE typing, analysis of virulence and resistance genes and patient relevant data from the hospital records.

Participants

Participants were patients admitted to the solid organ transplant unit between 15th November 2016 and 30th June 2017 with laboratory confirmation of VRE. Colonization was defined as laboratory confirmation of VRE in a sample of a patient from a non-sterile site without signs of infection such as fever > = 38.5 °C. Infection was defined as laboratory confirmation of VRE in a sample of a patient from a normally sterile site or signs of infection such as fever > = 38.5°.

Case definition

We defined a VRE case as a patient admitted to the transplant unit during the observation period with laboratory confirmation of VRE in at least one sample irrespective of the location or type of sampling. We defined a cluster case as a VRE case with the outbreak PFGE pattern A identified between December 2017 and June 2018 and admitted to the transplant unit.

Setting

The period of the outbreak lasted from 15 November 2016 until 30 June 2017.

The LKI is a 1600-bed tertiary-care hospital with several departments including a solid organ transplant unit.

The setting of the outbreak was the ward of the transplant unit consisting of 15 beds in seven rooms (one to four beds per room) and an adjacent intensive care unit (ICU) consisting of eight beds situated in three separate rooms. Patients were transferred between the standard care unit and the ICU depending on their medical condition. The ICT consisted of one senior hospital hygiene specialist and a local hygiene team.

Routine IPC protocol

The internal IPC protocol included the following recommendations: 1) twice daily unsupervised routine disinfection of inanimate surfaces of the patient close environment with an aldehyde-free-broad-spectrum disinfectant containing quaternary ammonium compounds (QACs, 2% TPH protect, Schülke & Mayr GmbH, Vienna, Austria) including once daily patient charts, 2) terminal cleaning and disinfection of patient rooms with the above mentioned disinfectant and 3) hand hygiene (HH) based on the WHO approach "My Five Moments for Hand Hygiene" [8] using alcohol-based detergents (Sterillium®, BODE Chemie GmbH, Hamburg, Germany). Surveillance of hand hygiene compliance is conducted through bi-annual audits based on the protocol from the Robert Koch Institute [9], measuring adherence to HH. The outcomes of the audits were categorized as sufficient or insufficient per unit but lacked a coding system to quantify the adherence to HH on an individual basis. Annual trainings of the IPC protocol through verbal presentations and ward round sessions were routinely conducted. Data on baseline IPC knowledge of HCW were not routinely collected. IPC guidelines did not require pre-admission VRE screening of patients, unless 1) patients had a positive history of exposure in a high endemic country, 2) were transferred from a long-term-care-facility or 3) were previously known having been infected or colonized with VRE.

According to the IPC protocol, each newly identified patient either colonized or infected by VRE irrespective of the patient being part of an outbreak, triggered a routine infection control response consisting of following measures: isolation precautions, defined as placement in a single room, if possible, and, contact precautions depending on the estimated potential for transmission including personal protective equipment.

Intervention during the outbreak

During the outbreak the following additional measures were implemented: Re-emphasizing strict adherence to HH and to environmental disinfection including unannounced microbiological monitoring of the environment and HCW's hands, repeated sampling of stool or rectal swabs of the VRE positive patients, newly admitted patients and rectal screening of HCWs. Rectal swabbing of patients was implemented as precautionary measure to limit the extent of the outbreak. Self-administered rectal swabbing of HCWs was conducted on voluntary basis upon the urgency of the situation. Thus informed consent was not obtained.

Frequency of ward round training was increased. The choice of HH antisepsis and environmental disinfection during the outbreak remained the same and compliance with HH was observed by the ICT. No additional decontamination procedures such as fogging or steaming were implemented.

Culturing and typing

Patient samples

We collected routine clinical samples and rectal screening swabs from patients according to the IPC protocol (no informed consent was requested for rectal sampling), cultivated them on blood agar (Becton Dickinson, Heidelberg, Germany) and selective ChromID VRE Agar (Biomerieux, Marcy-l'Étoile, France) and incubated them for 48 h at 37 °C under aerobic conditions. Suspect colonies were identified by matrix-assisted laser desorption ionization time-of-flight mass spectrometry (MALDI--TOF, Bruker, Bremen, Germany). Antibiotic susceptibility testing was performed according to the European Committee on Antimicrobial Susceptibility Testing (EUCAST version 6.0, 2016) protocol [10]. *Enterococci* were classified as VRE if the minimal inhibitory concentration of vancomycin was above 4 mg/L identified by E-Test (Biomerieux, Marcy-l'Étoile, France) [11]. Additional patient data such as diagnosis, duration of hospital stay, outcome, type and time of transplantation were obtained from the medical records of the LKI.

Environmental samples

Unheralded sampling of environment was conducted according to Galvins protocol (Galvin) using Columbia-III-Sheep blood agar 5% (Oxoid Limited, Basingstoke, UK) or Tryptic soy agar with neutralizers (VWR International, Radnor, USA) contact plates with a press on time of 10 seconds without any lateral movement. Surfaces were selected at different locations close and distant from the respective patients [12] during three occasions: immediately after the alert of the cluster on 18 January, and twice after enforcement of control measures (30th January and 2nd February 2017, respectively). Data recorded were date, type and location of sampling, laboratory findings and PFGE results. Direct unheralded observation of hygienic measures was conducted to identify potential gaps of adherence to infection control measures. Patient close samples were defined as samples obtained from the vicinity of patients such as the bedrail, bedframe, beside tables, clamps for urine-bags, drug perfusors, stethoscope and bedside monitors [13].

Microbial monitoring of HCWs hands was performed by imprinting all fingertips including the thumb onto Columbia agar containing 5% sheep blood (Becton, Dickenson and Company, Franklin Lakes, USA) for approximately 5 seconds [14, 15]. Confirmation of VRE was conducted as described above.

PFGE

Molecular Typing was performed using pulse field gel electrophoresis (PFGE) according to the protocols published by the Centers for Disease Control and Prevention [16]. Extracted bacterial DNA was restricted using SmaI enzyme. Strain typing was performed by manual PFGE restriction pattern analysis [17] and by computational analysis of band differences using GelJ Software Version 2 [18]. Dendrogram analysis of PFGE patterns was performed using Dice algorithm and Single Linkage clustering. Genotypically related strains with similarity > 90% were considered belonging to the same pattern.

Genetic analysis

Vancomycin resistance genotypes were determined according to the protocol from Jayaratne et al. [19]. The enterococcal surface antigen was identified according to the protocol by Toledo-Arana [20], the cytolysin activator according to Vankerckhoven [21] and the gelatinase E according to Hancock's protocol [22].

Infection related outcomes

Infection related outcomes, including colonization, infection and patient survival were assessed.

The specimen processing and turn-around time were performed according to local laboratory protocol from 2016.

Sample size

The sample size was limited to the number of identified patients ($n = 15$).

Statistical methods

Variables of interest were stored in excel database including age, gender, number of isolates obtained including positives, date of available laboratory result, source and material of samples, length of hospital stay, previous antibiotic treatment, previous confirmation of VRE in any sample, diagnosis, other identified pathogens, and patient outcome.

Descriptive analysis was performed using Epi info version 7.2.2.2. (CDC Atlanta). For comparison of medians the Mann-Whitney and for comparison of proportions the Fisher exact tests were used. A p-value of < 0.05 was considered statistically significant.

Results

Event description

On 7th January 2017 the outbreak response team of the LKI informed the transplant unit about a potential outbreak of VRE.

Analysis of historical data revealed that between May 2012 and October 2016, a total of 53 VRE cases were identified at this unit. The median incidence was one (0–3) case per month and the annual median incidence was 11 cases (6–16 cases) per year for the period 2013–2016. In comparison to previous years, the observed number of five VRE cases in a period of less than 2 months clearly exceeded the expected value suggesting an outbreak.

VRE cases

After a period of 4 months without any detection of VRE from the transplant unit, the potential index case was confirmed on 15th November 2016. He was a 58 year old male suffering from IgA Nephritis who received a kidney transplant on 12th November 2016, 3 days prior to the diagnosis of VRE in a single sample of a retroperitoneal surgical-site-drainage. The patient was classified as being infected.

Between 15th November 2016 and 30th June 2017, VRE was confirmed in at least one sample of 14 additional patients (Fig. 1). Of these, ten patients (66.7%) were males with a median age of 56.5 years (50–71 years). The five female patients showed a median age of 70 years (60–79 years) ($p = 0.003$) (Table 1).

VRE was first isolated twice from blood cultures, five times from urine samples, four times from wound drainage and once each from a tissue, stool, and rectal swab and from a broncho-alveolar lavage sample. Three of the patients were classified as being colonized, the remaining twelve as being infected with VRE. The median length of hospital stay was 24 days (10–112 days). All but one patient underwent transplantation and received immunosuppression. Twelve patients survived (80%) and three died (Table 1). In all patients *Enterococcus faecium* was identified, one patient harbored a tigecycline resistant, two a linezolid resistant and fourteen teicoplanin resistant strains.

PFGE patterns of cases

PFGE patterns were available for 13 of 15 patients (86.7%). Among those, five different PFGE patterns were identified and subsequently classified as patterns A to E. Nine of the thirteen cases (69.2%) were classified as PFGE pattern A (further called cluster strain, Table 1, Fig. 2).

All 10 of the 15 patient isolates (66.7%) available for vancomycin resistance genotyping (*van*R) revealed *van*A,

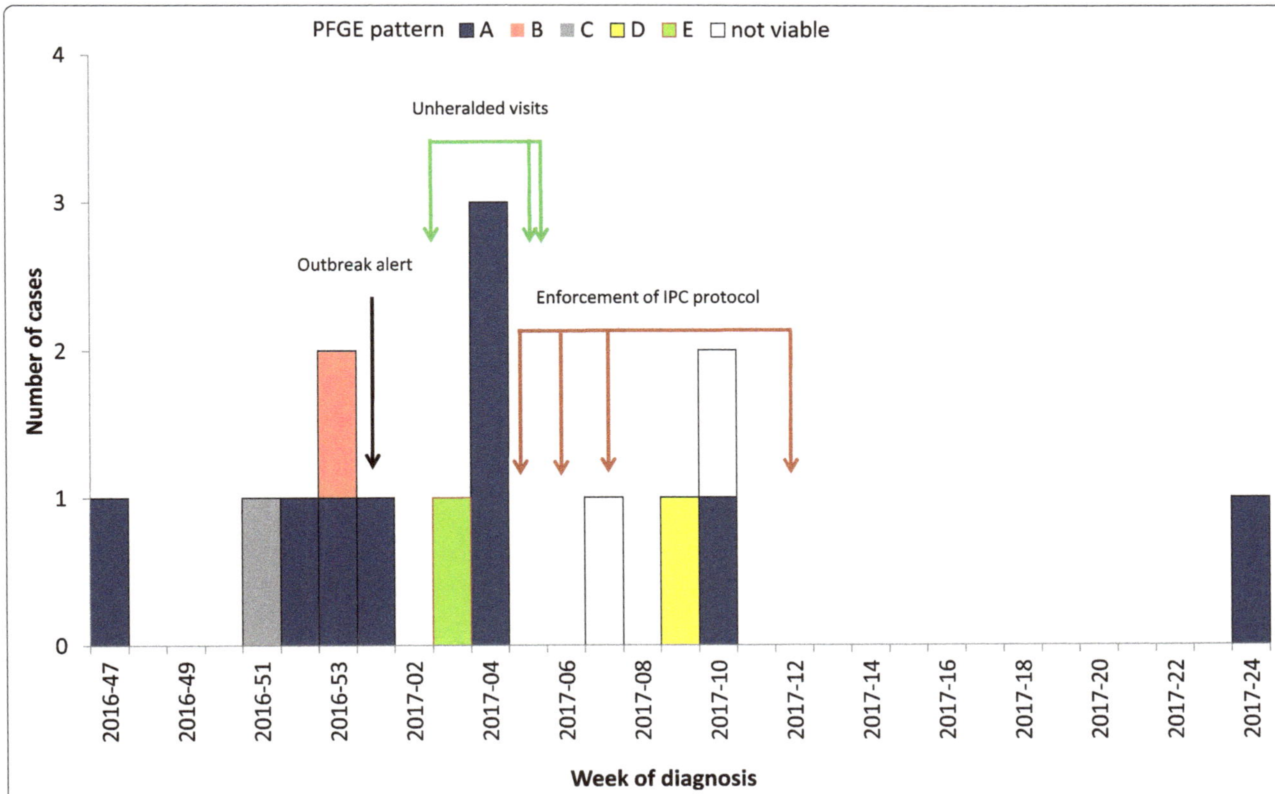

Fig. 1 Number of cases by PFGE pattern, week of diagnosis and main interventions ($n = 15$)

Table 1 Patient characteristics

	Categories	N/total or median (mean; range)	%
Demographic characteristics	Males	5/15	67
	Age	59 yrs. (61.3 yrs.; 50–79 yrs)	–
Clinical findings	Infected (versus colonized)	12/15	80
	Deceased	3/15	20
Laboratory sampling	Number of samples investigated per patient	24 (31; 8–105)	–
	Number of positive samples per patient	2 (6.1; 1–52)	–
Laboratory findings	PFGE pattern A (cluster strain)	9/13	69
	PFGE pattern E (environmental strain)	1/13	8
	other PFGE patterns	3/13 (one each)	23

irrespective of their PFGE pattern. The only patient isolate with pattern E, was not viable.

Cluster cases

In total, 194 patient samples were obtained from cluster cases, in 26 of them (13.4%) VRE was confirmed. The median number of samples investigated per cluster case was 20 (12–34) and the median number of positive samples was one (1–12). Five patients only had one sample positive for VRE. The median duration of confirmation between the first and the last positive sample was 4 days (1–33 days). The median interval between admission and first isolation of VRE was 13 days (same day-22 days) ($n = 14$). One additional patient already tested positive in another unit during the outbreak period, but the isolate was different from the cluster strain (PFGE C). From all other cases no information of previous VRE carriage was available as no routine VRE screening was conducted prior to this outbreak. VRE was first identified in following materials from the nine cluster cases: Blood ($n = 1$), (wound) drains ($n = 4$), rectal swab ($n = 1$), and urine ($n = 3$).

VRE screening

Pre-admission rectal screening was implemented after the outbreak alert. Among 169 patients screened until the end of 2017, only one was found to be VRE positive (0.6%).

Environmental and hand samples

A total of 139 hand ($n = 26$; 18.7%) and environmental ($n = 113$, 81.3%) samples were obtained during three unheralded on-site visits; nearly half of them ($n = 68$, 48.9%) were obtained prior to the first enforcement of control measures. More samples taken prior to enhanced disinfection ($n = 10$; 14.7%) were positive for VRE compared to post disinfection sampling ($n = 4$; 5.6%) ($p = 0.07$). Among the thirteen VRE positive environmental samples the cluster strain (PFGE A) was identified twice: once from a clamp of a urine-bag prior and once on a patients chart after the first enforcement of control measures. All other eleven VRE positive environmental samples revealed one identical PFGE pattern E which was distinct from the patient cluster strain (Fig. 2). Pattern E was confirmed only in one patient, who was admitted 2 days prior to the first environmental sampling. Eight of these positive non-cluster strains (PFGE E) were identified during the first on-site visit. Six of them were determined in the patient close environment and two outside patient rooms. During the third visit the environmental PFGE E strain was identified again three times. Once from the patient close environment (urine clamp bag) of the patient infected with PFGE E; and twice from a bed located in the corridor (Fig. 3). All tested environmental strains were *van*A positive.

One VRE positive hand sample of a HCW was not available for PFGE typing.

Virulence genes

Twenty three samples were available for virulence gene testing (13 environmental and 10 patient samples).

Two of nine (22.2%) PFGE A (six patient samples), but nine of 11 (81.2%) PFGE E (all environmental samples) were positive for gelatinase E ($p = 0.0123$). The two gelatinase E positive PFGE A samples were one human sample from a patient already discharged at the time of the environmental sampling and one environmental sample from a urinary bag clamp obtained during the first on-site visit which could not be linked to a specific patient.

All investigated samples were positive for enterococcal surface protein and negative for cytolysin activator.

Control measures

The first of the three unheralded on-site visit including environmental and hand sampling was undertaken on 18th January 2017. Lack of adherence to hand hygiene was observed and therefore enforcement of control measures was stressed by the infection control hygiene team. At the time of this first visit, five patients were admitted

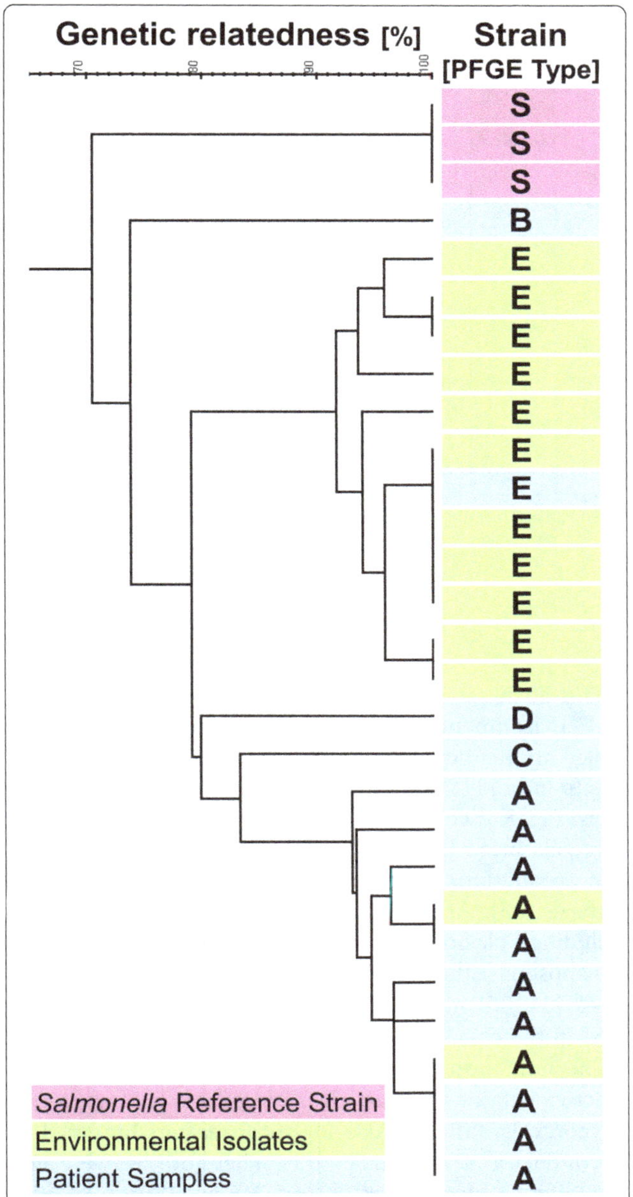

Fig. 2 Dendrogram of PFGE patterns of human ($n = 13$; pattern A = 9, one each pattern B, C, D, E and environmental VRE strains ($n = 13$; pattern E = 11, pattern A = 2) including 3 control strains

(two with PFGE A, one each with PFGE B and E and one without a viable isolate) and six already discharged (five of whom with PFGE A and one with PFGE C).

The second sampling on 30th January, performed after extended cleaning and disinfection procedures towards patients' distant zones did not detect any environmental contamination. Rectal screening targeting all staff was conducted the same day. The participation rate was 79% (94 of 119), all samples remained negative. Non-participation was mainly due to absence; No consent was obtained as participation was voluntary. In the current IPC protocol HCW hand sampling but no rectal swabbing is included.

During the last on-site visit on 2nd February, VRE was detected in four of 47 (8.51%) environmental samples. Three of those revealed PFGE E, all from patient-close sites of the patient infected with PFGE E, the cluster strain (PFGE A) was isolated from a patient chart. At the time of the third visit, five patients (two with PFGE A) were still admitted to the ward; four further cases, two with the cluster PFGE A were identified later. Enforcement of IPC measures was rigorously stressed again and four ward round sessions were conducted. Insufficient adherence to HH according to the IPC protocol was documented during the first visit. During the second and third visit the adherence to HH was evaluated to be sufficient. The terminal cleaning was audited by the ICT and adherence was defined as sufficient already at the first visit. The effect of teaching was not measured.

Discussion

We describe an outbreak of fifteen VRE cases in a solid organ transplant unit in late 2016 and early 2017, of which nine patients revealed an identical PFGE pattern A, further called the cluster strain.

During the first visit six VRE positive environmental samples were identified in the patient close environment which suggests lack of effective decontamination despite the audited terminal disinfection which was considered sufficient. Additionally, lack of adherence to strict hand hygiene was observed and compliance to HH was classified as insufficient. The two positive samples identified from a laundry rack suggest cross-contamination via HCW hands, as all patients were immobile. The fact, that the majority of environmental strains were identical - although distinct from the outbreak strain - may suggest that also prior to the first sampling environmental contamination via HCW hands may have occurred. HH adherence during audits improved from insufficient during the first visit to sufficient during the second and third visit.

Enforcement of ICP measures resulted in a decrease of the proportion of VRE contaminated environmental samples, although it was not significant (Fig. 3). Nevertheless, reconfirmation of the non-cluster strain during the third site visit may be due to recontamination and insufficient compliance to hand hygiene. In addition, the confirmation of the cluster strain on a patient chart after enforcement of control measures suggests the cross-contamination via HCW hands as well as ineffective decontamination of the patient chart. Decontamination of patient charts is described as effective measure to decrease horizontal transfer of organisms and to prevent transmission of health care associated infections [23, 24].

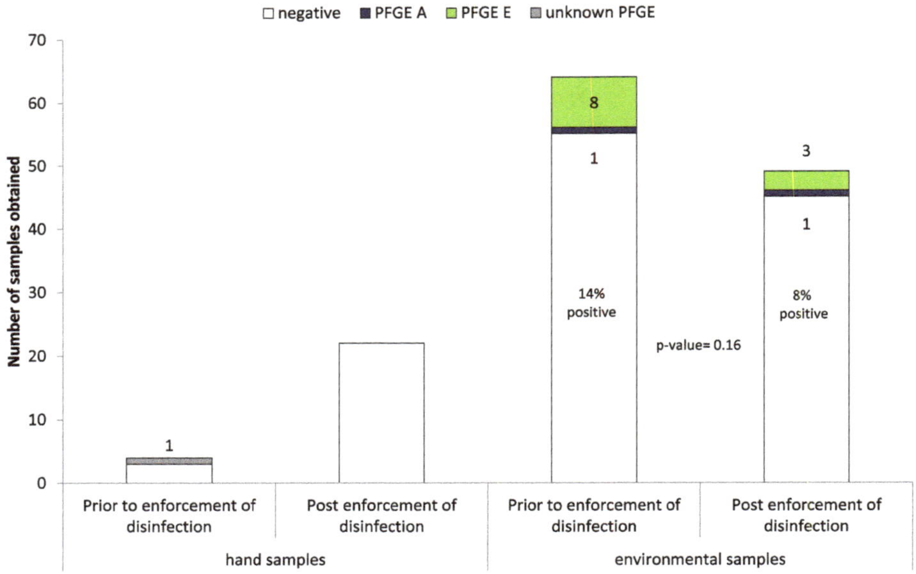

Fig. 3 Number and results of hand and environmental samples by intervention ($n = 139$)

We speculate that the lack of strict adherence to adequate hand hygiene might have led to contamination of the environment. This is supported by the facts that firstly, contamination was observed in patient distant areas such as laundry racks and secondly, that contaminated patient charts are described being a result of lack of adherence to recommended HH [25]. This may have played an important role in triggering the outbreak. Tight working spaces in the ICU unit favor the patient-to-patient contact [26] and may have resulted in a higher risk for transmission of VRE.

Hayden concludes that the role of environmental contamination in nosocomial cross-transmission of VRE is still unresolved but enforcement of environmental decontamination was both associated with reduction of surface contamination and contamination of HCWs' hands despite only moderate adherence to proper hand hygiene [27]. Proper environmental decontamination may reduce the risk of VRE outbreaks in hospital settings as suggested in previous studies. Dancer et al. [28] suggest to focus more on patient close hand-touch sites rather than on general surfaces and bathrooms.

The observed higher median age of male VRE patients rather reflects the distribution of admitted patients than being associated with VRE colonization or infection [29].

The pre-admission rectal screening implemented since the identification of the outbreak revealed less than one positive per hundred investigated patients. VRE screening in a tertiary hospital setting is suggested to decrease the incidence in routine patient care and even more important in an outbreak situation [30–32]. Therefore we speculate that most of the cluster cases acquired the VRE during the hospital stay.

The cluster strain PFGE A was identified only twice in the environment; all other environmental strains revealed an identical PFGE E pattern. This PFGE E pattern was found only in one patient. The fact, that significantly more PFGE E compared to PFGE A strains were producing gelatinase E, which is described as enhancing biofilm production, suggests a survival benefit on inanimate surfaces [33]. Accumulation of mobile genetic elements including plasmids, pathogenicity islands, resistance transposons other fitness islands, phages and surface types [34, 35] may also have contributed to better survival in the environment.

The limitations of our study are that we used retrospective data analysis which made selection of appropriate controls difficult. Also logistical reasons hindered us to conduct a case control study. Therefore we were neither able to identify risk factors for acquisition of VRE nor to identify the source of infection. Furthermore, neither retrospective data where patients were located within the ward at the time of admission nor information on staffing was available. A higher patient-staff ratio might have influenced the transmission risk. The only PFGE E strain from the patient could not be recovered from the archived skim-milk stock and was hence also not available for genotyping.

Conclusions

We conclude that enforcement of strict adherence to the existing IPC protocol and assessment of adherence are essential for controlling VRE outbreaks and reducing further transmission. We cannot exclude the role of other components in the multi-modal IPC plan instituted which ultimately may have played a role in the control of the outbreak. Unheralded visits are useful tools to further improve adherence to IPC protocols. Frequently touched surfaces such as patient charts are difficult to decontaminate and therefore require particular attention. We conclude that this outbreak has resulted in better control of future VRE outbreaks. HCWs reported a better understanding for the need of rigorous adherence to control measures. We expect further sporadic cases in future.

Abbreviations

CI: Confidence interval; EU/EEA: European Union and European Economic area; HCW: Health care worker; HH: Hand hygiene; ICT: Infection control team; ICU: Intensive care unit; IPC: Infection prevention and control; LKI: University Hospital Innsbruck (Landeskrankenhaus Innsbruck); PFGE: Pulse filed gel electrophoresis; VRE: Vancomycin resistant *enterococci*

Acknowledgements

The authors want to thank the staff of the unit and laboratory and the ICT for the good and transparent collaboration.

Authors' contributions

SE provided patient data regarding disease and transplant and reviewed the draft manuscript, MB and LK analyzed the patient samples and the antimicrobial susceptibility testing, SF and WP conducted the molecular examinations. AM and GH conducted and analyzed the environmental sampling, AO, CLF and DO reviewed the manuscript, PK analyzed and interpreted the data and drafted the manuscript. All authors read and approved the final manuscript.

Consent for publication

Not applicable

Competing interests

The authors declare that they have no competing interests.

Author details

[1]Department of Hygiene, Microbiology and Social Medicine, Division of Hygiene and Medical Microbiology, Medical University of Innsbruck, Innsbruck, Schoepfstr. 41, 6020 Innsbruck, Austria. [2]Department of Anesthesia and Critical Care, Centre of Operative Medicine, Medical University of Innsbruck, Anichstr. 35, 6020 Innsbruck, Austria. [3]Department of Neurosurgery, University Hospital of Innsbruck, Anichstr. 35, 6020 Innsbruck, Austria.

References

1. Gastmeier P, Schroder C, Behnke M, Meyer E, Geffers C. Dramatic increase in vancomycin-resistant enterococci in Germany. J Antimicrob Chemother. 2014;69(6):1660–4.
2. ECDC. Surveillance of antimicrobial resistance in Europe, 2016 2017 [cited 2018 13 Mar]. Available from: https://ecdc.europa.eu/en/publications-data/antimicrobial-resistance-surveillance-europe-2016.
3. Ulrich N, Gastmeier P. Where is the difference between an epidemic and a high endemic level with respect to nosocomial infection control measures? An analysis based on the example of vancomycin-resistant enterococcus faecium in hematology and oncology departments. GMS Hyg Infect Control. 2017;12:Doc14.
4. Hayden MK, Blom DW, Lyle EA, Moore CG, Weinstein RA. Risk of hand or glove contamination after contact with patients colonized with vancomycin-resistant enterococcus or the colonized patients' environment. Infect Control Hosp Epidemiol. 2008;29(2):149–54.
5. Brodrick HJ, Raven KE, Harrison EM, Blane B, Reuter S, Torok ME, et al. Whole-genome sequencing reveals transmission of vancomycin-resistant enterococcus faecium in a healthcare network. Genome Med. 2016;8(1):4.
6. Huang SS, Datta R, Platt R. Risk of acquiring antibiotic-resistant bacteria from prior room occupants. Arch Intern Med. 2006;166(18):1945–51.
7. Stone SP, Cooper BS, Kibbler CC, Cookson BD, Roberts JA, Medley GF, et al. The ORION statement: guidelines for transparent reporting of outbreak reports and intervention studies of nosocomial infection. J Antimicrob Chemother. 2007;59(5):833–40.
8. Organization WH. WHO Guidelines on Hand Hygiene in Health Care: First Global Patient Safety Challenge Clean Care is Safer Care 2009 [cited 2018 21 June]. Available from: http://apps.who.int/iris/bitstream/handle/10665/44102/9789241597906_eng.pdf;jsessionid=0353CC69A96F2B5A26F019487149B213?sequence=1.
9. Robert Koch Institute NRfSvnI. Hand-KISS 2017 [cited 2018 21 June]. Available from: http://www.nrz-hygiene.de/surveillance/kiss/hand-kiss/.
10. Testing TECoAS. Breakpoint tables for interpretation of MICs and zone diameters. Version 6.0, 2016.
11. Biomerieux. Gebrauchsfertige Teststreifen zur direkten Bestimmung der minimalen Hemmkonzentration [cited 2018 21 June]. Available from: http://www.biomerieux.de/klinische-diagnostik/etestr.
12. Galvin S, Dolan A, Cahill O, Daniels S, Humphreys H. Microbial monitoring of the hospital environment: why and how? J Hosp Infect. 2012;82(3):143–51.
13. Wille I, Mayr A, Kreidl P, Bruhwasser C, Hinterberger G, Fritz A, et al. Cross-sectional point prevalence survey to study the environmental contamination of nosocomial pathogens in intensive care units under real-life conditions. J Hosp Infect. 2018;98(1):90–5.
14. Bruhwasser C, Hinterberger G, Mutschlechner W, Kaltseis J, Lass-Florl C, Mayr A. A point prevalence survey on hand hygiene, with a special focus on Candida species. Am J Infect Control. 2016;44(1):71–3.
15. Creamer E, Dorrian S, Dolan A, Sherlock O, Fitzgerald-Hughes D, Thomas T, et al. When are the hands of healthcare workers positive for methicillin-resistant Staphylococcus aureus? J Hosp Infect. 2010;75(2):107–11.
16. CDC. Unified PulsedField Gel Electrophoresis (PFGE) Protocol for Gram Positive Bacteria 2012 [Available from: https://www.cdc.gov/hai/pdfs/labsettings/Unified_PFGE_Protocol.pdf.
17. Tenover FC, Arbeit RD, Goering RV, Mickelsen PA, Murray BE, Persing DH, et al. Interpreting chromosomal DNA restriction patterns produced by pulsed-field gel electrophoresis: criteria for bacterial strain typing. J Clin Microbiol. 1995;33(9):2233–9.
18. Heras J, Dominguez C, Mata E, Pascual V, Lozano C, Torres C, et al. GelJ--a tool for analyzing DNA fingerprint gel images. BMC Bioinformatics. 2015;16:270.
19. Jayaratne P, Rutherford C. Detection of clinically relevant genotypes of vancomycin-resistant enterococci in nosocomial surveillance specimens by PCR. J Clin Microbiol. 1999;37(6):2090–2.
20. Toledo-Arana A, Valle J, Solano C, Arrizubieta MJ, Cucarella C, Lamata M, et al. The enterococcal surface protein, Esp, is involved in enterococcus faecalis biofilm formation. Appl Environ Microbiol. 2001;67(10):4538–45.
21. Vankerckhoven V, Van Autgaerden T, Vael C, Lammens C, Chapelle S, Rossi R, et al. Development of a multiplex PCR for the detection of asa1, gelE, cylA, esp, and hyl genes in enterococci and survey for virulence determinants among European hospital isolates of enterococcus faecium. J Clin Microbiol. 2004;42(10):4473–9.
22. Hancock LE, Perego M. The enterococcus faecalis fsr two-component system controls biofilm development through production of gelatinase. J Bacteriol. 2004;186(17):5629–39.
23. Zimbudzi E, Stuart RL, Korman TM, Kotsanas D. Contamination of renal patients' hospital chart covers with vancomycin-- resistant enterococci: handle with care. Australas Med J. 2011;4(10):538–41.
24. Teng SO, Lee WS, Ou TY, Hsieh YC, Lee WC, Lin YC. Bacterial contamination of patients' medical charts in a surgical ward and the intensive care unit: impact on nosocomial infections. J Microbiol Immunol Infect. 2009;42(1):86–91.
25. Russotto V, Cortegiani A, Raineri SM, Giarratano A. Bacterial contamination of inanimate surfaces and equipment in the intensive care unit. J Intensive Care. 2015;3:54.
26. Ulrich N, Vonberg RP, Gastmeier P. Outbreaks caused by vancomycin-resistant enterococcus faecium in hematology and oncology departments: a systematic review. Heliyon. 2017;3(12):e00473.
27. Hayden MK, Bonten MJ, Blom DW, Lyle EA, van de Vijver DA, Weinstein RA. Reduction in acquisition of vancomycin-resistant enterococcus after enforcement

of routine environmental cleaning measures. Clin Infect Dis. 2006;42(11):1552–60.
28. Dancer SJ. The role of environmental cleaning in the control of hospital-acquired infection. J Hosp Infect. 2009;73(4):378–85.
29. Schold JD, Buccini LD, Goldfarb DA, Flechner SM, Hsich E, Mason D, et al. Patient participation in research among solid organ transplant recipients in the United States. Transplantation. 2011;91(12):1424–35.
30. Escaut L, Bouam S, Frank-Soltysiak M, Rudant E, Saliba F, Kassis N, et al. Eradication of an outbreak of vancomycin-resistant enterococcus (VRE): the cost of a failure in the systematic screening. Antimicrob Resist Infect Control. 2013;2(1):18.
31. Humphreys H. Controlling the spread of vancomycin-resistant enterococci. Is active screening worthwhile? J Hosp Infect. 2014;88(4):191–8.
32. Popiel KY, Miller MA. Evaluation of vancomycin-resistant enterococci (VRE)-associated morbidity following relaxation of VRE screening and isolation precautions in a tertiary care hospital. Infect Control Hosp Epidemiol. 2014; 35(7):818–25.
33. Banerjee T, Anupurba S. Prevalence of virulence factors and drug resistance in clinical isolates of enterococci: a study from North India. J Pathog 2015; 2015:692612.
34. Gaca AO, Gilmore MS. Killing of VRE enterococcus faecalis by commensal strains: evidence for evolution and accumulation of mobile elements in the absence of competition. Gut Microbes. 2016;7(1):90–6.
35. Hanczvikkel A, Toth A. Quantitative study about the role of environmental conditions in the survival capability of multidrug-resistant bacteria. J Infect Public Health. 2018;

18

In vitro and in vivo bactericidal activity of ceftazidime-avibactam against Carbapenemase–producing *Klebsiella pneumoniae*

Wenxia Zhang[1,2†], Yan Guo[1,4†], Jiayin Li[3†], Yiyuan Zhang[3], Yang Yang[1,4], Dong Dong[1,4], Demei Zhu[1,4], Ping He[3*] and Fupin Hu[1,4*]

Abstract

Background: In recent years, the incidence of carbapenem-resistant *Enterobacteriaceae* (CRE) infections has increased rapidly. Since the CRE strain is usually resistant to most of antimicrobial agents, patients with this infection are often accompanied by a high mortality. Therefore, it instigates a severe challenge the clinical management of infection. In this study, we study the in vitro and in vivo bactericidal activity of ceftazidime-avibactam administrated either alone or in combination with aztreonam against KPC or NDM carbapenemase-producing *Klebsiella pneumoniae*, and explore a new clinical therapeutic regimen for infections induced by their resistant strains.

Methods: The microdilution broth method was performed to analyze the minimal inhibitory concentration (MIC). The time-kill curve assay of ceftazidime-avibactam at various concentrations was conducted in 16 strains of KPC-2 and 1 strain of OXA-232 carbapenemase–producing *Klebsiella pneumoniae*. The in vitro synergistic bactericidal effect of ceftazidime-avibactam combined with aztreonam was determined by checkerboard assay on 28 strains of NDM and 2 strains of NDM coupled with KPC carbapenemase–producing *Klebsiella pneumoniae*. According to calculating grade, the drugs with synergistic bactericidal effect were selected as an inhibitory concentration index. The in vitro bactericidal tests of ceftazidime-avibactam combined with aztreonam were implemented on 12 strains among them. Effect of ceftazidime-avibactam antibiotic against KPC carbapenemase–producing *K. pneumoniae* strain Y8 Infection was performed in the mouse model.

(Continued on next page)

* Correspondence: hpatsh@sjtu.edu.cn; hufupin@fudan.edu.cn
†Wenxia Zhang, Yan Guo and Jiayin Li contributed equally to this work.
[3]Department of Medical Microbiology and Immunology, Shanghai Jiao Tong University School of Medicine, Shanghai 200025, China
[1]Institute of Antibiotics, Huashan Hospital, Fudan University, 12 M. Wulumuqi Rd, Shanghai 200040, China
Full list of author information is available at the end of the article

(Continued from previous page)

Results: The time-kill assays revealed that ceftazidime-avibactam at various concentrations of 2MIC, 4MIC and 8MIC showed significant bactericidal efficiency to the resistant bacteria strains. However, in 28 strains of NDM and 2 strains of NDM coupled with KPC carbapenemase- producing *Klebsiella pneumoniae*, only 7 strains appeared the susceptibility to ceftazidime-avibactam treatment, MIC_{50} and MIC_{90} were 64 mg/L and 256 mg/L, respectively. Antimicrobial susceptibility testing of ceftazidime-avibactam combined with aztreonam disclosed the synergism of two drugs in 90% (27/30) strains, an additive efficiency in 3.3% (1/30) strains, and irrelevant effects in 6.6% (2/30) strains. No antagonism was found. The subsequent bactericidal tests also confirmed the results mentioned above. Therapeutic efficacy of Ceftazidime-Avibactam against *K. pneumoniae* strain Y8 infection in mouse indicated 70% of infection group mice died within 4 days, and all mice in this group died within 13 days. Bacterial load testing results showed that there was no significant difference in the amount of bacteria in the blood between the infected group and the treatment group. However, the spleen and liver of treatment group mice showed lower CFU counts, as compare with infected group, indicating that ceftazidime-avibactam has a significant effect on the bacteria and led to a certain therapeutic efficacy.

Conclusion: This study indicated ceftazidime-avibactam therapy occupied significant bactericidal effects against KPC-2 and OXA-232 carbapenemase-producing *Klebsiella pneumoniae*. While combined with aztreonam, the stronger synergistic bactericidal effects against NDM carbapenemase-producing *Klebsiella pneumoniae* were achieved.

Keywords: *Klebsiella pneumoniae*, Carbapenemase, Ceftazidime-avibactam, Aztreonam, Time-kill curve assay

Background

Carbapenems are considered the most effective antibacterial agents against infections caused by multi-drug resistant gram-negative bacillus in clinical practice. However, with the broad use of carbapenems, and the emergence and wide-spread of carbapenem-resistant *Enterobacteriaceae* (CRE), in particular carbapenem-resistant *Klebsiella pneumoniae* (CR-KP), the clinical anti-infection treatment faces a drug-free dilemma [1–4]. Previous studies have shown that the most important resistant mechanism of CR-KP to carbapenems is production of carbapenemases including class A KPC carbapenemases, class B metallo-β-lactamases and class D OXA-48 family carbapenemases. Avibactam is a newly developed novel β-lactamase inhibitor in recent years and can efficiently inhibit class A and class D carbapenemases. As an inhibitor, avibactam can restore the antibacterial activity of ceftazidime to CR-KP. Nevertheless, it has less antibacterial efficiency against CR-KP with metallo-β-lactamase [5–7]. Knowing that aztreonam is stable against hydrolysis by class B metallo-β-lactamases, we hypothesized that supplement of aztreonam to the ceftazidime-avibactam would enhance the activity by "protecting" aztreonam from the "attack" of KPC type carbapenemase. This study aims to explore a new therapeutic regimen by administration of ceftazidime-avibactam alone or combined with aztreonam against carbapenemase-producing *Klebsiella pneumoniae*.

Materials and methods

Strains

A total of 47 non-repeated clinical strains of carbapenemase-producing *Klebsiella pneumoniae* were collected from 9 hospitals in 9 cities in China. Of these, 16 strains were bla_{KPC-2} positive, 1 was $bla_{OXA-232}$ positive, 28 were bla_{NDM} positive, and 2 were bla_{KPC2} coupled with bla_{NDM} positive *Klebsiella pneumoniae*. All strains were identified by mass spectrometry and the gene type of carbapenemases was analyzed by PCR amplification using primers previously described and DNA sequencing [8–10]. *E. coli* ATCC 25922 were used as quality control strain for antimicrobial susceptibility testing. One *K. pneumoniae* clinical strain Y8 was used for the Infection in the mouse model.

Antimicrobial susceptibility testing

The minimal inhibitory concentrations were determined by microbroth dilution according to Clinical and Laboratory Standards Institute (CLSI) guidelines [11]. The in vitro synergistic bactericidal effects of ceftazidime-avibactam combined with aztreonam against bla_{NDM}-positive strains were determined by checkerboard assay referred to the published reports [12, 13]. The calculation and interpretation of fractional inhibitory concentration (FIC) was referred to the document standards [14]. $FIC = MIC_{drug\ A} / MIC_{drug\ A\ plus\ drug\ B} + MIC_{drug\ B} / MIC_{drug\ A\ plus\ drug\ B}$. $FIC \leq 0.5$ was considered as a synergistic effect, $0.5 < FIC \leq 1$ was considered as an additive effect, $1 < FIC \leq 2$ was considered as an irrelevant effect, and > 2 was considered as an antagonism.

Time-kill assay

According to the minimal inhibitory concentration (MIC) of ceftazidime-avibactam to bla_{KPC-2} or $bla_{OXA-232}$ producers, the bactericidal effects of ceftazidime-avibactam at various concentrations of 0.5MIC, 1MIC, 2MIC, 4MIC and 8MIC were studied by time-kill assay. In line with the results of antimicrobial susceptibility testing of ceftazidime-avibactam combined with aztreonam, and following the methods recommended in literatures [15, 16], 10 *Klebsiella pneumoniae* strains with bla_{NDM} and 2 *Klebsiella pneumoniae* strains with bla_{NDM} coupled with bla_{KPC-2} were randomly selected for synergistic bactericidal effects. The operation procedure is briefly described as follows: Mueller-hinton broth containing 1×10^5 CFU/mL bacteria is mixed with single or combined antimicrobial agents incubated overnight with consecutive shacking at 35 °C in an atmospheric environment. Meanwhile, the same broth without antibiotics was served as a growth control. Broth samples were serially diluted at times of 0, 2, 4, 6, 8 and 10 h and smeared on a mueller-Hinton plate respectively. After overnight incubation at 35 °C, the colonies were counted. If the reduction of bacterial survival amount in sample treated with combined antibiotics was ≥2 log10 CFU/mL than those in the sample treated by single drug, it was considered to have a synergistic bactericidal effect.

Effect of ceftazidime-avibactam against *K. pneumoniae* strain Y8 infection in the mouse model

Six-week-old BALB/c mice (female) were bought from Shanghai Laboratory Animal Company (SLAC), China. Animal experiments were performed in accordance with the Animal Ethics Committee of Shanghai Jiao Tong University. Groups of 10 mice were infected with 2.5×10^6 CFU of strain Y8 via the intraperitoneal (ip) route. Then mice were treated with PBS (infection group) or ceftazidime-avibactam (treatment group) (0.375 mg/g of body weight in 0.1 ml PBS) by subcutaneous injection 4 h post infection and given every 8 h for 10 days. The survival rates of mice were measured at desired time point to assess the therapeutic efficacy of ceftazidime-avibactam. Survival curves were monitored for 15 days.

Bacterial load in the blood and tissues of mice

To measure the efficacy of this drug, the bacterial load was measured in the blood and tissues of mice. Groups of 8 mice were infected with 2.5×10^6 CFU of strain Y8 via the ip and then treated with PBS or ceftazidime-avibactam by subcutaneous injection. The antibiotic dosage and administration were same as the survival experiment mentioned above. At 3 days post infection (dpi), mice in treatment and infected group were euthanized, and the blood and tissues of mice were removed to determine the bacterial burden through bacterial dilution-plate method.

Results

Antimicrobial susceptibility testing

All 16 *Klebsiella pneumoniae* strains with bla_{KPC-2} were susceptible to ceftazidime-avibactam with MIC range for 4–8 mg/L. However, all of strains were resistant to ceftazidime with MIC_{50} of 32 mg/L and MIC_{90} of > 256 mg/L. The resistance rate of imipenem was 93.8% with MIC_{50} and MIC_{90} for 64 mg/L and 128 mg/L, respectively. The resistance rate of meropenem was 93.8% with MIC_{50} and MIC_{90} for 64 mg/L and 256 mg/L, respectively (Table 1).

Table 1 Minimal inhibitory concentration (MIC) of ceftazidime-avibactam against KPC-2 or OXA-232 carbapenemase-producing *Klebsiella pneumoniae*

Strain no.	Bacteria	β-lactamase	MIC (mg/L)				Associated β-lactamase
			CAZ-AVI	CAZ	IPM	MEM	
R16- Hefei	*K. pneumoniae*	KPC-2	8	128	64	64	CTX-M-14, SHV-11, DHA-1
R18- Hefei	*K. pneumoniae*	KPC-2	4	128	8	16	SHV-28, DHA-1
R19- Hefei	*K. pneumoniae*	KPC-2	4	128	16	16	SHV-12, DHA-1
R31- Beijing	*K. pneumoniae*	KPC-2	8	128	64	256	SHV-11, DHA-1
R35- Beijing	*K. pneumoniae*	KPC-2	8	128	128	256	SHV-11, DHA-1
R39-Fuzhou	*K. pneumoniae*	KPC-2	8	> 256	32	64	CTX-M-14, SHV-12, DHA-1
R42- Fuzhou	*K. pneumoniae*	KPC-2	8	> 256	32	64	CTX-M-14, SHV-12, DHA-1
R44- Fuzhou	*K. pneumoniae*	KPC-2	8	> 256	64	128	CTX-M-14, SHV-12, DHA-1
R46- Fuzhou	*K. pneumoniae*	KPC-2	8	> 256	64	64	SHV-12, DHA-1
R52- Fuzhou	*K. pneumoniae*	KPC-2	8	> 256	64	128	CTX-M-14, SHV-12, DHA-1
R53- Fuzhou	*K. pneumoniae*	KPC-2	8	> 256	64	128	CTX-M-14, SHV-12, DHA-1
R59- Hangzhou	*K. pneumoniae*	KPC-2	8	32	8	16	CTX-M-14, SHV-11, DHA-1
R60- Hangzhou	*K. pneumoniae*	KPC-2	4	32	4	4	CTX-M-14, SHV-11, DHA-1
JSD-Shanghai	*K. pneumoniae*	KPC-2	8	128	128	512	CTX-M-14, SHV-11, DHA-1
WJQ-Shanghai	*K. pneumoniae*	KPC-2	8	> 256	128	256	CTX-M-14, SHV-11, DHA-1
LDX-Shanghai	*K. pneumoniae*	KPC-2	8	> 256	32	64	CTX-M-55, SHV-31, DHA-1
PED-Shanghai	*K. pneumoniae*	OXA-232	2	> 32	1	4	CTX-M-15, SHV-1

Note: *CAZ-AVI* Ceftazidime-avibactam, *CAZ* Ceftazidime, *IPM* Imipenem, *MEM* Meropenem

The MIC of ceftazidime-avibactam to one OXA-232 carbapenemase-producing *Klebsiella pneumoniae* was 2 mg/L. The resistance rate of ceftazidime-avibactam to 30 bla_{NDM} (including NDM plus KPC-2) positive *Klebsiella pneumoniae* strains was 76.7% with MIC range for 0.5~ 256 mg/L, MIC_{50} and MIC_{90} for 64 mg/L and 256 mg/L, respectively. The MIC range of aztreonam was 8~ > 256 mg/L with MIC_{50} and MIC_{90} were 128 mg/L and > 256 mg/L, respectively. Ceftazidime-avibactam combined with aztreonam showed synergistic effects to 90% (27/30) of strains with bla_{NDM}, 3.3% (1/30) showed additive effects and 6.6%(2/30) showed unrelated effects. No antagonism was found for ceftazidime-avibactam combined with aztreonam (Table 2).

Time-kill assay

The results of time-kill assays showed that all bla_{KPC-2} or $bla_{OXA-232}$ positive *K. pneumoniae* strains rebounded to grow 4 to 6 h at 0.5 MIC of ceftazidime-avibactam. At the concentration of 1 MIC ceftazidime-avibactam, 23.5% (4/17) of strains declined stably 2 h after dosing and no colonies were detected at 24 h, however, 76.5% (13/17) of strains rebounded to grow in 4–6 h. At the concentrations of 2MIC, 4MIC or 8MIC of ceftazidime-avibactam, it

Table 2 Results of MIC and antimicrobial susceptibility testing of ceftazidime-avibactam single dosing and combined with aztreonam against NDM + KPC-2 carbapenemase-producing *Klebsiella pneumoniae* in 30 strains

Strain no.	Bacteria	β-lactamase	MIC(mg/L) single dosing		MIC(mg/L) Combined dosing		FIC value	Associated β-lactamase
			ATM	CAZ-AVI	ATM	CAZ-AVI	ATM + CAZ-AVI	
R078 Anhui	*K. pneumoniae*	NDM	256	32	8	1	0.06	SHV-28, DHA-1, CTX-M-15
R080 Hainan	*K. pneumoniae*	NDM	128	4	32	0.25	0.31	SHV-11, DHA-1, CTX-M-14
R081 Hainan	*K. pneumoniae*	NDM	1024	8	64	2	0.31	SHV-11, DHA-1, CTX-M-14
R082 Hainan	*K. pneumoniae*	NDM	256	64	16	1	0.08	SHV-11, DHA-1, CTX-M-15, CTX-M-14
R083 Hainan	*K. pneumoniae*	NDM	128	64	32	0.5	0.26	SHV-12, DHA-1, CTX-M-15
R084 Hainan	*K. pneumoniae*	NDM	512	64	16	1	0.05	SHV-12, DHA-1
R085 Hainan	*K. pneumoniae*	NDM	1024	128	32	2	0.05	SHV-12, DHA-1, CTX-M-15
R086 Hainan	*K. pneumoniae*	NDM	128	64	16	0.5	0.13	SHV-12, DHA-1, CTX-M-15
R088 Hainan	*K. pneumoniae*	NDM	32	2	4	0.5	0.38	SHV-11, DHA-1, CTX-M-14
R093 Hebei	*K. pneumoniae*	NDM	32	64	4	0.5	0.13	SHV1, DHA-1, CTX-M-14
R094 Hebei	*K. pneumoniae*	NDM	32	64	8	0.25	0.25	SHV-12, DHA-1, CTX-M-14
R095 Hebei	*K. pneumoniae*	NDM	32	2	8	0.25	0.38	SHV-12, DHA-1, CTX-M-15
R096 Henan	*K. pneumoniae*	NDM	16	64	16	0.5	1.01	SHV1, DHA-1, CTX-M-15
R097 Henan	*K. pneumoniae*	NDM	8	256	4	128	1.00	SHV1, DHA-1, CTX-M-14
R098 Henan	*K. pneumoniae*	NDM	256	64	32	1	0.14	DHA-1
R100 Shanxi	*K. pneumoniae*	NDM	8	32	4	32	1.50	SHV-78, DHA-1, CTX-M-14
R101 Shanxi	*K. pneumoniae*	NDM	256	128	16	1	0.07	SHV-78, DHA-1, CTX-M-14
R102 Shanxi	*K. pneumoniae*	NDM	32	256	4	1	0.13	SHV-78, DHA-1, CTX-M-14
R103 Shanxi	*K. pneumoniae*	NDM	128	64	32	0.25	0.25	SHV1, DHA-1, CTX-M-15
R106 Sanxi	*K. pneumoniae*	NDM	128	64	8	1	0.08	SHV-12, DHA-1
R110 Sanxi	*K. pneumoniae*	NDM	128	256	8	1	0.07	SHV-12, DHA-1
R113 Sanxi	*K. pneumoniae*	NDM	128	64	16	0.5	0.13	SHV-12, DHA-1
R122 Tianjin	*K. pneumoniae*	NDM	32	1	4	0.25	0.38	SHV-12, DHA-1, CTX-M-14
R126 Tianjin	*K. pneumoniae*	NDM	512	64	16	1	0.05	SHV-12, DHA-1, CTX-M-14
R127 Tianjin	*K. pneumoniae*	NDM	256	128	32	1	0.13	SHV2, DHA-1
R128 Zhejiang	*K. pneumoniae*	NDM	128	256	8	2	0.07	SHV1, DHA-1
R129 Zhejiang	*K. pneumoniae*	NDM	4	0.5	0.5	0.125	0.38	SHV-12, DHA-1, CTX-M-15
R136 Zhejiang	*K. pneumoniae*	NDM	256	64	16	1	0.08	SHV-12, DHA-1
R148 Tianjing	*K. pneumoniae*	KPC-2,NDM	2048	8	256	2	0.38	SHV-12, DHA-1, CTX-M-14
R153 Henan	*K. pneumoniae*	KPC-2,NDM	2048	128	128	8	0.13	SHV-12, DHA-1

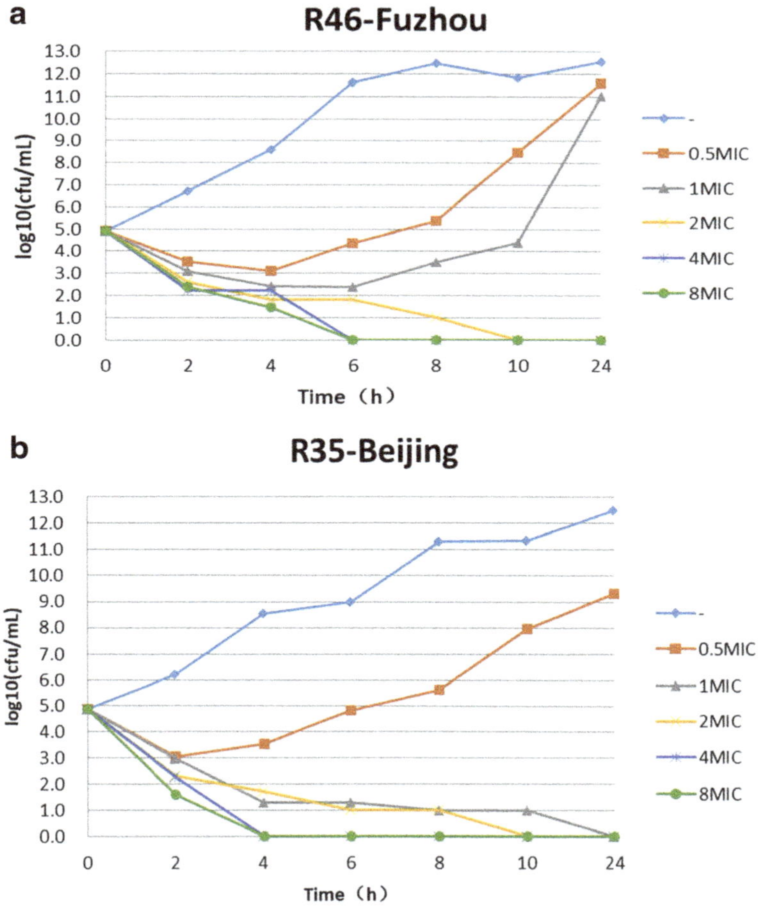

Fig. 1 Bactericidal curve plots of ceftazidime-avibactam at various concentrations against KPC-2 carbapenemase-producing *Klebsiella pneumoniae*

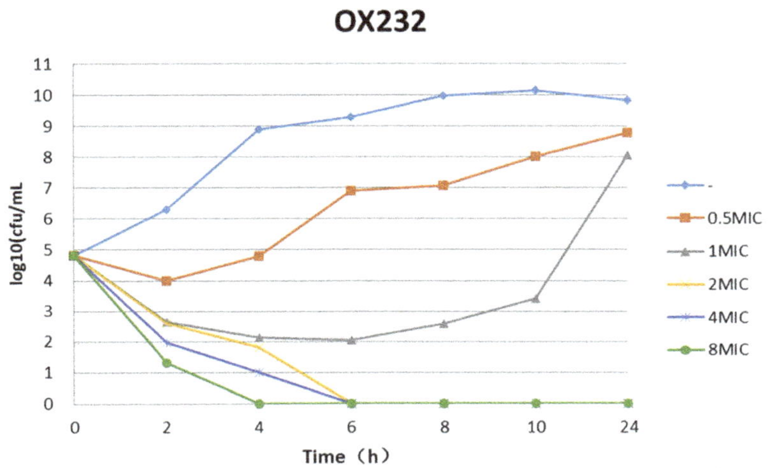

Fig. 2 Bactericidal curve plots of ceftazidime-avibactam at various concentrations against OXA-232 carbapenemase-producing *Klebsiella pneumoniae*

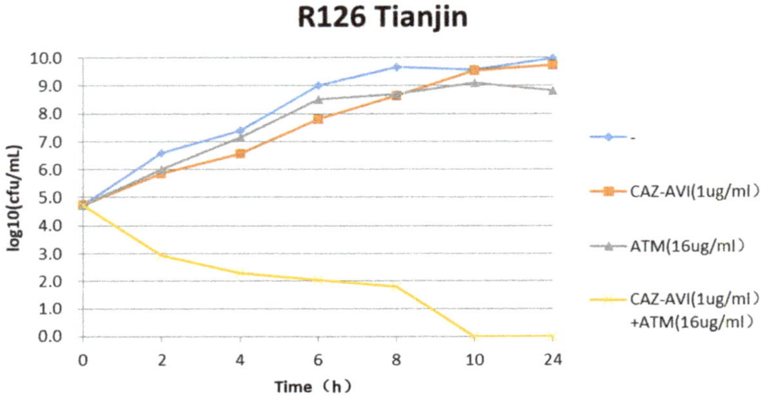

Fig. 3 Bactericidal curve plots of ceftazidime-avibactam combined with aztreonam against NDM carbapenemase-producing *Klebsiella pneumoniae*

showed a significant bactericidal effectiveness for either bla_{KPC} or $bla_{OXA-232}$ positive *K. pneumoniae* and the colony growth was undetected after 24 h incubation for most of strains (Fig. 1 and Fig. 2). For bla_{NDM} positive *K. pneumoniae*, ceftazidime-avibactam combined with aztreonam showed a significant bactericidal effectiveness and the colony growth was undetected after 10 h incubation (Fig. 3).

Therapeutic efficacy of ceftazidime-avibactam against *K. pneumoniae* strain Y8 infection in mouse

Mice were infected with 2.5×10^6 CFU of strain Y8 and treated with PBS or ceftazidime-avibactam for 10 days. 70% of infection group mice died within 4 days, and all mice in this group died within 13 days (Fig. 4). All treatment group mice survived at 10 dpi with the antibiotic applied every 8 h, whereas 100% of mice in this group died within 4 days after the antibiotic treatment stopped (Fig. 4).

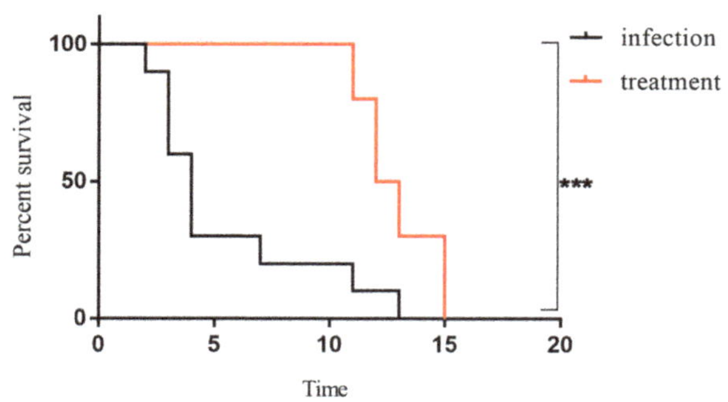

Fig. 4 Therapeutic efficacy of ceftazidime-avibactam against *K. pneumoniae* strain Y8 infection in mouse. Mice were infected with 2.5×10^6 CFU of strain Y8 via the ip route and then treated with PBS or ceftazidime-avibactam by subcutaneous injection. Their survival was assessed daily for 15 days ($n = 10$). $*P < 0.05$; $***P < 0.001$

Bacterial load in the blood and tissues of mice

Mice were infected with 2.5×10^6 CFU of strain Y8 via the ip and then treated with PBS or ceftazidime-avibactam. The viable bacteria were quantified in blood, liver and spleen at 3 dpi. The results showed that there was no significant difference in the amount of bacteria in the blood between the infected group and the treatment group. However, the spleen and liver of treatment group mice showed lower CFU counts, as compare with that of infected group, indicating that the antibiotic has significant effect on the bacteria and ceftazidime-avibactam led to a certain therapeutic efficacy (Fig. 5).

Discussion

In the recent decade, the prevalence and dissemination of CR-KP has posed a serious challenge in healthcare facilities in the world. The data from the Centers for Disease Control, USA disclosed the infection incidence of CR-KP increased from 1.2% in 2001 to 4.2% in 2011. In annual of 140,000 cases with *Enterobacteriaceae* infections, 9300 cases (6.6%) were infected by these multidrug-resistant bacteria [17]. According to CHINET surveillance data, the resistance rate of *Klebsiella pneumoniae* to carbapenems were significantly increasing from 3% in 2005 to 20% in 2017 [18]. Due to lack of effective antibacterial agents, infections due to CR-KP especially for hypervirulent *Klebsiella pneumoniae* usually accompany with high mortality [19, 20]. Carbapenemases are the major resistance mechanism of *Klebsiella pneumoniae* to carbapenems. Currently, the common carbapenemase among *K. pneumoniae* clinical strains include Ambler class A, Ambler class B and Ambler class D (eg. bla_{OXA-48}, and $bla_{OXA-232}$). bla_{KPC-2} is the most common carbapenemase in class A enzymes which can hydrolyze almost all of β-lactam antibiotics. bla_{NDM} is the most common carbapenemase in class B metallo-β-lactamase which can hydrolyze all β-lactam antibiotics except aztreonam. Previous studies have shown the CR-KP strains isolated from children in China mainly

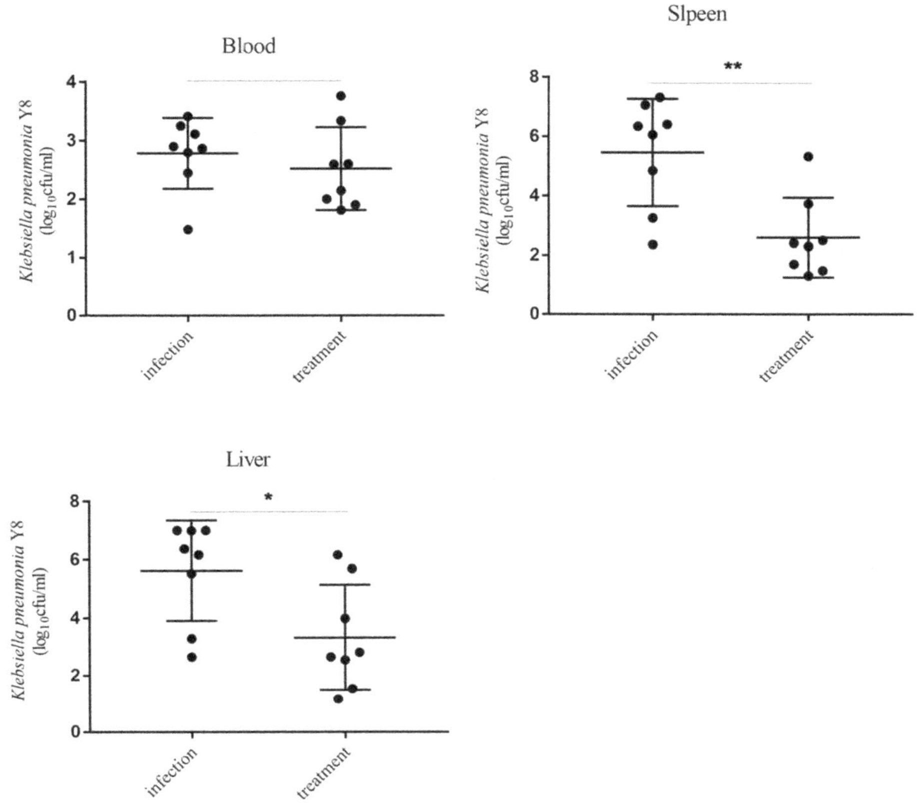

Fig. 5 Bacterial burden in blood, spleen and liver of mice at 3 days post infection (dpi). Mice were infected with 2.5×10^6 CFU of strain Y8 via the ip route and then treated with PBS or ceftazidime-avibactam by subcutaneous injection. At 3dpi, the viable bacteria of blood, spleen and liver was determined by plating serial dilutions on agar plates ($n = 8$). $*P < 0.05$; $**P < 0.01$

produce bla_{NDM} [21]. bla_{OXA-48} carbapenemase are predominantly existent in *Klebsiella pneumoniae* isolated in Tokyo and Europe [22]. In China, $bla_{OXA-181}$ and $bla_{OXA-232}$ have also been detected among *Klebsiella pneumoniae* clinical strains [23, 24].

Since CRE are usually extensively drug resistant, infections due to CRE are often associated with a high mortality. Therefore, a serious challenge of anti-infection therapy for CRE has been raised in clinical practice. Studies have revealed that compared to use carbapenems antibiotics alone, in the combination of carbapenems with other antibacterial agents such as tigecycline or polymyxin [25–28], amikacin [29] or fosfomycin [30] can considerably improve the outcomes of patient with CR-KP infection. Laurent adopted a combined pharmacotherapy regimen of dual carbapenems to provide a new approach in the treatment of CRE-induced infections [31]. As a novel β-lactam/β-lactamase inhibitor, studies have shown that ceftazidime-avibactam can successfully cure the infections due to *Enterobacteriaceae* with bla_{KPC} [32–35]. Nevertheless, it is worth to be noticed that with the increasing application of ceftazidime-avibactam, the resistant strains and failed cases have been reported [6, 7, 36]. Our results showed that all of 16 bla_{KPC-2} positive and 1 of $bla_{OXA-232}$ positive *Klebsiella pneumoniae* were susceptible to ceftazidime-avibactam with MIC_{50} and MIC_{90} for both 8 mg/L. Time-kill assays demonstrated that it showed a significant bactericidal effectiveness for either bla_{KPC} or $bla_{OXA-232}$ positive *K. pneumoniae* at the concentrations of 2MIC, 4MIC or 8MIC of ceftazidime-avibactam. 1 and Fig. 2). At 1 MIC of ceftazidime-avibactam, most of *K. pneumoniae* strains started to regrowth within 4–6 h. These results mean that the dosage of ceftazidime-avibactam is very important in the treatment of infections caused by bla_{KPC} or $bla_{OXA-232}$ positive *K. pneumoniae* [37].

In this study, 76.7% of bla_{NDM} positive *Klebsiella pneumoniae* were resistance to ceftazidime-avibactam with MIC_{50} and MIC_{90} for 64 mg/L and 256 mg/L, respectively. Because avibactam can not inhibit the activity of metallo-β-lactamase, ceftazidime-avibactam monotherapy was ineffective for infections caused by bla_{NDM-1} positive *Klebsiella pneumoniae* [38]. According to the results of time-kill assay, ceftazidime-avibactam combined with aztreonam is necessary for the treatment of infection due to bla_{NDM} positive *K. pneumoniae* based on the characteristics of weak hydrolysis capacity of metallo-β-lactamases to aztreonam. Eric Wenzler et al. also demonstrated that the combination of ceftazidime-avibactam and aztreonam had a synergistic bactericidal effect against class B metallo-β-lactamase-producing gram-negative bacteria [39]. Simultaneously, Benjamin Davido et al. reported that two cases infected either with metallo-β-lactamase-producing *Klebsiella pneumoniae* or *Pseudomonas aeruginosa* were successfully cured by combined administration of ceftazidime-avibactam and aztreonam [40]. The results of antimicrobial susceptibility testing indicated 90% (27/30) strains showed a synergistic effect for ceftazidime-avibactam combined with aztreonam. After combined with aztreonam, the MICs of ceftazidime-avibactam for 27 strains were reduced 4–256 times than ceftazidime-avibactam alone and all of them were susceptible to ceftazidime-avibactam with MIC ≤8 mg/L. Subsequently, the bactericidal curve tests performed on 12 strains of *Klebsiella pneumoniae* with a synergistic effect were also shown the consistent synergistic bactericidal effects. The reduction of bacterial colonies number was >2 $\log_{10}$ CFU/ mL compared with monotherapy and no colonies were detected after 24 h. In addition to strain of R148 showing the synergism 8 h after combined therapy, three bla_{NDM} positive *Klebsiella pneumoniae* clinical strains of R96, R97 and R100 did not demonstrate the synergistic effects after combined use with aztreonam, implying the other mechanisms of drug resistance may exist and require the further investigation in the future.

Conclusions

In summary, as a compound preparation of novel enzyme inhibitor, ceftazidime-avibactam possesses visible advantages in the treatment of class A and class D type carbapenemase–producing *Klebsiella pneumoniae* clinical isolates. In addition, if combined with aztreonam, it can also play a synergetic bactericidal effects against infections caused by bla_{NDM} positive *Klebsiella pneumoniae* clinical strains.

Abbreviations

CAZ: Ceftazidime; CAZ-AVI: Ceftazidime-avibactam; CRE: Carbapenem-resistant *Enterobacteriaceae*; CR-KP: Carbapenem-resistant *Klebsiella pneumoniae*; FIC: Fractional inhibitory concentration; IPM: Imipenem; MEM: Meropenem; MIC: Minimal inhibitory concentration

Acknowledgements

We thank all the laboratories for contributing data to this analysis.

Funding

This work was supported by the National Natural Science Foundation of China (grant no. 81871690).

Authors' contributions

PH, and FPH designed the study. WXZ, YG, JYL and YYZ performed the experimental work. YY, DD, and DMZ collected the data. FPH analysed the data. All authors read and approved the final manuscript.

Consent for publication

Not applicable.

Competing interests

The authors declare that they have no competing interests.

Author details

[1]Institute of Antibiotics, Huashan Hospital, Fudan University, 12 M. Wulumuqi Rd, Shanghai 200040, China. [2]Department of Clinical Laboratory, Shuguang Hospital Affiliated to Shanghai University of Traditional Chinese Medicine, 528 Zhangheng Rd, Shanghai 201203, China. [3]Department of Medical Microbiology and Immunology, Shanghai Jiao Tong University School of Medicine, Shanghai 200025, China. [4]Key Laboratory of Clinical Pharmacology of Antibiotics, Ministry of Health, Shanghai, China.

References

1. Ducomble T, Faucheux S, Helbig U, Kaisers UX, Konig B, Knaust A, Lubbert C, Moller I, Rodloff AC, Schweickert B, Eckmanns T. Large hospital outbreak of KPC-2-producing *Klebsiella pneumoniae*: investigating mortality and the impact of screening for KPC-2 with polymerase chain reaction. J Hosp Infect. 2015;89:179–85.
2. Kim JO, Song SA, Yoon EJ, Shin JH, Lee H, Jeong SH, Lee K. Outbreak of KPC-2-producing *Enterobacteriaceae* caused by clonal dissemination of *Klebsiella pneumoniae* ST307 carrying an IncX3-type plasmid harboring a truncated Tn4401a. Diagn Microbiol Infect Dis. 2017;87:343–8.
3. Yang J, Ye L, Guo L, Zhao Q, Chen R, Luo Y, Chen Y, Tian S, Zhao J, Shen D, Han L. A nosocomial outbreak of KPC-2-producing *Klebsiella pneumoniae* in a Chinese hospital: dissemination of ST11 and emergence of ST37, ST392 and ST395. Clin Microbiol Infect. 2013;19:E509–15.
4. Liu J, Yu J, Chen F, Yu J, Simner P, Tamma P, Liu Y, Shen L. Emergence and establishment of KPC-2-producing ST11 *Klebsiella pneumoniae* in a general hospital in Shanghai, China. Eur J Clin Microbiol Infect Dis. 2018;37:293–9.
5. Zasowski EJ, Rybak JM, Rybak MJ. The beta-lactams strike Back: ceftazidime-avibactam. Pharmacotherapy. 2015;35:755–70.
6. Shields RK, Nguyen MH, Chen L, Press EG, Kreiswirth BN, Clancy CJ. Pneumonia and renal replacement therapy are risk factors for ceftazidime-avibactam treatment failures and resistance among patients with carbapenem-resistant *Enterobacteriaceae* infections. Antimicrob Agents Chemother. 2018;62:e02497–17.
7. Shields RK, Chen L, Cheng S, Chavda KD, Press EG, Snyder A, Pandey R, Doi Y, Kreiswirth BN, Nguyen MH, Clancy CJ. Emergence of ceftazidime-avibactam resistance due to plasmid-borne blaKPC-3 mutations during treatment of Carbapenem-resistant *Klebsiella pneumoniae* infections. Antimicrob Agents Chemother. 2017;61(3):e02097–16.
8. Zhu J, Sun L, Ding B, Yang Y, Xu X, Liu W, Zhu D, Yang F, Zhang H, Hu F. Outbreak of NDM-1-producing *Klebsiella pneumoniae* ST76 and ST37 isolates in neonates. Eur J Clin Microbiol Infect Dis. 2016;35(4):611–8.
9. Woodford N, Fagan EJ, Ellington MJ. Multiplex PCR for rapid detection of genes encoding CTX-M extended-spectrum (beta)-lactamases. J Antimicrob Chemother. 2006;57(1):154–5.
10. Poirel L, Walsh TR, Cuvillier V, Nordmann P. Multiplex PCR for detection of acquired carbapenemase genes. Diagn Microbiol Infect Dis. 2011;70(1):119–23.
11. Clinical and Laboratory Standards Institute. Performance Standards for Antimicrobial Susceptibility Testing[S]: Twenty-seventh Informational Supplement. PA: CLSI; 2017.
12. Bercot B, Poirel L, Dortet L, Nordmann P. In vitro evaluation of antibiotic synergy for NDM-1-producing *Enterobacteriaceae*. J Antimicrob Chemother. 2011;66:2295–7.
13. Elemam A, Rahimian J, Doymaz M. In vitro evaluation of antibiotic synergy for polymyxin B-resistant carbapenemase-producing *Klebsiella pneumoniae*. J Clin Microbiol. 2010;48:3558–62.
14. Gunderson BW, Ibrahim KH, Hovde LB, Fromm TL, Reed MD, Rotschafer JC. Synergistic activity of colistin and ceftazidime against multiantibiotic-resistant Pseudomonas aeruginosa in an in vitro pharmacodynamic model. Antimicrob Agents Chemother. 2003;47:905–9.
15. Paevskii SA. A means for determining the bactericidal activity of the tissues during the treatment of orthopedic patients by transosseous osteosynthesis methods. Klin Lab Diagn. 1993:25–9.
16. Norden CW, Wentzel H, Keleti E. Comparison of techniques for measurement of in vitro antibiotic synergism. J Infect Dis. 1979;140:629–33.
17. US Centers for Disease Control and Prevention. Antibiotic Resistance Theats in the United States. 2013. https://www.cdc.gov/drugresistance/threat-report-2013/pdf/ar-threats-2013-508.pdf.

18. Hu FP, Guo Y, Zhu DM, Wang F, Jiang XF, Xu YC, Zhang XJ, Zhang CX, Ji P, Xie Y, Kang M, Wang CQ, Wang AM, Xu YH, Shen JL, Sun ZY, Chen ZJ, Ni YX, Sun JY, Chu YZ, Tian SF, Hu ZD, Li J, Yu YS, Lin J, Shan B, Du Y, Han Y, Guo S, Wei LH, Wu L, Zhang H, Kong J, Hu YJ, Ai XM, Zhuo C, Su DH, Yang Q, Jia B, Huang W. Resistance trends among clinical isolates in China reported from CHINET surveillance of bacterial resistance, 2005-2014. Clin Microbiol Infect. 2016;22(Suppl 1):S9–14.
19. Chew KL, Lin RTP, Teo JWP. *Klebsiella pneumoniae* in Singapore: Hypervirulent infections and the Carbapenemase threat. Front Cell Infect Microbiol. 2017;7:515.
20. Kohler PP, Volling C, Green K, Uleryk EM, Shah PS, McGeer A. Carbapenem resistance, initial antibiotic therapy, and mortality in *Klebsiella pneumoniae* bacteremia: a systematic review and meta-analysis. Infect Control Hosp Epidemiol. 2017;38:1319–28.
21. Javed H, Ejaz H, Zafar A, Rathore AW, Ikram ul H. Metallo-beta-lactamase producing Escherichia coli and *Klebsiella pneumoniae*: a rising threat for hospitalized children. J Pak Med Assoc. 2016;66:1068–72.
22. Ma L, Wang JT, Wu TL, Siu LK, Chuang YC, Lin JC, Lu MC, Lu PL. Emergence of OXA-48-producing *Klebsiella pneumoniae* in Taiwan. PLoS One. 2015;10: e0139152.
23. Liu Y, Feng Y, Wu W, Xie Y, Wang X, Zhang X, Chen X, Zong Z. First report of OXA-181-producing *Escherichia coli* in China and characterization of the isolate using whole-genome sequencing. Antimicrob Agents Chemother. 2015;59(8):5022–5.
24. Yin D, Dong D, Li K, Zhang L, Liang J, Yang Y, Wu N, Bao Y, Wang C. Hu F. clonal dissemination of OXA-232 Carbapenemase-producing *Klebsiella pneumoniae* in neonates. Antimicrob Agents Chemother. 2017;61(8): e00385–17.
25. Tzouvelekis LS, Markogiannakis A, Piperaki E, Souli M, Daikos GL. Treating infections caused by carbapenemase-producing *Enterobacteriaceae*. Clin Microbiol Infect. 2014;20:862–72.
26. Qureshi ZA, Paterson DL, Potoski BA, Kilayko MC, Sandovsky G, Sordillo E, Polsky B, Adams-Haduch JM, Doi Y. Treatment outcome of bacteremia due to KPC-producing *Klebsiella pneumoniae*: superiority of combination antimicrobial regimens. Antimicrob Agents Chemother. 2012;56:2108–13.
27. Zhang Y, Li P, Yin Y, Li F, Zhang Q. In vitro activity of tigecycline in combination with rifampin, doripenem or ceftazidime against carbapenem-resistant *Klebsiella pneumoniae* bloodstream isolates. J Antibiot (Tokyo). 2017;70:193–5.
28. Machuca I, Gutierrez-Gutierrez B, Gracia-Ahufinger I, Rivera Espinar F, Cano A, Guzman-Puche J, Perez-Nadales E, Natera C, Rodriguez M, Leon R, Caston JJ, Rodriguez-Lopez F, Rodriguez-Bano J, Torre-Cisneros J. Mortality associated with bacteremia due to Colistin-resistant *Klebsiella pneumoniae* with high-level Meropenem resistance: importance of combination therapy without Colistin and Carbapenems. Antimicrob Agents Chemother. 2017;61:e00406–17.
29. Hajjej Z, Gharsallah H, Naija H, Boutiba I, Labbene I, Ferjani M. Successful treatment of a Carbapenem-resistant *Klebsiella pneumoniae* carrying Bla OXA-48 , Bla VIM-2 , Bla CMY-2 and Bla SHV- with high dose combination of imipenem and amikacin. IDCases. 2016;4:10–2.
30. Albiero J, Sy SK, Mazucheli J, Caparroz-Assef SM, Costa BB, Alves JL, Gales AC, Tognim MC. Pharmacodynamic evaluation of the potential clinical utility of Fosfomycin and Meropenem in combination therapy against KPC-2-producing *Klebsiella pneumoniae*. Antimicrob Agents Chemother. 2016;60:4128–39.
31. Poirel L, Kieffer N, Nordmann P. In vitro evaluation of dual carbapenem combinations against carbapenemase-producing *Enterobacteriaceae*. J Antimicrob Chemother. 2016;71:156–61.
32. Gugliandolo A, Caio C, Mezzatesta ML, Rifici C, Bramanti P, Stefani S, Mazzon E. Successful ceftazidime-avibactam treatment of MDR-KPC-positive *Klebsiella pneumoniae* infection in a patient with traumatic brain injury: a case report. Medicine (Baltimore). 2017;96:e7664.
33. Temkin E, Torre-Cisneros J, Beovic B, Benito N, Giannella M, Gilarranz R, Jeremiah C, Loeches B, Machuca I, Jimenez-Martin MJ, Martinez JA, Mora-Rillo M, Navas E, Osthoff M, Pozo JC, Ramos Ramos JC, Rodriguez M, Sanchez-Garcia M, Viale P, Wolff M, Carmeli Y. Ceftazidime-avibactam as salvage therapy for infections caused by Carbapenem-resistant organisms. Antimicrob Agents Chemother. 2017;61:e01964–16.
34. Holyk A, Belden V, Lee JJ, Musick W, Keul R, Britz GW, Lin J. Ceftazidime/avibactam use for carbapenem-resistant *Klebsiella pneumoniae* meningitis: a case report. J Antimicrob Chemother. 2018;73:254 6.
35. van Duin D, Lok JJ, Earley M, Cober E, Richter SS, Perez F, Salata RA, Kalayjian RC, Watkins RR, Doi Y, Kaye KS, Fowler VG, Jr., Paterson DL, Bonomo RA, Evans S, Antibacterial Resistance Leadership G. Colistin versus ceftazidime-avibactam in the treatment of infections due to Carbapenem-resistant *Enterobacteriaceae*. Clin Infect Dis. 2018;66:163–71.
36. Barnes MD, Winkler ML, Taracila MA, Page MG, Desarbre E, Kreiswirth BN, Shields RK, Nguyen MH, Clancy C, Spellberg B, Papp-Wallace KM, Bonomo RA. *Klebsiella pneumoniae* Carbapenemase-2 (KPC-2), substitutions at ambler position Asp179, and resistance to ceftazidime-avibactam: unique antibiotic-resistant phenotypes emerge from beta-lactamase protein engineering. MBio. 2017;8:e00528–17.
37. Bensman TJ, Wang J, Jayne J, Fukushima L, Rao AP, D'Argenio DZ, Beringer PM. Pharmacokinetic-Pharmacodynamic target attainment analyses to determine optimal dosing of ceftazidime-avibactam for the treatment of acute pulmonary exacerbations in patients with cystic fibrosis. Antimicrob Agents Chemother. 2017;61:e00988–17.
38. Davido B, Senard O, de Truchis P, Salomon J, Dinh A. Monotherapy of ceftazidime-avibactam and ceftolozane-tazobactam: two effective antimicrobial agents against multidrug-resistant organisms except for NDM-1 isolates. Int J Infect Dis. 2017;62:124–5.
39. Wenzler E, Deraedt MF, Harrington AT, Danizger LH. Synergistic activity of ceftazidime-avibactam and aztreonam against serine and metallo-beta-lactamase-producing gram-negative pathogens. Diagn Microbiol Infect Dis. 2017;88:352–4.
40. Davido B, Fellous L, Lawrence C, Maxime V, Rottman M, Dinh A. Ceftazidime-avibactam and Aztreonam, an interesting strategy to overcome beta-lactam resistance conferred by Metallo-beta-lactamases in *Enterobacteriaceae* and *Pseudomonas aeruginosa*. Antimicrob Agents Chemother. 2017;61:e01008–17.

Neisseria Gonorrhoae and their antimicrobial susceptibility patterns among symptomatic patients from Gondar town, north West Ethiopia

Addisu Gize Yeshanew* and Rozina Ambachew Geremew

Abstract

Background: *Neisseria gonorrhoeae*, the causative agent of gonorrhoea, is a Gram negative, coffee-bean shaped facultative intracellular diplococcus bacterium, the classical sexually transmitted bacteria. Nowadays, *N. gonorrhoeae* has developed high-level resistance to all traditional antimicrobials used for the treatment of gonorrhoea and makes the treatment complicated. So, the aim of this study was to determine magnitude and antimicrobial resistance patterns of *N. gonorrhoeae*.

Methods: A cross sectional study was conducted between April and August 2016 among STI clinic clients in Gondar town hospitals and health centers. Urethral swab and cervical swab specimens were inoculated to Thayer Martin media (OXOID, UK) plates. Observation of Gram-negative intracellular diplococcic was a presumptive diagnosis of gonococcal infection. Finally, antimicrobial susceptibility was assessed by using a modified Kirby-Bauer disk diffusion test, with results indicating susceptible, intermediate or resistant. Data were entered and analyzed using SPSS version 20.

Results: The overall prevalence of laboratory confirmed N. *gonorrhoeae* was 25(20.8%). The isolated N. *gonorrhoeae* was resistant 100% to tetracycline, penicillin and 80% percent was multidrug resistant.

Conclusion: Prevalence and drug resistance of *N. gonorrhoeae* were high in the study area. A large study is needed in order to know the magnitude in the community as well as to increase awareness of both regional health bureaus and the Ministry of Health about the treatment guide-lines.

Keywords: *N. Gonorrhoeae*, Antimicrobial sensitivity test

Background

Neisseria gonorrhoeae is a Gram negative, coffee-bean shaped intracellular diplococcus bacterium responsible for gonorrhoea which is one of the classical sexually transmitted infections (STIs) [1]. The causative organism is highly adapted to the genital tract and often causing asymptomatic and undetected infection [2]. Gonorrhoea is acquired by unsafe sex practices and also can be transmitted from mother to child during delivery [1], which has medically significant implications if not treated early. Untreated gonorrhoea can lead infertility, inflammation leading to acute and chronic abdominal pain in women, ectopic pregnancy and maternal death, first trimester abortion, severe neonatal eye infection that lead to blindness, a fivefold increase in HIV transmission, disseminated gonococcal infection which results in localized septic arthritis, endocarditis, and meningitis [1, 3, 4]. Therefore, accurate efforts should be made to offer routine endocervical cultures for *N. gonorrhoeae* to all women who have risk behavior of STIs to prevent this infection [5]. Gonorrhoea treatment is complicated by *N.gonorrhoeae's* ability to develop antimicrobial resistance [6]. Since the introduction of antimicrobials to treat *N. gonorrhoeae* infection 70–80 years ago, *N. gonorrhoeae*

* Correspondence: addisu.gize@sphmmc.edu.et; konjoaddisu@gmail.com
Department of Microbiology, St. Paul's Hospital Millennium Medical College,

has progressively developed resistance to most antimicrobial previously recommended for treatment, including sulfonamides, penicillin, tetracycline, and fluoroquinolone antibiotics [7]. In European Surveillance of combined antimicrobial susceptibility data, the resistance was found to be high to ciprofloxacin (30.9%), penicillin (21.3%) and tetracycline (59.8%), and Neisseria gonorrhoeae strain (H041) that is highly resistant to the extended-spectrum cephalosporin (ESC) ceftriaxone [8, 9].

In many parts of the developing world, the absence of etiologic diagnostic capacity due to constraints imposed by cost, lack of equipment or trained personnel, and time management has forced health care providers to rely on a syndrome based approach to STI management, because many STIs have common symptoms or are asymptomatic and therefore undetected and untreated [10]. Therefore, this study primarily aimed to determine the prevalence *N. gonorrhoeae* and their antimicrobial susceptibility pattern among STI clinics attendants at Gondar town, North West of Ethiopia.

Materials and methods

A cross-sectional study was conducted from April 1 to August 30, 2016 in Gondar town hospitals and health centers, Gondar town, Northwest Ethiopia. The Town is 725 km away from Addis Ababa, Ethiopia, located in the North Gondar Zone of the Amhara Region. Based on figures from 2011 Central Statistical Agency (CSA) of Ethiopia, Gondar town has a total population of 207,044, of whom 98,120 are men and 108,924 women. There are two hospital (1 governmental and 1 private) and 5 health centers in the town.

Patients who visited Gondar town hospitals and health centers during the study period serve as the source population, whereas, all STI suspected patients attending in the STI clinic were included as the case of the study. However, patients under antibiotic treatment during 7 days before the enrolment and female patients who were on menstruation at the time of examination were excluded from the study. Descriptive statistics, including socio-demographics factors and known risk factors for STI were performed.

Sample size and sampling technique

Sample size was calculated based on the single population proportion formula considering the prevalence rate of 8.5% from the previous study conducted in Bahirdar, Northwest Ethiopia. Expected margin of error (d) was 0.05 and confidence interval (z) was 95%. One hundred twenty consecutive consenting patients, who attended Gondar town hospitals and health centers STI clinic, with one or more of the complaints as stated by WHO in its syndrome approach for the diagnosis of STI were included [5].

Data collection procedure

Socio-demographic characteristics

After taking written informed consent from each study participant, a semi-structured questionnaire was used to collect socio-demographic and clinical data needed in this study. Data were collected by trained nurses.

Sample collection

Urethral and cervical specimen

External inspections of the genital area were made, and the characteristics of any local changes such as; erythema, abrasions, ulceration, urethral discharge and vaginal discharge were noted, including color, amount, odor and consistency. In the absence of visible urethral discharge, the patient was asked to milk the urethra. Specimens of discharge were obtained at or just within the urethral meatus for male and cervical swabs were taken for female. Two swabs were taken; one for Gram staining and the other were put on Amies transport media for *N. gonorrhoeae* culture at Gondar University Hospital laboratory. This laboratory, according to Ethiopian National Accreditation Office (ENAO), which established the Stepwise Laboratory (Quality) Improvement Process towards Accreditation (SLIPTA), has got 3 stars (75–84%) ranked from 5 stars (≥95%). ENAO gives recognition based on progress towards meeting requirements set by international standards and on laboratory performance during the 12 months preceding the SLIPTA audit, relying on complete and accurate data, to improve quality of public health laboratories in developing countries to achieve ISO 15189 standards.

Laboratory method

Isolation and identification of N. Gonorrhoeae

Identification was made by observing polymorphonuclear leucocytes (PMNLs) with Gram-negative intracellular diplococci as a presumptive diagnosis of gonococcal infection. Specimens inoculated directly into the modified Thayer Martin medium (MTM) (OXOID, UK) plates contained vancomycin, colistin, nistatin and trimetoprin and incubated at 36.5 °C for 24–48 h. Then isolates was identified as *N. gonorrhoeae* on the basis of colony morphology, Gram staining, oxidase test, and carbohydrate utilization test [11]. *N. gonorrhoeae* is observed as Gram negative diplococci when Gram stained, positive for oxidase, ferments only glucose, and is resistant to colisin [12].

Antibiotic susceptibility testing

From a pure culture, 3–5 selected colonies of bacteria were transferred to a tube with a straight wire and prepared in a suspension of 2.5 ml normal saline and incubated at 36.5 °C until the turbidity of the suspension become adjusted to a McFarland 0.5. A sterile swab was used to distribute the bacteria evenly over the entire surface of MTM agar. The susceptibility to the following antimicrobial agents (OXOID, UK) were assessed: penicillin (P 10 IU), tetracycline (TE 30 μg), ciprofloxacin (CIP 5 μg), ceftriaxone (CRO 30 μg), Cefotaxime (30 μg), Cefoxitin (FOX 30 μg), Clindmycin (CLI 2 μg). The criteria used to select the antimicrobial agents tested were based on their availability and frequent prescriptions for the management of gonococcal infection and the national list of medicines by Food, Medicine and Health- Care Administration and Control Authority (FMHACA) Ethiopia in 2010 to treat infections, and the syndromic management package for the management of sexually transmitted infections guideline from the Federal Ministry of Health.

Finally, antimicrobial susceptibility testing was performed for all isolates according to the criteria of Clinical and Laboratory Standard Institute (CLSI) by the modified Kirby-Bauer disk diffusion method on Thayer Martin medium plates, results as to susceptible or resistant were based on the M100-S24 Performance Standards for Antimicrobial Susceptibility Testing [12].

Data quality control

The questionnaire was pre-tested on 15 outpatient department patients for comprehensiveness, effectiveness, reliability and validity. Training was given for data collectors on data collection procedures with support from an investigator, venereologist and gynecologist. Culture media sterility was ensured by incubating 5% of each batch of the prepared media at 37°c for 24 h. Performance of prepared media was also checked by inoculating with control strains *N. gonorrhoeae ATCCTM* 49226 (10) [13].

Data analysis

Data were entered and analyzed using SPSS version 20. Descriptive statistics was applied to determine the distribution of the socio-demographic and clinical characteristics.

Ethical consideration

The proposed study was approved by the research and ethics committee of the School of Biomedical and Laboratory Sciences of the University of Gondar. Official permission was obtained from each of the health facilities. The aim and details of the study was explained to each study participant before obtaining their written consent for specimen collection. Confidentiality was maintained at all levels of the study by using codes rather than names of the study participants. The results of all positive individuals were reported to the respective health facilities for better management of the patients.

Results

Socio-demographic characteristics

A total of 120 patients, 21 (17.5%) males and 99 (82.5%) females, were enrolled in the study. The mean ± SD age of the study participants was 27.8 ± 7.2 years. The majority (66.6%) of the study participants were in the age group below 30 years old. Fifty eight (48.3%) were married. The majority of the patients 74 (61.7%) were literate. Regarding their occupation, house wives numbered 26(21.7%), and in terms of economic status, 37 (30.8%) participants reported not to receiving income of their own (Table 1).

Prevalence of N. Gonorrhoeae

The overall prevalence of laboratory confirmed *N. gonorrhoeae* pathogens among suspected attendees of Gondar town hospitals and health centers was 25(20.8%). N. *gonorrhoeae* infections were higher among females and age groups 15-29 yrs. The majority of the respondents 82(68.3%) had multiple sexual partners, and 69(57.5%) had never used condoms (Table 1).

.Antimicrobial susceptibility pattern of N. Gonorrhoeae strains

The antimicrobial susceptibility pattern of all isolates of *N. gonorrhoeae* is shown in Table 2. All isolates of *N. gonorrhoeae* showed resistance to at least one antimicrobial agent. The susceptibility pattern of isolates shows there were a hundred percent non-susceptibility for tetracycline, 76% non-susceptibility and 24% intermediate resistant for penicillin. The isolated *N. gonorrhoeae* was resistant 52% to ciprofloxacin, 48% to ceftriaxone, 44% to cefoxitin, 29% to cefotaxime, and 28% to clindmycin. Most of the isolates (80%) showed multiple drug resistance and 11(44%) of the isolates showed non-susceptibility to both ciprofloxacin and ceftriaxone.

Discussion

The overall prevalence of laboratory confirmed *N. gonorrhoeae* was 25(20.8%). This prevalence rate was comparable with studies from Mozambique (22.5%) [14], Egypt (26%) [15] and southwestern Nigeria (25%) [16]. However it was higher than the value reported from previous findings of studies done in Hawassa, Southern Ethiopia (5.1%) [2] as well as the Northern part of Ethiopia [17]. Again the present finding was higher than the studies conducted in other countries: for example, 11% in Mongolia [18], 6% United States [19], 1.4% in Colombia [20], 6% in India and 1% from Nigeria [21]. These discrepancies might be due to the lack of advancement in both early diagnosis and treatment in our country, which can lead to an increased number of untreated patients. A lack of differential diagnosis for resource poor settings can lead to an increased number of untreated patients

Table 1 Prevalence of *N. gonorrhoeae* described by socio-demographic characteristics and known risk factors for STI, Gondar town, North West Ethiopia from April–August 2016

Characteristics	Total N (%), $n = 120$	*N. gonorrhoeae* + ve (%),$n = 25$	*N. gonorrhoeae* - ve (%), $n = 95$
Sex			
Male	21(17.5)	6 (29)	15 (71)
Female	99(82.5)	19(19)	80(81)
Age			
15–29	80(66.7)	17(21)	63(79)
30–45	40(33,3)	8(20)	32(80)
Marital status			
Single	62(51.7)	14(23)	48(77)
Married	58(48.3)	11(19)	47(81)
Educational status			
Illiterate	46(38.3)	9(20)	37(80)
Literate	74(61.7)	16(22)	58(78)
Occupation			
Government employed	31(25.8)	7(23)	24(77)
House wife	26(21.7)	3(11)	23(89)
CSW	11(9.2)	2(18)	9(82)
No	23(19.2)	5(22)	18(78)
Self-employed	29(24.1)	8(18)	21(72)
Income			
No	37(30.8)	7(19)	30(81)
< 800	25(20.8)	7(18)	18(72)
801–1600	31(25.8)	5(16)	26(84)
> 1600	27(22.5)	6(22)	21(78)
Knowledge about STI			
No	54(45)	10(19)	44(81)
Yes	66(55)	15(23)	51(77)
Alcohol use			
No	39(32.5)	5(13)	34(87)
Yes	81(67.5)	20(25)	61(75)
Khat chewing			
No	102(86)	21(21)	81(79)
Yes	18(14)	4(28)	13(72)
Smoking			
No	111(93)	22(20)	89(80)
Yes	9(7.5)	3(33)	6(67)
History of abortion			
No	55(55.5)	12(22)	43(78)
Yes	44(44.5)	7(15)	37(84)
Sexual partner			
One partner	38(31.6)	7(18)	31(82)
More than one partner	82(68.3)	18(22)	64(78)

Table 1 Prevalence of *N. gonorrhoeae* described by socio-demographic characteristics and known risk factors for STI, Gondar town, North West Ethiopia from April–August 2016 *(Continued)*

Characteristics	Total N (%), *n* = 120	*N. gonorrhoeae* + ve (%),*n* = 25	*N. gonorrhoeae* - ve (%), *n* = 95
Condom use			
Never	69(57.5)	13(19)	56(81)
S/Rarely	38(32)	9(24)	29(76)
Always	13(10.5)	3(15)	11(85)
Males sexual contact with prostitute women			
No	16(13)	1(6)	15(94)
S/Rarely	100(83)	21(21)	79(79)
Yes	5(4)	3(60)	2(40)
History of STI			
No	53(44.2)	9(17)	44(83)
Yes	67(55.8)	16(24)	51(76)
Commonly using toillet & washing materials			
No	81(67.5)	19(23)	62(77)
Yes	39(32.5)	6(15)	33(85)
Contact new person the last 3 months			
No	78(65)	16(21)	62(79)
Yes	42(35)	9(21)	33(79)
HIV status			
Positive	17(14.2)	1(6)	16(94)
Negative	103(86)	24(23)	79(77)

+ *ve* infected with N. gonorrhoeae, , *ve* non-infected with N. gonorrhoeae, *S/Rarely* sometimes or rarely, *CSW* Commercial Sex Workers, *STI* Sexual Transmitted Infection, *HIV* Human Immunodeficiency Virus

and a poor partner tracing system and using a syndromic approach, especially in the study area, might be the possible causes for this high prevalence rate.

The main reason for the rapid increase of *N. gonorrhoeae* resistance rates to Penicillin, Tetracycline and Ciprofloxacin after they had been recommended for clinical use is likely their indiscriminate use. Patients tend to administer antimicrobial treatment by themselves or visit non-formal medical institutions such as unregistered private clinics.

Table 2 Antimicrobial susceptibility pattern of *N. gonorrhoeae* isolates from STI clinic attendants in Gondar town, North West Ethiopia from April–May 2016

Antibiotic	#S (%)	# I (%)	# R (%)
Penicillin	0(0)	6(24)	19(76)
Tetracycline	0(0)	0(0)	25(100)
Ciprofloxacin	4(16)	8(32)	13(52)
Ceftriaxone	13(52)	*	12(48)
Cefotaxime	17(71)	*	7(29)
Cefoxitin	14(56)	*	11(44)
Clindmycin	18(72)	*	7(28)

\# *S* number of sensitive, # *I* number of intermediate, # *R* number of resistance, * have no intermediate range

Moreover, some patients do not complete the full treatment course, increasing the chance for antimicrobial resistance to develop. For example, patients could buy antimicrobials in drug stores without a prescription. Indeed, an association between self-prescribed antimicrobial use and gonococcal AMR may be high.

Gonococcal infection was observed in 6(29%) of males and, patients having multiple sexual partners 18(22%) and previous history of STI 16(24%). This prevalence rate may be attributed to less condom usage by females and having a history of STI which leads to the infection. The same factors were shown to increase the exposure and prevalence rate of gonococcal infection in other studies as well [22, 23].

In addition, it was observed infection in both the age groups of 15–29 & 30–45 years old. The finding on the target group was also supported by other studies [24, 25].

The antimicrobial resistance patterns ranged from 7(28%) for Cefotaxime and Clindmycin up to 100% in Tetracycline. This Tetracycline resistance pattern was similar with the study done in Gambella hospital, Ethiopia [1]. The present study showed a high level of resistance to Tetracycline 25(100%) and Ciprofloxacin 13(52%) compared to the study done in North West

Ethiopia (92.6, 40.9%) (15), Southern Ethiopia (55, 18%) [2] and United States (25.3, 19.2%) [4].

Most researchers are worried gonorrhoea will soon become untreatable with those antibiotics. This may be true in resource limited countries because of a lack of proper usage of antibiotics and application of antimicrobials as therapeutic agents for syndromatic treatment or may be due to the emergence of new resistant beta-lactamase producing strains over a period of time.

The resistance of Cefotaxime 7(28%) and Cefoxitin 11(44%) in the current study is also higher than the study conducted in Gambella hospital, Ethiopia [1] and Southern Ethiopia [2] but lower as compared to Tetracycline, Penicillin, Ciprofloxacin. The reason might be these drugs are expensive, not intensively used and not easily available outside the health institution, plus these drugs are newer compared to the others. Low resistance pattern of these drugs in our study may make these drugs excellent choices as first-line treatment.

Conclusion

High prevalence of *N. gonorrhoeae* and drug resistance among symptomatic clients who attended the STI clinics in the study area was observed. This should cause alarm and should lead to a large community based study and increased awareness of both regional health bureaus and the Ministry of Health about the treatment guide-lines.

Abbreviations

AMR: Antimicrobial Resistance; CLSI: Clinical and Laboratory Standards Institute; ESBL: Extended-spectrum β-lactamase; FDA: US Food and Drugs Administration; HIV: Human Immunodeficiency Virus; SPSS: Statistical Packages for Social Sciences.; STI: Sexually Transmitted Infections

Acknowledgements

We acknowledge the staff of the STI clinics of Gondar town for their cooperation during data collection. We would like to thank Professor Moges Tiruneh and Dr. Kassahun Tameyalew for their advice and suggestions. Our acknowledgment also extends our manuscript grammatical and topographical editors, **Meron Begashaw,** Human Resource Strategies Fellow and last but not least we would like to acknowledge **Amy Vercler,** admin assistant of the SPHMMC for her language edition of the manuscripts.

Funding

This research work was financed by Amhara Regional Health Bureau, Ethiopia. The funder had no role in study design, data collection and analysis, decision to publish, or preparation of the manuscript.

Authors' contributions

AGY was involved in study conception, data analysis, drafting the manuscript and critically reviewing the manuscript. RAG was involved in the study conception and design, data analysis, and drafting the manuscript. Both authors have read, edited and approved the manuscript.

Consent for publication

Not applicable. This study does not contain any individual or personal data.

Competing interests

The authors declare that they have no competing interests.

References

1. Ali S, Sewunet T, Sahlemariam Z, Kibru G. Neisseria gonorrhoeae among suspects of sexually transmitted infection in Gambella hospital, Ethiopia: risk factors and drug resistance. BMC Res Notes. 2016 Sep 13;9(1):439.
2. Hailemariam M, Abebe T, Mihret A, Lambiyo T. Prevalence of Neisseria gonorrhoeae. And their antimicrobial susceptibility patterns among symptomatic women attending gynecology outpatient department in Hawassa Referral Hospital, Hawassa, Ethiopia. Ethiop J Health Sci. 2013 Jan 1; 23(1):10–8.
3. Fingerhuth SM, Bonhoeffer S, Low N, Althaus CL. Antibiotic-resistant Neisseria gonorrhoeae spread faster with more treatment. Not More Sexual Partners PLoS Pathog. 2016 May;12(5):e1005611.
4. Kirkcaldy RD, Harvey A, Papp JR, Del Rio C, Soge OO, Holmes KK, et al. Neisseria gonorrhoeae Antimicrobial Susceptibility Surveillance - The Gonococcal Isolate Surveillance Project, 27 Sites, United States, 2014. Morb Mortal Wkly Rep Surveill Summ Wash DC 2002. 2016 Jul 15;65(7):1–19.
5. Organization WH, others. Management of patients with sexually transmitted diseases: report of a WHO Study Group [meeting held in Geneva from 3 to 6 July 1990]. 1991 [cited 2016 Oct 31]; Available from: http://apps.who.int/iris/handle/10665/40873
6. Organization WH. Global action plan to control the spread and impact of antimicrobial resistance in Neisseria gonorrhoeae. 2012 [cited 2016 Dec 28]; Available from: http://www.who.int/iris/handle/10665/44863
7. Kidd S, Moore PC, Kirkcaldy RD, Philip SS, Wiesenfeld HC, Papp JR, et al. Comparison of antimicrobial susceptibility of urogenital Neisseria gonorrhoeae isolates obtained from women and men. Sex Transm Dis. 2015 Aug;42(8):434–9.
8. Martin IMC, Hoffmann S, Ison CA. European surveillance of sexually transmitted infections (ESSTI): the first combined antimicrobial susceptibility data for Neisseria gonorrhoeae in Western Europe. J Antimicrob Chemother. 2006 Sep 1;58(3):587–93.
9. Ohnishi M, Golparian D, Shimuta K, Saika T, Hoshina S, Iwasaku K, et al. Is Neisseria gonorrhoeae initiating a future era of untreatable gonorrhea?: detailed characterization of the first strain with high-level resistance to ceftriaxone. Antimicrob Agents Chemother. 2011 Jul 1;55(7):3538–45.
10. Verma R, Sood S. Gonorrhoea diagnostics: An update. Indian J Med Microbiol. 2016 Apr 1;34(2):139.
11. Juayang AC, Lim JPT, Acosido MAD, Jr DGM, Gallega CT. Antibiotic Susceptibility of Neisseria gonorrhoeae in Bacolod City, Philippines. Br Microbiol Res J [Internet]. 2015 [cited 2016 Oct 31];10(2). https://doi.org/10.9734/BMRJ/2015/19641.
12. Wkler MA, Cockerill FR, Bush K, Dudely MN, Etiopoule GM, Hardy DJ, et al. Clinical and Laboratory Standard Institute. Performance standards for antimicrobial disc susceptibility tests; Approved standard, 10th edn. Available from: http://www.clsi.org/source/orders/free/ m02-a10.pdf.
13. Organization WH, others. WHO global strategy for containment of antimicrobial resistance. 2001 [cited 2016 Dec 28]; Available from: http://apps.who.int/iris/handle/10665/66860
14. Zimba TF, Apalata T, Sturm WA, Moodley P. Aetiology of sexually transmitted infections in Maputo. Mozambique J Infect Dev Ctries. 2010; 5(01):041–7.
15. Ali F, Aziz AA, Helmy MF, Mobdy AA, Darwish M. Prevalence of certain sexually transmitted diseases in Egypt. J Egypt Public Health Assoc. 1995; 71(5_6):553–75.
16. Bersoff-Matcha SJ, Horgan MM, Fraser VJ, Mundy LM, Stoner BP. Sexually transmitted disease acquisition among women infected with human immunodeficiency virus type 1. J Infect Dis. 1998;178(4):1174–7.
17. Tibebu M, Shibabaw A, Medhin G, Kassu A. Neisseria gonorrhoeae non-susceptible to cephalosporins and quinolones in Northwest Ethiopia. BMC Infect Dis. 2013 Sep 5;13:415.
18. Garland SM, Tabrizi SN, Chen S, Byambaa C, Davaajav K. Prevalence of sexually transmitted infections (Neisseria gonorrhoeae, chlamydia trachomatis, trichomonas vaginalis and human papillomavirus) in female attendees of a sexually transmitted diseases clinic in Ulaanbaatar. Mongolia Infect Dis Obstet Gynecol. 2001;9(3):143–6.
19. Kent CK, Chaw JK, Wong W, Liska S, Gibson S, Hubbard G, et al. Prevalence of rectal, urethral, and pharyngeal chlamydia and gonorrhoeae. Detected in

2 clinical settings among men who have sex with men: San Francisco, California, 2003. Clin Infect Dis. 2005;41(1):67–74.
20. Ángel-Müller E, Rodríguez A, Núñez-Forero LM, Moyano LF, González P, Osorio E, et al. The prevalence of and factors associated with C. Trachomatis, N. Gonorrhoeae, t. Vaginalis, C. Albicans infection, syphilis, HIV and bacterial vaginosis in females suffering lower genital tract infection symptoms in three healthcare attention sites in Bogotá, Colombia, 2010. Rev Colomb Obstet Ginecol. 2012;63(1):14–24.
21. Okonko IO, Okerentugba PO, Adejuwon AO, Onoh CC. Prevalence of sexually transmitted infections (STIs) among attendees of lead city university medical Centre in Ibadan, southwestern. Nigeria Arch Appl Sci Res. 2012; 4(2):980–7.
22. Taffa N, Bjune G, Sundby J, Gaustad P, Alestrøm A. Prevalence of gonococcal and chlamydial infections and sexual risk behavior among youth in Addis Ababa. Ethiopia Sex Transm Dis. 2002;29(12):828–33.
23. Duncan ME, Reimann K, Tibaux G, Pelzer A, Mehari L, Lind I. Seroepidemiological study of gonorrhoea in Ethiopian women. 1. Prevalence and clinical significance. Genitourin Med. 1991;67(6):485–92.
24. Workowski KA, Berman SM. Centers for Disease Control and Prevention Sexually Transmitted Diseases Treatment Guidelines. Clin Infect Dis. 2007 Apr 1;Supplement_3(44):S73–6.
25. Force USPST. Screening for gonorrhoeae: recommendation statement. Ann Fam Med. 2005 May 1;3(3):263–7.

20

Intra-hospital differences in antibiotic use correlate with antimicrobial resistance rate in *Escherichia coli* and *Klebsiella pneumoniae*

Alexia Cusini[1,5*], David Herren[1], Lukas Bütikofer[3], Catherine Plüss-Suard[4], Andreas Kronenberg[1,2†] and Jonas Marschall[1†]

Abstract

Background: Monitoring antimicrobial use and resistance in hospitals are important tools of antimicrobial stewardship programs. We aimed to determine the association between the use of frequently prescribed antibiotics and the corresponding resistance rates in *Escherichia coli* and *Klebsiella pneumoniae* among the clinical departments of a tertiary care hospital.

Methods: We performed a retrospective observational study to analyse the use of nine frequently prescribed antibiotics and the corresponding antimicrobial resistance rates in hospital acquired *E. coli* and *K. pneumoniae* isolates from 18 departments of our institution over 9 years (2008–2016). The main cross-sectional analysis assessed the hypothetical influence of antibiotic consumption on resistance by mixed logistic regression models.

Results: We found an association between antibiotic use and resistance rates in *E. coli* for amoxicillin-clavulanic acid (OR per each step of 5 defined daily dose/100 bed-days 1.07, 95% CI 1.02–1.12; $p = 0.004$), piperacillin-tazobactam (OR 2.11, 95% CI 1.45–3.07; $p < 0.001$), quinolones (OR 1.52, 95% CI 1.25–1.86; $p < 0.001$) and trimethoprim-sulfamethoxazole (OR 1.59, 95% CI 1.19–2.13; $p = 0.002$). Additionally, we found a significant association when all nine antibiotics were combined in one analysis. The association between consumption and resistance rates was stronger for nosocomial than for community strains. In *K. pneumoniae*, we found an association for amoxicillin-clavulanic acid (OR 1.07, 95% CI 1.01–1.14; $p = 0.025$) and for trimethoprim-sulfamethoxazole (OR 2.02, 95% CI 1.44–2.84; $p < 0.001$). The combined analysis did not show an association between consumption and resistance (OR 1.06, 95% CI 0.99–1.14; $p = 0.07$).

Conclusions: We documented an association between antibiotic use and resistance rate for amoxicillin-clavulanic acid, piperacillin-tazobactam, quinolones and trimethoprim-sulfamethoxazole in *E. coli* and for amoxicillin-clavulanic acid and trimethoprim-sulfamethoxazole in *K. pneumoniae* across different hospital departments. Our data will support stewardship interventions to optimize antibiotic prescribing at a department level.

Keywords: *E. coli*, *K. pneumoniae*, Antibiotic resistance, Antibiotic use, Correlation

* Correspondence: alexia.cusini@ksgr.ch
[†]Andreas Kronenberg and Jonas Marschall contributed equally to this work.
[1]Department of Infectious Diseases and Hospital Epidemiology, Bern University Hospital and University of Bern, Bern, Switzerland
[5]Infectious Diseases Unit, Cantonal Hospital, 7000 Chur, Switzerland
Full list of author information is available at the end of the article

Background

Antibiotic resistance in gram-negative bacteria has increased worldwide [1]. Infections with resistant gram-negative bacteria are a particularly serious threat to public health because they are difficult to treat and are associated with high morbidity and mortality, and great healthcare costs [2].

Escherichia coli (*E. coli*) and *Klebsiella pneumoniae* (*K. pneumoniae*) are among the most important gram-negative pathogens in the hospital setting, accounting for around one fifth of all pathogens causing healthcare-associated infections in the USA [3]. These two pathogens are frequent causes of catheter-associated urinary tract infections (CAUTI), surgical site infections (SSI) and ventilator-associated pneumonia (VAP) [3]. Risk factors for the emergence of infections with resistant gram-negative bacteria include existing comorbidities, presence of medical devices, previous invasive procedures and admission from a long-term care facility [4]. Despite the widespread belief that the most important driver in the selection of bacterial resistance is the use of antimicrobials, the relationship between antibiotic use and resistance rates across individual departments within a single hospital is not well studied. Willemsen et al. comprehensively investigated this relationship in a teaching hospital in the Netherlands and showed a correlation between ward-specific use and resistance rates for ciprofloxacin and amoxicillin-clavulanic acid in *E. coli* [5]. Compared to Willemsen et al. we have investigated resistance data for *K. pneumoniae* in addition to *E. coli*, included more antibiotics and used the annual antibiotic consumption per 100 bed-days per department over 9 years (2008–2016). Our objective was to identify antibiotics associated with a higher risk of resistance development in order to optimise the antibiotic prescribing practice particularly in those departments in our hospital with the highest antibiotic consumption.

Methods

Study aim

We aimed to determine the association between the use of frequently prescribed antibiotics and the corresponding resistance rates in *E. coli* and *K. pneumoniae* among the clinical departments of a tertiary care hospital.

Study design

We performed a retrospective observational study of antibiotic use and antibiotic resistance rates of *E. coli* and *K. pneumoniae* across 18 departments at the Bern University Hospital in Bern, Switzerland, between January 1st 2008 and December 31st 2016.

Hospital setting

Bern University Hospital is a 950-bed tertiary care teaching hospital that covers all medical specialties and includes a 30-bed mixed intensive care unit (ICU). There are around 40'000 admissions annually, resulting in 290'000 patient-days. The following 18 departments were included in the study: abdominal surgery and medicine, cardiology, cardiovascular surgery, critical care, dermatology, general internal medicine, gynecology and obstetrics, nephrology, neurology, neurosurgery, oncology and hematology, ophthalmology, orthopedics, otorhinolaryngology, plastic and hand surgery, rheumatology and clinical immunology, thoracic surgery and pulmonology, and urology.

Data collection

Data was extracted from Anresis [6], the national surveillance program that collects data on antibiotic resistance and antibiotic consumption in all Swiss hospitals, including Bern University Hospital.

Antimicrobial susceptibility testing (AST) for the following frequently prescribed antibiotics active against wild type *E. coli* and *K. pneumoniae* were included: amoxicillin (only active against *E. coli*), amoxicillin-clavulanic acid, ceftriaxone, cefepime, piperacillin-tazobactam, meropenem, ciprofloxacin, norfloxacin, trimethoprim-sulfamethoxazole and gentamicin. Antibiotics mainly prescribed for perioperative prophylaxis (e.g. cefuroxime) were not included. All *E. coli* and *K. pneumoniae* isolates originated from routine clinical diagnostics. AST for isolates from urine was routinely performed only for amoxicillin, amoxicillin-clavulanic acid, quinolones and trimethoprim-sulfamethoxazole; all other isolates were tested for all listed antibiotics. Therefore, the number of tested samples varies for each of the antibiotics. AST was performed at the Institute for Infectious Diseases of the University of Bern and was based on breakpoints for inhibitory zone diameters (disk diffusion method) according to the guidelines of the Clinical and Laboratory Standards Institute (CLSI). Over the study period the approved version of the 9th, 10th and 11th CLSI edition were adopted by the laboratory. Intermediate susceptibility was recorded as resistance. Quinolone resistance was defined as resistance to at least one of the substances in this group (e.g. norfloxacin and/or ciprofloxacin). We included only the last sample per patient per calendar year. In the main analysis, we included only hospital-acquired samples, i.e. samples that had been isolated more than 2 days after hospital admission. In subsequent sensitivity analyses for community-acquired samples, only samples isolated during the first two hospitalization days were analysed. In addition, we repeated the analysis using a stricter definition of hospital-acquired infection including only the bacterial isolates that had been detected more than 5 days after hospital admission.

The hospital pharmacy provided data on antibiotic consumption in numbers of packages delivered to each department from 2008 to 2016. We assumed that deliveries to the departments reflected consumption as all unused antibiotics were returned to the pharmacy and subtracted for our analyses. All departments used the same delivery system without significant storage and without shifting of antibiotics from one department to another. In the Anresis database the aggregated data were converted into defined daily doses (DDD) using the ATC/DDD system promoted by the World Health Organization [7]. The DDD is the assumed average maintenance dose per day for an antimicrobial used for its main indication in adults.

We obtained annual bed-days per department from the finance and controlling department of Bern University Hospital. In their calculation, the day of admission and the day of discharge were counted together as one bed-day. Annual Antibiotic use in DDD/100 bed-days was calculated for each of the 18 departments.

Statistical analyses

Antibiotic use across the departments was summarized by median, interquartile range (IQR, lower quartile-upper quartile) and total range (minimum-maximum) of the time-averaged data. The change in antibiotic use over time within each department was analysed with a linear regression model with year, department and the interaction of year and department as covariates. The marginal mean per department and the change per year and department are presented as DDD/100 bed-days with 95% confidence intervals (CI).

We used mixed logistic regression to model antibiotic resistance in dependence of consumption. The main analysis was cross-sectional (i.e. consumption and resistance were assessed at the same time) and was restricted to nosocomial strains. We fitted antibiotic-specific models that only considered resistance towards and use of a specific antibiotic and a combined model that considered data from all antibiotics and treated the antibiotic as random effect. The antibiotic-specific model included a fixed effect for antibiotic use and random intercepts for department and year (nested within department). The combined model included a fixed effect for antibiotic use and random intercepts for antibiotic, department (nested within antibiotic), and year (nested within antibiotic and department). Overall resistance proportions and corresponding 95% CI were obtained by marginal predictions. The association of consumption and resistance is expressed as an odds ratio (OR) per each step of 5 DDD/100 bed-days (i.e. referring to the incremental change in the odds for resistance for an increase in consumption by 5 DDD/100 bed-days) with corresponding 95% CI.

We performed four sensitivity analyses. First, resistance was regressed on the antibiotic use of the preceding year to investigate a potential temporal relation. Second, we repeated the analysis for community-acquired bacterial strains to check for a potential spillover of the (hospital) consumption effect. The strength of the association was compared with that found for nosocomial strains by fitting models using both nosocomial and community data with an additional random intercept for the mode of acquisition. We compared models with and without the interaction of antibiotic use and the site of acquisition using likelihood ratio tests; the p-value is reported as p-value for interaction. Third, we performed the analysis using a stricter definition of hospital-acquired infection including only the strains that were obtained more than 5 days after hospital admission in the analysis. Fourth, we performed separate analyses for isolates from urine, blood and other sites of origin. We calculated a p-value for interaction from likelihood ratio tests of models with and without an interaction for consumption and the origin of the sample. All analyses were done with Stata version 15 (StataCorp. 2017. Stata Statistical Software: Release 15. College Station, TX.)

Results

Antibiotic consumption in 18 individual hospital departments

The average use of the antibiotics selected for this study was 48.5 DDD/100 bed-days, corresponding to 62% of the total antibiotic use in the study departments between 2008 and 2016.

The annual use of these antibiotics varied widely between the 18 departments, from a mean of 19.4 (95% CI: 14.7–24.2) DDD/100 bed-days in neurology to a mean of 117 (95% CI: 112–122) DDD/100 bed-days in urology (Fig. 1 and Additional file 1: Table S1). Within the departments the antibiotic use changed unequally over the study period. It decreased significantly in critical care, gynecology and obstetrics, nephrology, thoracic surgery/pulmonology and urology departments, and increased significantly in the orthopedics, plastic and hand surgery departments. The trends in antibiotic use within each department are illustrated by fitted lines in Fig. 1 and summarised in Additional file 1: Table S1.

Overall, amoxicillin-clavulanic acid was by far the most frequently used antibiotic with a median use of 19.0 DDD/100 bed-days (IQR: 10.0–26.5), followed by cefepime with 3.9 DDD/100 bed-days (IQR 1.7–5.2) and ceftriaxone with 2.6 DDD/100 bed-days (IQR: 2.0–5.3) (Table 1).

Antibiotic resistances in *E. coli* isolates

The different origins (urine, blood, respiratory tract, wound swabs and other) of the *E. coli* isolates, the number of AST performed for each antibiotic and the time point of sampling during the hospital stay are shown in Table 2. Sixty-five percent of the isolates originated from urine and 11% from blood. For amoxicillin/ampicillin, amoxicillin-clavulanic acid, quinolones and

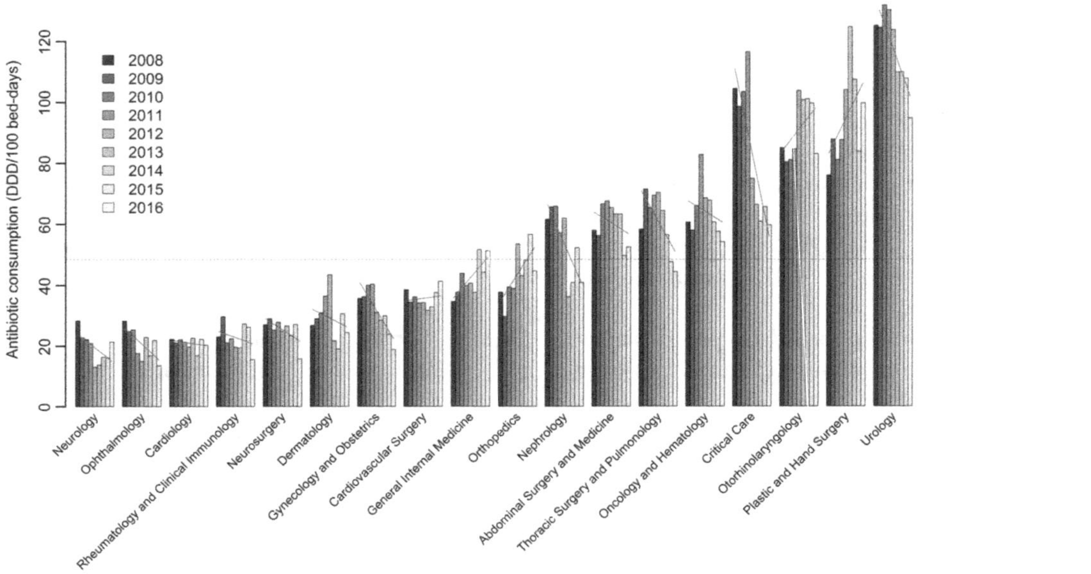

Fig. 1 Annual use of the study antibiotics in DDD/100 bed days in 18 departments for the period between 2008 and 2016. The red lines indicate fitted values from a linear regression model, the dashed line the overall average

trimethoprim-sulfamethoxazole, 139 department-years with 2329 (trimethoprim-sulfamethoxazole) and 2330 (other antibiotics) samples, were analysed. For ceftriaxone, cefepime, piperacillin-tazobactam and gentamicin we analyzed 119 department-years with 1083 (cefepime) and 1085 (other antibiotics) samples. The resistance rate was highest for amoxicillin/ampicillin at 62% (95% CI 55–69%), followed by amoxicillin-clavulanic acid at 39% (95% CI 35–44%), and trimethoprim-sulfamethoxazole at 32% (95% CI 27–37%) (Table 3). For all tested antibiotics the resistance rates for hospital-acquired samples was higher than for community-acquired samples (Additional file 1: Table S3).

Association of antibiotic consumption and resistance in *E. coli* isolates

We found a significant positive association between use and resistance rates in *E. coli* for amoxicillin-clavulanic acid (OR per each step of 5 DDD/100 bed-days 1.07, 95% CI 1.02–1.12; $p = 0.004$), piperacillin-tazobactam (OR 2.11, 95% CI 1.45–3.07; $p < 0.001$), quinolones (OR 1.52, 95% CI 1.25–1.86; $p < 0.001$) and trimethoprim-sulfamethoxazole (OR 1.59, 95% CI 1.19–2.13; $p = 0.002$). An association between antibiotic use and antimicrobial resistance was also found in the combined analysis (OR 1.09, 95% CI 1.04–1.14; $p < 0.001$). No significant association between use and resistance rates in *E. coli* were found for amoxicillin/ampicillin, ceftriaxone, cefepime or gentamicin. (Table 3, Fig. 2). Due to the absence of meropenem-resistant strains of *E. coli* the association between meropenem use and the resistance rate could not be studied.

The association between antimicrobial resistance and the preceding year's antibiotic consumption was similar to the analysis for all study antibiotics (Additional file 1: Table S2). The association of antibiotic use and

Table 1 Annual antibiotic consumption (DDD/100 bed-days) summarized across 18 departments in the years 2008–2016

	Median	Interquartile range	Total range
Amoxicillin/Ampicillin	2.7	1.2–5.2	0.3–8.4
Amoxicillin-clavulanic acid	19.0	10.0–26.5	6.4–85.3
Ceftriaxone	2.6	2.0–5.3	0.5–8.7
Cefepime	3.9	1.7–5.2	0.1–30.2
Piperacillin-tazobactam	0.9	0.4–1.8	0.0–11.1
Meropenem	1.2	0.3–2.7	0.1–9.8
Quinolones	2.4	1.8–3.5	0.8–15.4
Trimethoprim-sulfamethoxazole	1.7	1.0–3.2	0.2–13.3
Gentamicin	0.2	0.1–0.5	0.0–2.4

Table 2 Number of *E. coli* samples with antimicrobial susceptibility testing (AST) by origin across 18 departments in the years 2008–2016

Origin of the samples	Tested for	All nosocomial samples ($N = 2330$)	Samples obtained after 2 to 5 hospital days ($N = 525$)	Samples obtained after 5 hospital days ($N = 1805$)
Urine	AM-CL, Amox/AMP, Quinolones, TMP-SMX	1503 (65%)	377 (72%)	1126 (62%)
	CFP	256 (11%)	53 (10%)	203 (11%)
	CFT, Gent, MER[a], PIP-TZ,	258 (11%)	55 (10%)	203 (11%)
Blood	AM-CL, Amox/AMP, CFP, CFT, Gentamicin, MER[a], PIP-TZ, Quinolones, TMP-SMX	264 (11%)	32 (6%)	232 (13%)
Respiratory -tract	AM-CL, Amox/AMP, CFP, CFT, Gent, MER[a], PIP-TZ, Quinolones, TMP-SMX	86 (4%)	29 (6%)	57 (3%)
Wound swabs	AM-CL, Amox/AMP, CFP, CFT, Gent, MER[a], PIP-TZ, Quinolones	83 (4%)	12 (2%)	71 (4%)
	TMP-SMX	82 (4%)	12 (2%)	70 (4%)
Other	AM-CL, Amox/AMP, CFP, CFT, Gent, MER[a], PIP-TZ, Quinolones, TMP-SMX	394 (17%)	75 (14%)	319 (18%)

Abbreviations: *Amox* amoxicillin, *AMP* ampicillin, *AM-CL* amoxicillin-clavulanic acid, *CFP* cefepime, *CFT* ceftriaxone, *Gent* gentamicin, *MER* meropenem, *PIP-TZ* piperacillin-tazobactam, *TMP-SMX* trimethoprim-sulfamethoxazole
[a]Not included in the models for resistance because all samples were susceptible to Meropenem

resistance appeared to be stronger in hospital-acquired than in community-acquired strains for most antibiotics and a significant effect of resistance on consumption in community strains was only found for trimethoprim-sulfamethoxazole However, we could hardly prove systematic differences and a significant interaction was only found for piperacillin-tazobactam ($p = 0.034$) (Additional file 1: Table S3).

Using a stricter definition for hospital-acquired strains — by only considering samples obtained more than 5 days after hospital admission — did not have significant influence on the results and all main findings were identical (Additional file 1: Table S4). Analysis of subgroups according to sample origin confirmed an association of antibiotic use and resistance for amoxicillin/clavulanic acid, quinolones, trimethoprim-sulfamethoxazole and for the combined analysis in urine. An association for piperacillin-tazobactam was only found in the samples other than urine and blood (Additional file 1: Table S5). However, we did not find much evidence for systematic differences and a significant p-value for interaction was only observed for gentamicin.

Antibiotic resistance in *K. pneumoniae* isolates

For amoxicillin-clavulanic acid, quinolones and trimethoprim-sulfamethoxazole we included 115 department-years with 648 samples; for cefepime, ceftriaxone, gentamicin and piperacillin-tazobactam 92 department-years with 369 samples. Fifty one percent of the *K. pneumoniae* samples were isolated from urine, 14% from blood and 11% from the respiratory tract (Table 4). The resistance rate was highest for piperacillin-tazobactam at 21% (95% CI 17–25%), followed by amoxicillin-clavulanic acid at 17% (95% CI 14–21%)

Table 3 Antibiotic resistance and association with antibiotic use for *E. coli*

	Resistance		Association with antibiotic use	
	No. of tests/strata	Proportion resistant (95% CI)	Odds ratio (95% CI)	p-value
Amoxicillin/Ampicillin	2330 / 139	62 (55–69)	1.08 (0.84–1.40)	0.53
Amoxicillin-clavulanic acid	2330 / 139	39 (35–44)	1.07 (1.02–1.12)	0.004
Ceftriaxone	1085 / 119	18 (13–24)	1.10 (0.68–1.76)	0.71
Cefepime	1083 / 119	8 (6–12)	1.06 (0.90–1.25)	0.49
Piperacillin-tazobactam	1085 / 119	17 (13–21)	2.11 (1.45–3.07)	< 0.001
Quinolones	2330 / 139	20 (17–23)	1.52 (1.25–1.86)	< 0.001
Trimethoprim-sulfamethoxazole	2329 / 139	32 (27–37)	1.59 (1.19–2.13)	0.002
Gentamicin	1085 / 119	18 (14–22)	1.30 (0.45–3.71)	0.63
Combined	13,657 / 1032	24 (15–36)	1.09 (1.04–1.14)	< 0.001

Results from logistic mixed models for antibiotic resistance in relation to consumption. Odds ratios represent the change in the odds for resistance per increase in antibiotic use by 5 DDD/100 bed-days. Strata refer to year/department combinations
CI confidence interval

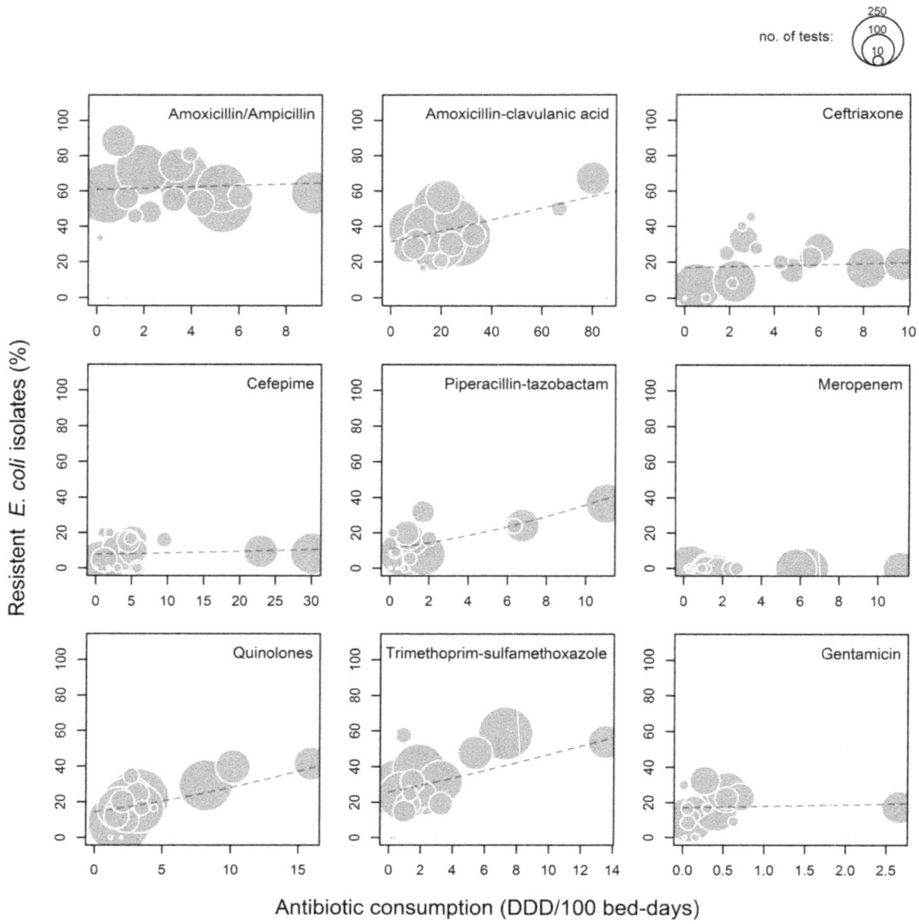

Fig. 2 Comparison of the proportions of resistant nosocomial *E. coli* and antibiotic use. Each point indicates the time-averaged values for an individual department for the period between 2008 and 2016. The size corresponds to the number of bacteria tested for resistance, i.e. reflects the precision of the resistance estimate. The dashed lines indicate the fitted value from the logistic mixed models

Table 4 Number of *K. pneumoniae* samples with antimicrobial susceptibility testing (AST) by origin across 18 departments in the years 2008–2016

Origin of the samples	Tested for	All nosocomial samples ($N = 648$)	Samples obtained after 2 to 5 hospital days ($N = 124$)	Samples obtained after 5 hospital days ($N = 524$)
Urine	AM-CL, Amox/AMP[b], Quinolones, TMP-SMX	329 (51%)	72 (58%)	257 (49%)
	CFP, CFT, Gent, MER[a], PIP-TZ	51 (8%)	12 (10%)	39 (7%)
Blood	AM-CL, Amox/AMP[b], CFP, CFT, Gent, MER[a], PIP-TZ, Quinolones, TMP-SMX	89 (14%)	9 (7%)	80 (15%)
Respiratory samples	AM-CL, Amox/AMP[b], CFP, CFT, Gent, MER[a], PIP-TZ, Quinolones, TMP-SMX	69 (11%)	16 (13%)	53 (10%)
Wound swabs	AM-CL, Amox/AMP[b], CFP, CFT, Gent, MER[a], PIP-TZ, Quinolones, TMP-SMX	22 (3%)	3 (2%)	19 (4%)
Other	AM-CL, Amox/AMP[b], CFP, CFT, Gent, MER[a], PIP-TZ, Quinolones, TMP-SMX	139 (21%)	24 (19%)	115 (22%)
	PIP-TZ	138 (21%)	24 (19%)	114 (22%)

Abbreviations: *Amox* amoxicillin, *AMP* ampicillin, *AM-CL* amoxicillin-clavulanic acid, *CFP* cefepime, *CFT* ceftriaxone, *Gent* gentamicin, *MER* meropenem, *PIP-TZ* piperacillin-tazobactam, *TMP-SMX* trimethoprim-sulfamethoxazole

[a]Not included in the models for resistance because only two samples were resistant to Meropenem

[b]Not included in the models for resistance because all samples were resistant to Amoxicillin/Ampicillin

and trimethoprim-sulfamethoxazole at 15% (95% CI 12–19%) (Table 5).

Association of antibiotic consumption and resistance in *K. pneumoniae* isolates

There was a significant association between use and resistance rates for amoxicillin-clavulanic acid (OR per 5 DDD/100 patient-days 1.07, 95% CI 1.01–1.14; $p = 0.025$) and trimethoprim-sulfamethoxazole (OR 2.02, 95% CI 1.44–2.84; $p < 0.001$) No association between use and resistance rates were found for ceftriaxone, cefepime, piperacillin-tazobactam, quinolones or gentamicin. The combined analysis did not show an overall association between consumption and resistance (Table 5, Fig. 3).

We did not analyse meropenem and amoxicillin/ampicillin because only two meropenem-resistant strains were observed and *K. pneumoniae* has an intrinsic resistance to amoxicillin/ampicillin.

Using last year's antibiotic use did not show any major differences to the main analysis (Additional file 1: Table S6). In community strains, we observed an association between antibiotic use and resistance for trimethoprim-sulfamethoxazole (OR 1.62, 95% CI 1.08–2.42; $p = 0.021$) and for quinolones (OR 1.42, 95% CI 1.04–1.96; $p = 0.029$). Evidence for an interaction was not found (Additional file 1: Table S7).

Using a stricter definition for hospital-acquired strains largely confirmed the main analysis but the ORs tended to be increased and the combined analysis was now significant (OR 1.09, 95% CI 1.02–1.18; $p = 0.012$) (Additional file 1: Table S8). In the sample origin subgroups, we only found significant associations for trimethoprim-sulfamethoxazole use and resistance in urine and blood samples. We did not observe much evidence for an influence of sample origin on the relationship of use and resistance (Additional file 1: Table S9).

Discussion

Our analysis showed an association between use and resistance for amoxicillin-clavulanic acid, piperacillin-tazobactam, quinolones and trimethoprim-sulfamethoxazole in *E. coli* and for amoxicillin-clavulanic acid and trimethoprim-sulfamethoxazole in *K. pneumoniae* across different hospital departments.

It is intuitive that antibiotic resistance emerges predominantly in environments with high antibiotic consumption. This has been shown for individual countries [8] and individual hospitals [9–11]. It is however conceivable that even antibiotic prescription within individual departments of the same hospital may affect bacterial resistance in the patients sharing the same environment, as bacteria can be transmitted from patient to patient and antibiotic resistance can spread between bacteria. In this regard, the results of our study confirmed the main findings reported by Willemsen et al. demonstrating that a higher use of amoxicillin-clavulanic acid and quinolones was associated with higher antimicrobial resistance in *E. coli*.

Interestingly, we only found associations between antibiotic use and resistance for some antibiotics and different associations between *E. coli* and *K. pneumoniae*.

A plausible explanation is the considerable difference in the quantitative use of the antibiotics studied across our hospital's departments. Considering the substantial use of amoxicillin-clavulanic acid at our institution, it is not surprising that its use was associated with resistance in both microorganisms analysed. A wide quantitative range of antibiotic use across different departments may also facilitate the detection of an association, as observed for piperacillin/tazobactam, where the median consumption was low, but the range was very wide.

However, the resistance barrier of the individual antibiotics may also be relevant for the emergence of resistance. For cefepime, which is recommended in our

Table 5 Antibiotic resistance and association with antibiotic use for *K. pneumoniae*

	Resistance		Association with antibiotic use	
	No. of tests/strata	Proportion resistant (95% CI)	Odds ratio (95% CI)	*p*-value
Amoxicillin-clavulanic acid	648 / 115	17 (14–21)	1.07 (1.01–1.14)	0.025
Ceftriaxone	369 / 92	10 (5–18)	1.12 (0.52–2.45)	0.77
Cefepime	369 / 92	3 (1–9)	0.86 (0.59–1.25)	0.43
Piperacillin-tazobactam	369 / 92	21 (17–25)	0.84 (0.61–1.18)	0.32
Quinolones	648 / 115	6 (3–9)	1.37 (0.94–2.01)	0.10
Trimethoprim-sulfamethoxazole	648 / 115	15 (12–19)	2.02 (1.44–2.84)	< 0.001
Gentamicin	369 / 92	8 (4–16)	1.82 (0.13–25.42)	0.66
Combined	3420 / 713	12 (8–16)	1.06 (0.99–1.14)	0.07

Results from logistic mixed effects models. The odds ratios represent the relative change in the odds for resistance for an increase in antibiotic use by 5 DDD/100 bed-days. Strata refers to year/department combinations
CI confidence interval

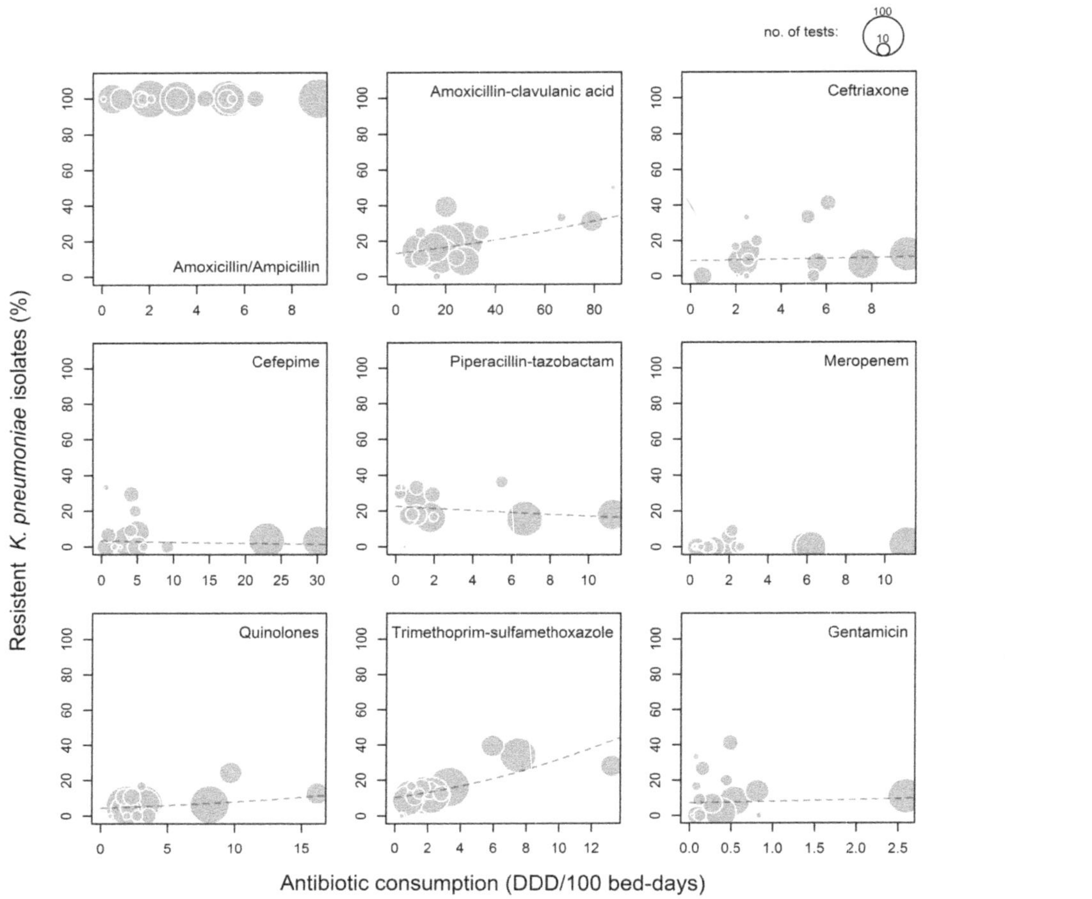

Fig. 3 Comparison of the proportions of resistant nosocomial K. pneumoniae and antibiotic use. Each point indicates the time-averaged values for an individual department for the period between 2008 and 2016. The size corresponds to the number of bacteria tested for resistance, i.e. reflects the precision of the resistance estimate. The dashed lines indicate the fitted value from the logistic mixed models

internal antibiotic guidelines [12] as first-line antibiotic for several nosocomial infections (e.g. pneumonia and fever in neutropenia), we did not find an association between use and resistance, even though it was the second most frequently used antibiotic overall. Cefepime is a robust fourth generation cephalosporin, which is relatively stable against β-lactamases and maintains activity even against difficult organisms. In contrast, *Enterobacteriaceae* may acquire resistance to quinolones and trimethoprim-sulfamethoxazole more readily and we indeed observed significant associations between their use and resistance in *E. coli.*

Results for *K. pneumoniae* were less clear than for *E. coli*, mainly because the sample size was much smaller. In particular, for ceftriaxone, cefepime, piperacillin-tazobactam and gentamicin the number of susceptibility tests performed for *K. pneumoniae* ($n = 369$) was substantially lower than for *E. coli* ($n = 1085$).

Our first sensitivity analysis examined the potential temporal relationship between the consumption of antibiotics and the development of resistance a year later. However, the last year's use did not have a stronger influence than the current use. Possible explanations are the relatively stable antibiotic use over time in our setting or a different timing of the emergence of resistance. Even a reverse causation is possible — the reduction in use due to the emergence of resistance.

The antibiotic use varied widely between the different departments and within the individual departments; there were significant variations in antibiotic use over time. Notably, the antibiotic use was high in predominantly surgical departments like urology, plastic and hand surgery, and otorhinolaryngology. Even though cefuroxime, which is recommended for perioperative prophylaxis, was not included in the analysis the high antibiotic use of these departments is probably due to the frequent use of amoxicillin-clavulanic acid and quinolones (urology) for perioperative prophylaxis that in some cases is given longer than suggested by international guidelines. During the study period, there were no specific antimicrobial stewardship interventions in any hospital department. Improving perioperative prophylaxis in the mentioned surgical departments will be a priority in the future.

To address the specificity of the association we compared nosocomial and community strains, given that the latter was not exposed to antibiotic use in the hospital. As expected, the association between antibiotic consumption and resistance tended to be systematically stronger for nosocomial strains than for community strains in *E. coli* even though we did not always find significant interactions. This result is consistent with another Swiss study showing that strains isolated ≥48 h after admission were less susceptible than those stemming from the community [13]. The same pattern was not found for *K. pneumoniae*, mainly because we did not observe many clear associations in the first place. Trimethoprim-sulfamethoxazole, for which the association persisted in community-acquired *K. pneumoniae* strains, is also frequently prescribed in the outpatient setting [14]. Furthermore, we could not distinguish patients with previous contacts with the healthcare system and some community-acquired infections could actually be healthcare-associated.

The accuracy of distinguishing community- from hospital-acquired pathogens plays an important role in our analyses. We chose a 2-day cut-off according to the Centers for Disease Control and Prevention (CDC) definition [15]. A stricter definition for hospital-acquired samples (i.e. a cut-off of five instead of 2 days after hospital admission) did not change any of the main findings, as the vast majority of samples (79% for *E. coli* and 81% for *K. pneumoniae*) was obtained after 5 days of hospital admission.

In recent years, several studies have analyzed the relationship between antibiotic use and development of resistance in *Enterobacteriaceae*. Consistent with our findings, several studies have described an association between in-hospital antibiotic use and resistance to quinolones in *E. coli* [16–18]. This association may be particularly relevant for Switzerland with its comparatively higher quinolone consumption than other European countries [19].

Two other studies have reported associations in *E. coli* between amoxicillin-clavulanic acid [5, 20] and piperacillin-tazobactam [21, 22]. The main discrepancy between our results and those of other studies is the absence of an association between the use of ceftriaxone and the emergence of third-generation cephalosporin resistance in our study [20, 23, 24]. This may be due to a relatively low median use of ceftriaxone of 2.6 DDD/100 patient days compared to other studies.

Our study has several limitations. First, the number of AST available differed considerably among the antibiotics and the sample size was low for some. The majority of samples (65% of *E. coli*, and 51% of *K. pneumoniae*) originated from urine and a complete AST of these samples is only performed if routine testing shows several resistances. Therefore, the resistance data for cefepime, ceftriaxone, piperacillin-tazobactam and gentamicin was only available in one sixth of the urine samples. The low sample size reduces the power of the analysis, which was particularly problematic for *K. pneumoniae* where it severely hampered the conclusions. Moreover testing some antibiotics only in higher resistant isolates may lead to an overestimation of resistance in urinary samples against these antibiotics, due to sampling bias. Second, this was a single-centre study, therefore our results may not be generalizable to other contexts with potential differences in case-mix and epidemiologic characteristics. Third, we could not take into account individual risk factors for infections with resistant microorganisms (such as underlying diseases or previous antimicrobial therapy), because of the anonymization of the samples. Fourth, we did not analyse the association between the use of one particular antibiotic and the resistance to a second antibiotic. Fifth, the antibiotic consumption expressed in DDD per 100 bed-days does not reflect the adequacy of treatment in terms of proper dosage and duration. Sixth, we calculated antibiotic use based on deliveries to the hospital departments rather than administration to the patients. The departments of our hospital are advised to order only those antibiotics that are needed for daily use. Antibiotics that are delivered to the departments but are for some reason not administrated to the patients must be returned to the hospital pharmacy. We subtracted the returned antibiotics from the deliveries and are confident that our data reflect the real antibiotic administration to the patients.

However, to the best of our knowledge, our study is the first comprehensive analysis of the use of the most important antibiotics for the treatment of gram-negative bacteria and corresponding antimicrobial resistance across multiple departments within one institution. We included all clinical *E. coli* and *K. pneumoniae* samples isolated across 18 departments at our institution over the study period of 9 years and used the well-established, standardized ATC/DDD system. The study therefore has important relevance for clinical practice.

Conclusions

We have demonstrated that antibiotic use in different hospital departments is associated with resistance rates in *E. coli* and in *K. pneumoniae* for some but not all antibiotics and antibiotics differ in the strength of the association. Despite a high consumption of cefepime we could not demonstrate an association between its use and resistance rates. We will therefore continue to promote the use of cefepime over piperacillin/tazobactam as an empiric broad-spectrum antibiotic in our guidelines.

Keeping resistance in *Enterobacteriaceae* in check requires a comprehensive approach including infection control strategies and an antibiotic stewardship program. Our data support targeted antibiotic stewardship interventions, such as department-specific or antimicrobial agent-specific interventions, to improve antimicrobial prescribing and reduce the development of antimicrobial resistance.

Additional file

Additional file 1: Table S1. Mean antibiotic use and change per year in 18 departments in years 2008-2016. **Table S2.** Antibiotic resistance and association with last year's antibiotic use for *E. coli*. **Table S3.** Antibiotic resistance and association with antibiotic use for nosocomial and community *E. coli*. **Table S4.** Antibiotic resistance and association with antibiotic use for *E. coli* with an alternative definition of nosocomial. **Table S5.** Antibiotic resistance in *E. coli* and association with antibiotic use according to the origin of the sample. **Table S6.** Antibiotic resistance and association with last year's antibiotic use for *K. pneumoniae*. **Table S7.** Antibiotic resistance and association with antibiotic use for nosocomial and community *K. pneumoniae*. **Table S8.** Antibiotic resistance and association with antibiotic use for *K. pneumoniae* with an alternative definition of nosocomial. **Table S9.** Antibiotic resistance in *K. pneumoniae* and association with antibiotic use according to the origin of the sample.

Abbreviations

AM-CL: Amoxicillin-clavulanic acid; Amox: Amoxicillin; AMP: Ampicillin; AST: Antimicrobial susceptibility testing; CAUTI: Catheter-associated urinary tract infections; CDC: Centers for Disease Control and Prevention; CFP: Cefepime; CFT: Ceftriaxone; CI: Confidence interval; CLSI: Clinical and Laboratory Standards Institute; DDD: Defined daily doses; *E. coli*: *Escherichia coli*; ESBL: Extended-spectrum beta lactamase; Gent: Gentamicin; ICU: Intensive care unit; IQR: Interquartile range; *K. pneumoniae*: *Klebsiella pneumoniae*; MER: Meropenem; OR: Odds ratio; PIP-TZ: Piperacillin-tazobactam; SSI: Surgical site infections; TMP-SMX: Trimethoprim-sulfamethoxazole; VAP: Ventilator-associated pneumonia; WHO: World Health Organisation

Acknowledgements

We would like to acknowledge Roswitha Halder Tobler of the Bern University Hospital pharmacy department for providing the antibiotic consumption data and Bettina Bächler from our hospital's medical controlling for providing the annual bed days data.

Funding

We did not receive any dedicated financial support for performing the study.

Authors' contributions

AC was involved in concept, design, data analysis and interpretation and writing of the article. DH contributed to data collection, data analysis and interpretation, and writing of the article. AK contributed to concept and design and data collection. LB performed data analysis and statistics. CPS contributed to data collection. JM contributed to data analysis and critical revision of the article. All authors read and approved the final manuscript.

Consent for publication

Not applicable

Competing interests

A.C. received travel grants and meeting expenses from Abbott, MSD, BMS, Gilead and Astellas. A. K. received travel grants and meeting expenses from Gilead, Viofor and the World Health Organisation (WHO). A.K. is advisor of the Swiss Federal Office of Public Health concerning antibiotic resistance epidemiology in Switzerland. He provides annual resistance data without commentary to pharmaceutical company LEO and the Swiss government. J.M. received travel grants from Gilead and served on an advisory board for Astellas Switzerland and is co-applicant for SNSF grant 153,377 (PI: Andrea Endimiani) on carriage of resistant Enterobacteriaceae. D.H., L.B. and C.P.S. have no competing interest.

Author details

[1]Department of Infectious Diseases and Hospital Epidemiology, Bern University Hospital and University of Bern, Bern, Switzerland. [2]Institute for Infectious Diseases, University of Bern, Bern, Switzerland. [3]CTU Bern, and Institute of Social and Preventive Medicine (ISPM), University of Bern, Bern, Switzerland. [4]Service of Hospital Preventive Medicine, Lausanne University Hospital, Lausanne, Switzerland. [5]Infectious Diseases Unit, Cantonal Hospital, 7000 Chur, Switzerland.

References

1. Vincent J-L, Rello J, Marshall J, et al. International study of the prevalence and outcomes of infection in intensive care units. JAMA. 2009;302:2323–9.
2. Evans HL, Lefrak SN, Lyman J, et al. Cost of gram-negative resistance. Crit Care Med. 2007;35:89–95.
3. Sievert DM, Ricks P, Edwards JR, et al. Antimicrobial-resistant pathogens associated with healthcare-associated infections: summary of data reported to the National Healthcare Safety Network at the Centers for Disease Control and Prevention, 2009-2010. Infect Control Hosp Epidemiol. 2013;34:1–14.
4. Kaye KS, Pogue JM. Infections caused by resistant gram-negative Bacteria: epidemiology and management. Pharmacotherapy. 2015;35:949–62.
5. Willemsen I, Bogaers-Hofman D, Winters M, Kluytmans J. Correlation between antibiotic use and resistance in a hospital: temporary and ward-specific observations. Infection. 2009;37:432–7.
6. Startseite - Main. Available at: http://www.anresis.ch/. Accessed 15 Apr 2017.
7. WHOCC - ATC/DDD Index. Available at: https://www.whocc.no/atc_ddd_index/. Accessed 15 Apr 2017.
8. Kahlmeter G, Menday P, Cars O. Non-hospital antimicrobial usage and resistance in community-acquired Escherichia coli urinary tract infection. J Antimicrob Chemother. 2003;52:1005–10.
9. Rogues AM, Dumartin C, Amadéo B, et al. Relationship between rates of antimicrobial consumption and the incidence of antimicrobial resistance in Staphylococcus aureus and Pseudomonas aeruginosa isolates from 47 French hospitals. Infect Control Hosp Epidemiol. 2007;28:1389–95.
10. Plüss-Suard C, Pannatier A, Kronenberg A, Mühlemann K, Zanetti G. Impact of antibiotic use on carbapenem resistance in Pseudomonas aeruginosa: is there a role for antibiotic diversity? Antimicrob Agents Chemother. 2013;57:1709–13.
11. Gbaguidi-Haore H, Dumartin C, L'Hériteau F, et al. Antibiotics involved in the occurrence of antibiotic-resistant bacteria: a nationwide multilevel study suggests differences within antibiotic classes. J Antimicrob Chemother. 2013;68:461–70.
12. Universitätsklinik für Infektiologie: Antibiotikarichtlinien. Available at: http://www.infektiologie.insel.ch/de/antibiotikarichtlinien/. Accessed 15 Apr 2017.
13. Lamoth F, Wenger A, Prod'hom G, et al. Comparison of hospital-wide and unit-specific cumulative antibiograms in hospital- and community-acquired infection. Infection. 2010;38:249–53.
14. Swiss Antibiotic Resistance Report 2016. Available at: https://www.bag.admin.ch/bag/de/home/service/publikationen/broschueren/publikationen-uebertragbare-krankheiten/publikation-swiss-antibiotic-resistance-report-2016.html. Accessed 15 Apr 2017.
15. Horan TC, Andrus M, Dudeck MA. CDC/NHSN surveillance definition of health care-associated infection and criteria for specific types of infections in the acute care setting. Am J Infect Control. 2008;36:309–32.
16. Jensen US, Skjøt-Rasmussen L, Olsen SS, Frimodt-Møller N, Hammerum AM, DANRES Study Group. Consequences of increased antibacterial consumption and change in pattern of antibacterial use in Danish hospitals. J Antimicrob Chemother. 2009;63:812–5.

17. Hsu L-Y, Tan T-Y, Tam VH, et al. Surveillance and correlation of antibiotic prescription and resistance of gram-negative bacteria in Singaporean hospitals. Antimicrob Agents Chemother. 2010;54:1173–8.
18. Tammer I, Geginat G, Lange S, et al. Antibiotic consumption and the development of antibiotic resistance in surgical units. Zentralbl Chir. 2016;141:53–61.
19. Plüss-Suard C, Pannatier A, Kronenberg A, Mühlemann K, Zanetti G. Hospital antibiotic consumption in Switzerland: comparison of a multicultural country with Europe. J Hosp Infect. 2011;79:166–71.
20. Wattal C, Joshi S, Sharma A, Oberoi JK, Prasad KJ. Prescription auditing and antimicrobial resistance at a tertiary care hospital in New Delhi, India. J Hosp Infect. 2005;59:156–8.
21. Sedláková MH, Urbánek K, Vojtová V, Suchánková H, Imwensi P, Kolář M. Antibiotic consumption and its influence on the resistance in Enterobacteriaceae. BMC Res Notes. 2014;7:454.
22. Lai C-C, Wang C-Y, Chu C-C, et al. Correlation between antibiotic consumption and resistance of gram-negative bacteria causing healthcare-associated infections at a university hospital in Taiwan from 2000 to 2009. J Antimicrob Chemother. 2011;66:1374–82.
23. Lee H-S, Loh Y-X, Lee J-J, Liu C-S, Chu C. Antimicrobial consumption and resistance in five gram-negative bacterial species in a hospital from 2003 to 2011. J Microbiol Immunol Infect Wei Mian Yu Gan Ran Za Zhi. 2015;48:647–54.
24. Meyer E, Gastmeier P, Deja M, Schwab F. Antibiotic consumption and resistance: data from Europe and Germany. Int J Med Microbiol. 2013;303:388–95.

21

The acceptability of screening for Carbapenemase Producing *Enterobacteriaceae* (CPE): cross-sectional survey of nursing staff and the general publics' perceptions

Kay Currie[1*], Caroline King[1], Kareena McAloney-Kocaman[1], Nicola J. Roberts[1], Jennifer MacDonald[1], Adele Dickson[1], Shona Cairns[2], Nitish Khanna[3], Paul Flowers[1], Jacqui Reilly[1,2] and Lesley Price[1]

Abstract

Background: Carbapenemase Producing *Enterobacteriaceae* (CPE) has spread rapidly and presents a growing challenge in antimicrobial resistance (AMR) management internationally. Screening for CPE may involve a rectal swab, there are limited treatment options for affected patients, and colonised patients are cared for in isolation to protect others. These measures are sound infection prevention precautions; however, the acceptability of CPE screening and its consequences are currently unknown.
The aim of this study was 'To determine factors influencing acceptability of CPE screening from the perspectives of nursing staff and the general public.'

Methods: National cross-sectional surveys of nursing staff ($n = 450$) and the general public ($n = 261$). The Theoretical Domains Framework (TDF) guided data collection and analysis. Regression modelling was used to identify factors that predicted acceptability of CPE screening.

Results: For nursing staff, the following predictor variables were significant: intention to conduct CPE screening (OR 14.19, CI 5.14–39.22); belief in the severity of the consequences of CPE (OR 7.13, CI 3.26–15.60); knowledge of hospital policy for screening (OR 3.04, CI 1.45–6.34); preference to ask patients to take their own rectal swab (OR 2.89, CI 1.39–6.0); awareness that CPE is an organism of growing concern (OR 2.44, CI 1.22–4.88). The following predictor variables were significant for the general public: lack of knowledge of AMR (β − .11, $p = .01$); social influences (β .14, $p = .032$); social norms (β .21$p = .00$); acceptability of being isolated if colonised (β .22, $p = .000$), beliefs about the acceptability of rectal swabbing (β .15, p = .00), beliefs about the impact of careful explanation about CPE screening from a health professional (β .32, p = .00).
Integrating results from staff and public perspectives points to the importance of knowledge of AMR, environmental resources, and social influences in shaping acceptability.

Conclusions: This is the first study to systematically examine the acceptability of CPE screening across nursing staff and the public. The use of TDF enabled identification of the mechanisms of action, or theoretical constructs, likely to be important in understanding and changing CPE related behaviour amongst professionals and public alike.

Keywords: CPE screening, Acceptability, Public perceptions, Staff perceptions, Theoretical domains framework

* Correspondence: k.currie@gcu.ac.uk
[1]School of Health & Life Sciences, Glasgow Caledonian University, Cowcaddens Road, Glasgow, Scotland G4 0BA, UK
Full list of author information is available at the end of the article

Background

The World Health Organisation [1, 2] has characterised antimicrobial resistance (AMR) as a global threat to public health, with Carbapenemase Producing *Enterobacteriaceae* (CPE) identified as a growing challenge. Increases in CPE have been reported internationally, with endemic situations in the USA, India, and Greece and predictions of forthcoming worldwide epidemics [3]. In the USA, some forms of CPE infections have increased from 2 to 10% in the last decade [4]. The EUScape survey [5] highlighted the significant spread of CPE across Europe, with an endemic situation now common in the southern Mediterranean region. Within the UK, there have been isolated outbreaks reported [6]; however, significant concern exists regarding spread across geographical boundaries into areas of currently low prevalence [5]. A report published by the Centre for Disease Control pooled the results of international studies to evaluate deaths attributable to carbapenem resistant *enterobacteriaceae* infections, as opposed to carbapenem susceptible infections; the authors concluded that the number of deaths was significantly higher in resistant infections [7]. Thus, CPE is a significant and growing problem. To reduce the risk of transmission of CPE, international guidelines recommend active surveillance by rectal screening of any patient deemed 'at risk' of CPE carriage [8–11].

Microbiological testing for CPE normally involves obtaining a rectal swab, which may be considered more invasive and more embarrassing than testing for other organisms associated with healthcare associated infection (HAI), for example, nasal swabs for Meticillin-resistant *Staphylococcus aureus* (MRSA). Anecdotal evidence suggested that nursing staff were uncomfortable asking patients for a rectal swab to screen for CPE. In addition, there are currently no decolonisation protocols for clearing CPE and relatively few treatment options for patients should they develop a CPE infection; once admitted to hospital, patients colonised with CPE are managed in isolation for the protection of other patients. All of these factors may affect the acceptability of CPE screening from the perspectives of patients and staff. It is a well-established public health principle that if we are to expect routine implementation of any screening intervention, then it should be acceptable to all stake-holders, in this case, clinical staff implementing the CPE screening programme as well as patients being screened [12, 13]. Whilst Dyakova et al [14] have recently highlighted factors associated with patients who refused to provide a rectal swab as part of a prevalence study of ESBLs, at the time our study commenced (2016), we were unable to locate any published evidence on behavioural or attitudinal factors which influenced the acceptability of routine CPE screening from the perspectives of either nursing staff or the general public.

This paper reports findings from two national cross-sectional surveys of the acceptability of CPE screening; one from the perspective of Scottish nursing staff and the other from the general public. The aim of the study was to determine those factors which may predict acceptability of CPE screening.

Methodology

As our interest was in exploring those factors which might influence staff and patient attitudes and behaviours related to the acceptability of CPE screening, we sought an appropriate theoretical framework from implementation science to guide study design, data collection, and analysis. The Theoretical Domains Framework enables exploration of psychosocial constructs across 14 distinct 'domains' and can explain an individual's decisions to act or behave in specific situations [15, 16]. In our case, constructs from the TDF were used to develop survey items which were analysed to predict individual psychosocial factors that would influence the acceptability of CPE screening, from both nursing staff and general public perspectives. By identifying the antecedents, or influencing factors, that are central to implementing screening, it is possible to direct future behaviour change intervention development.

The study was reviewed and approved by the School of Health and Life Sciences Ethics Committee at Glasgow Caledonian University (HLS/NCH/15/18). Access permission to NHS Nursing staff was granted by all 15 Scottish Regional Board Executive Leads for healthcare associated infection.

Data collection

Data was collected via two cross-sectional surveys (Additional file 1). Participants were asked to indicate their level of agreement with a series of statements on a Likert type scale from strongly disagree to strongly agree. The dependent variable for the clinical staff survey was "I believe that CPE screening is acceptable" and for the public survey, "If I were to be admitted to hospital I would find CPE screening acceptable". Independent variables were aligned with relevant TDF constructs to enable subsequent interpretation of results in light of this theoretical framework. Survey tools were piloted with a small group of members of the public and with nursing educators; minor changes were made to questions to enhance ease of understanding.

A paper questionnaire was distributed via hospital based link co-ordinators to 588 nursing staff working in different clinical areas in acute hospitals expected to screen for CPE, across all 15 Scottish health boards. Three paper-based questionnaires were distributed to selected areas in every acute hospital: one to be completed by the nurse in charge and two by other nurses. Completed questionnaires were sealed, then collected and returned to the research team via the link co-ordinator.

For the public component, a paper-based questionnaire was distributed to a random sample of 1000 names selected from the open electoral rolls of four diverse geographical regions of Scotland. Given the recognised limitations of postal survey recruitment [17], an electronic questionnaire was also made available via SurveyMonkey© and distributed via email link to local University students and promoted via social media networks.

Data analysis

Survey data was entered into SPSS (Version 23)© for analysis. For the clinical staff survey, each questionnaire item related to participants' responses was collapsed into dichotomous variables; agree versus all other responses (do not agree, don't know and neither). The general public questionnaire items collected responses using a 10 point scale, where scores of 1 indicated strongly disagreeing with a statement and a score of 10 indicated strong agreement. Any responses for questionnaire items using this scale were coding accordingly from 1 to 10. Additionally participants were asked to respond to a number of categorical response items about demographics, their awareness of antimicrobial resistance and CPE itself, and experiences of and preferences for screening. Descriptive analysis and univariate inferential testing (Chi-Square, Mann-Whitney, Kruskall-Wallis and correlation analyses) were undertaken for both nursing staff and general public samples, to explore relationships with the respective dependent variables ('I believe that CPE screening is acceptable' and 'If I were to be admitted to hospital I would find CPE screening acceptable'), and for the purpose of variable reduction in regression modelling. For the nursing staff survey a multiple logistic model was estimated, and for the general public survey a multiple linear regression model. In the multiple logistic regression model the Wald statistic provides an indication of whether the variables in the model contribute significantly to the dependent variable. Odds ratios and 95% confidence intervals of the odds ratios are provided as an indication of the effect size of the association between the dependent and independent variables. For the multiple linear regression model the t-statistic is reported as an indication of the reliability of the regression co-efficient, and the regression co-efficient is reported as standardised beta.

Finally, the resultant significant predictor variables in each model were then mapped against TDF [15] constructs to interpret findings in light of the mechanisms important in influencing behaviour related to the acceptability of screening for CPE.

Results

The survey response rate for nursing staff was 86% (505/588). A final sample of 450 viable responses were included in descriptive analysis. As there were 14 missing responses to the screening dependant variable questions, 436 participants were included in the inferential analysis and modelling; sample sizes met power calculation requirements (minimum sample size of 350 respondents) specifically for a logistic regression [18].

It was not possible to calculate a response rate for the general public survey as the number of recipients of the online questionnaire distributed via social media is unknown. Therefore emphasis was placed on achieving a sample size that met the power calculation requirements for the multiple linear regression. Ninety-two out of 1000 (9.2%) responses from the paper based general public survey were combined with 216 responses from the online survey, giving a total of 308 public survey responses; 47 were excluded due to incomplete data, which left a sample of 261 viable responses. This exceeded the power calculation requirements of 220 participants for the range of planned analyses [19].

Sample characteristics

Among the nursing staff 30.7% were senior nurses, 60% were staff nurses and 9.3% health cares assistants. Clinical areas represented by the nursing staff were renal (8.7%), care of the elderly (9.3%), pre-admission (9.6%), orthopaedics (17.8%), general surgery (11.3%), general medical (17.1%), vascular (3.8%), and receiving (3.8%) the remaining 2.8% reported either another clinical areas or no clinical area was reported.

Acceptability of CPE screening

Whilst the majority ($n = 303$, 67.3%) of nursing staff agreed 'I believe that CPE screening is acceptable', perhaps more notably, 1/3 nursing staff did not agree that CPE screening is acceptable. Table 1 reports the frequencies of agreement with the CPE items for nursing staff.

Among the general public, while there was a high prevalence of awareness of antibiotic resistance, there was low reported knowledge of CPE specifically. Table 2 reports descriptive statistics of the general publics' understanding and awareness of CPE.

Median scores for the general public for the dependent variable 'If I were to be admitted to hospital I would find CPE screening acceptable' indicated high levels of agreement (Median = 9, IQR = 3). Similarly, high levels of general public agreement were demonstrated in relation to the acceptability of having a rectal swab taken (Median = 9, IQR = 3) or being cared for in isolation as a consequence of a positive screen (Median = 8, IQR = 4). For the general public, there were no significant differences

Table 1 Frequency of agreement to survey items among nursing staff

Survey Questions	Agree N (%)
I am aware that CPE is an emerging multi-drug resistant bacteria of growing concern. (CPE1)	68.4
I have been informed about my hospital's policy and processes for screening patients for CPE. (CPE2)	55.1
Screening for CPE is undertaken in the clinical area I work in (CPE3)	76.2
The consequences of CPE infection for the patients I care for is/will be so severe that screening will always be a priority. (CPE5)	46.9
Screening patient for CPE would be/is embarrassing for them if a rectal swab is/was required. (CPE6)	66.9
If a rectal swab is/was required as part of CPE screening for the patient I care for they should be asked to do this themselves, if they are able.(CPE7)	74.0
Screening patient for CPE is/would be embarrassing for me as I may need to ask to take a rectal swab (CPE8)	20.0
I intend to conduct CPE screening, on patients on admission, according to my hospital policy. (CPE9)	79.0
I believe that CPE screening is acceptable. (CPE10)	67.3

between acceptability according to age or gender (see Table 3).

Univariate analysis

Univariate analysis indicated that there was significant variation in the acceptability of CPE screening among nursing staff across independent variables reflecting TDF domains of 'intentions to screen'; 'environmental context and resources'; 'knowledge'; 'social influences'; 'beliefs about the severity of consequences of CPE'; and, 'emotion' (embarrassment for patients in being asked for rectal swab). For the pubic data, univariate analysis revealed significant variations in acceptability of CPE screening across experience of health care employment, the acceptability of being cared for in isolation and the TDF domains of 'knowledge'; 'social influences'; and 'beliefs about the severity of consequences of CPE'. All significant predictors were subsequently entered into regression models. (univariate results available in Additional file 2).

Results of regression modelling

The following section presents the results of the modelling for the nursing staff (Table 4) and general public (Table 5), aligned with the respective theoretical domain.

For nursing staff, logistic regression analysis resulted in a well-fitting model (H-L $\chi^2 = 9.96$, df = 8, $p = 0.27$) accounting for 57% of the variance in the outcome (Nagelkereke R^2). Five predictors emerged as significantly associated with acceptability in the model, in the theoretical domains: 'intentions to screen'; 'beliefs about the severity of consequences of CPE'; 'environmental

Table 2 Descriptive statistics of the general publics' understanding and awareness of CPE

Question	N (%)
Have you heard about the problem of some bacteria becoming resistant to antibiotics	
Yes	214 (83.9)
No	41 (16.1)
Have you heard of CPE ($n = 256$)	
Yes	59 (23.0)
No	197 (77.0)
Have you been screened for CPE (n = 256)	
Yes	2 (0.8)
No	191 (74.6)
Don't know	63 (24.6)
Have you ever had a rectal swab or rectal examination by a Doctor or Nurse? ($n = 254$)	
Yes	61 (24.0)
No	193 (76.0)
Have you ever provided a stool sample ($n = 253$)	
Yes	124 (49.0)
No	129 (51.0)
If I needed to be tested for CPE, I would prefer to provide? ($n = 254$)	
Rectal swab	34 (13.4)
Stool specimen	107 (42.1)
I have no preference	113 (44.5)
If a rectal swab was required to test you for CPE, would you prefer ($n = 250$)	
A nurse took the swab	47 (18.8)
You did this yourself	111 (44.4)
I have no preference	92 (36.8)

Table 3 Associations between age and gender and acceptability

Variable	Median (IQR)	Test Statistic	P
Gender			
Male	8.00 (3.00)	5388[a]	0.12
Female	9.00 (3.00)		
Age			
16–24	9.00 (3.00)	7.21[b]	0.07
25–40	8.00 (3.25)		
41–64	9.00 (2.00)		
65 and over	9.00 (2.00)		

[a]Mann-Whitney U test
[b]Kruskall Wallis test

Table 4 Nursing staff results for logistic regression model

TDF Domain	Significant predictors			
	Questionnaire Item[a]	Wald	OR	95% CI
1. Intentions	I intend/ would intend to conduct CPE screening, on patients on admission, according to my hospital policy. (79% nursing staff agree)	26.17***	14.2	5.1–39.2
2. Beliefs about the severity of consequences	The consequences of CPE infection for the patients I care for is/will be so severe that screening will always be a priority. (47% nursing staff agree)	24.15***	7.1	3.26–15.6
3. Knowledge, and Environmental context and resources	I have been informed about my hospital's policy and processes for screening patients for CPE. (55% nursing staff agree)	8.70**	3.04	1.45–6.3
4. Social influences	If a rectal swab is/was required as part of CPE screening for the patient I care for they should be asked to do this themselves, if they are able. (74% nursing staff agree)	8.12**	2.89	1.39–6.0
5. Knowledge	I am aware that CPE is an emerging multi-drug resistant bacterium of growing concern. (68% nursing staff agree)	6.36*	2.44	1.22–4.9

Adjusted odds ratios, controlling for Health Board and reported CPE screening undertaken in the clinical area
* = $p < 0.05$, ** = $p < 0.01$; *** = $p < 0.001$; Wald reported to 2 significant places [27]; OR and 95% CI reported in line with rule of four [28]
[a]In all cases 'Not agreeing' with the statement is the reference category

context and resources'; 'social influences'; and 'knowledge' (Table 4).

For the general public, a multiple linear regression model explained over 68% of the variance in acceptability of CPE screening ($R^2 = 0.68$), and was significant ($F = 26.9$, $p < 0.001$). Acceptability of CPE screening was significantly associated with six key predictors related to the theoretical domains of 'knowledge' and 'social influences' (Table 5). Not having heard of the problem of bacteria becoming resistant to antibiotics was associated with lower ratings of CPE screening acceptability. Higher scores on the social influence scale, as well as explanations from health care professionals, were associated with higher ratings of acceptability (scale items related to concern about transmission to others; beliefs about family norms; sense of responsibility to be screened). Higher acceptability ratings of items related to components of CPE management (rectal screening, isolation in single room) were also associated with higher ratings of acceptability of CPE.

Discussion

To the authors' knowledge, this is the first study to have investigated factors which influence the acceptability of CPE screening and management from the perspectives of both nursing staff and the general public, using the TDF. Given the global threat of CPE, and the continued emergence of new multi-drug resistant organisms, understanding those barriers and enablers which may influence the acceptability of screening is fundamental to improving screening uptake and thereby reducing the risk of CPE transmission in hospitals. Using TDF to guide the research means that influencing factors can be mapped to specific behaviour change interventions to guide future recommendations.

Whilst regression modelling identifies specific variables found to predict the acceptability of CPE screening, of particular interest to this discussion is the influence of the theoretical domains of 'knowledge', 'environmental resources', and 'social influences', which were

Table 5 General public results for linear regression model

TDF Domain	Significant predictors	Beta	t
	Questionnaire Item[a]		
1. Knowledge:	Are you aware of the problem of some bacteria becoming resistant to antibiotics	−.11*	−2.54
2. Social influences	Composite item of transmission and screening responsibility	.14*	2.16
3. Social influences	I would find rectal swabbing for CPE acceptable	.15**	2.99
4. Social influences	I believe that CPE screening would be acceptable to most people being admitted to hospital	.21***	4.03
5. Social influences	I would find being place in a single room acceptable	.22***	4.36
6. Knowledge: Social influences	Careful explanation about CPE screening from a health professional would make screening more acceptable to me	.32***	5.85

[a]Note: All predictors except the first (Knowledge) entered as scale variables; model includes controls for health care profession experience, screening experience, and TDF items identified as significant at univariate analysis but not significant in the model (full table available on request)
* = $p < 0.05$, ** = $p < 0.01$; *** = $p < 0.001$; standardised beta reported to 2 significant places [27]

common to both nursing staff and general public groups.

For both nursing staff and the general public, knowledge and awareness of AMR in general and CPE in particular were associated with greater acceptability of CPE screening. For nursing staff, knowledge may lead to greater appreciation of the potential severity of consequences of CPE infection and possibly shape attitudes towards the acceptability of screening procedures. However, fewer than half of the nursing staff respondents agreed that the consequences of CPE would be severe. If, as we found, greater acceptability is influenced by belief in the severity of consequences, then nursing staff must be supported to develop greater understanding of the potential severity of CPE. However, providing opportunities to develop staff knowledge and awareness can be challenging. Similarly, whilst the 'intention to conduct screening in line with hospital policy and procedure' was an important predictor in explaining staff perceptions of CPE screening acceptability, just over half of respondents agreed they had been made aware of hospital policy. This emphasises the pivotal link between 'environmental resources', as an enabler, and nursing staff 'knowledge'; resources are required to facilitate staff training about CPE policies and thus influence staff attitudes towards the acceptability of screening. This finding echoes the work of Parker et al. [20], who also report the challenges in addressing low staff awareness of CPE and providing educational opportunities across intensive care units in three New York hospitals.

Knowledge about AMR was also one of the most important factors in understanding the public's acceptability of CPE screening. The O'Neill Report [21] highlights the 'urgent priority' of a global public awareness campaign as a means of tackling AMR. A recent systematic review [22] considered 54 studies and concluded that the public have an incomplete understanding of antibiotic resistance, misconceptions about its causes, and do not believe they contribute to its development. However, there is some evidence from systematic reviews that by increasing awareness and knowledge of AMR, demand for and prescription of unnecessary antibiotics shows decline [23, 24]. In the context of the acceptability of CPE screening, our results indicate that knowledge of AMR enables a broader understanding of why CPE screening, and rectal swabbing in particular, is important. Therefore, increasing public knowledge about AMR more broadly is likely to increase personal acceptability of CPE screening, and associated consequences of being cared for in isolation, for patients. Thus, the issue of public awareness of AMR, in general, requires to be addressed.

The fact that 'careful explanation of CPE screening from a healthcare professional' also predicts personal acceptability indicates the 'social influence' that nurses may have on patients' attitudes. This finding has parallels with the recent work of Dyakova et al [14], who reported a reduction in the number of research study participants who refused to consent to a rectal swab after the explanation of the procedure had been simplified to focus on providing a consistent message around potential benefits to patients and their peers. The influence of the nurse in this situation also underlines the importance of nurses having adequate knowledge themselves, in order to explain the reasons for screening to patients. This point reiterates the link between nursing 'knowledge' and their capability to exert 'social influence' in this situation.

Other social influences are at play from both staff and patient perspectives. Beliefs regarding asking patients to self-swab also made a notable contribution to explaining the variance in CPE screening acceptability for nursing staff. Staff appear to believe that the procedure is embarrassing for patients and consequently think it would be more acceptable if those patients that were able to, self-swabbed. This is a concern, as the effectiveness of rectal self-swabbing has not yet been shown to be reliable in the context of CPE screening. A study of the sensitivity of rectal versus perineal swabs for detecting ESBL *Enterobacteriaceae* [14] showed that rectal swabs were around two times more sensitive than perineal swabs for detecting the organism and that staff-collected swabs resulted in higher detection rates than patient-collected swabs. Unfortunately that study gave patients the option for staff or self-swab, but did not compare staff and self-swabbing in the same patient. Further research to assess the reliability of self-swabbing in this context is required. Conversely, despite the concerns expressed by nursing staff, the general public survey demonstrated high levels of 'strong agreement' that rectal swabbing was acceptable.

Wider 'social influences' also predicted the personal acceptability of CPE screening for the public. This variable captured people's perceptions of social responsibility regarding screening (they felt it was their and other people's social duty to be screened). The role of such social norms in determining behaviour is debated in the literature; for example, a meta-analysis of 196 studies undertaken by Manning [25] suggests that whilst there is a relationship between injunctive norms (a behaviour perceived to be approved of by others in a social group) and actual behaviour, this is not always strong. However, our findings suggest that providing the public with information about social norms, noting that most people find screening acceptable, as well as focusing attention on ideas of collective action or the public good, may well increase the personal acceptability of CPE screening; further research is required in this area.

Whilst views from across a range of ages and geographical distribution of the public were obtained we make no claims on the representativeness of the general public sample. However, the sample sizes did meet power calculation requirements for both nursing staff and the general public. A key strength of the study is the integration of psychological theory, in the form of TDF [15], which enables the development of targeted, psychologically based interventions. Work by Mitchie et al. [26], based on the TDF, has identified a wide range of potential interventions, or taxonomy of Behaviour Change Techniques (BCTs), which can be proposed in response to identified barriers or enablers within specific theoretical domains. This means that future interventions to address the barriers and enablers to the acceptability of CPE screening (knowledge, environmental resources, social influences) can be determined on the basis of well-established behaviour change principles.

Conclusions

This report provides original evidence of barriers and enablers to the acceptability of CPE screening from the perspectives of nursing staff from 15 Scottish regional Health Boards and the Scottish general public. Developing knowledge and understanding of AMR, providing adequate environmental resources and capitalising on social norms to influence behaviour are all enablers which may enhance the acceptability of CPE screening.

Understanding the nature of AMR in general and CPE in particular creates the foundation for acceptability of CPE screening for both nursing staff and the public. With knowledge and appreciation of the consequences of CPE, at both local and global health levels, staff are better equipped to provide appropriate information to patients. Staff could then also appreciate the importance of reliable swabbing for microbiological testing and overcome potential socially based barriers regarding patient embarrassment. However, staff require the environmental context to deliver resources, in terms of time and training opportunities, to enable the development and sharing of this knowledge. For the public, greater knowledge regarding the importance of reducing the transmission of infection and recognition of the social influences of responsibility for self and others, would enable the acceptability of CPE screening and its consequences.

In considering both staff and general public perspectives, the concern expressed by nursing staff that patients would find being asked for a rectal swab embarrassing appears to be unfounded. This is an important message to share with nursing staff, as careful explanation about CPE screening from a healthcare professional makes CPE screening more acceptable to the public.

This study has identified the range of factors which present as barriers and enablers to the acceptability of CPE screening. Interventions based on psychological theory, such as the behaviour change wheel [26], should be adopted to systematically identify key intervention components based on the specific barriers and enablers within the domains of knowledge, social influence, and environmental resources.

Acknowledgements

We would like to acknowledge the contribution of the Project Advisory Group in supporting the conduct of this study.

Funding

This study was funded by NHS Health Protection Scotland and the Scottish Infection Research Network. Additional support was provided by the Scottish HAI Prevention Institute (SHAIPI).

Authors' contributions

The conception and design of the study (KC, LP, PF, SC, JR). acquisition of data, or analysis and interpretation of data (KC, CK, KMcA-K, NJR, JMcD, AD, PF, LP). drafting the article or revising it critically for important intellectual content (KC, CK, KMcA-K, NJR, JMcD, AD, SC, NK, PF, LP). All authors read & approved the final manuscript (KC, CK, KMcA-K, NJR, JMcD, AD, SC, NK, PF, JR, LP).

Consent for publication

Not applicable.

Competing interests

The authors declare that they have no competing interests.

Author details

[1]School of Health & Life Sciences, Glasgow Caledonian University, Cowcaddens Road, Glasgow, Scotland G4 0BA, UK. [2]NHS Health Protection Scotland, Glasgow, UK. [3]NHS Greater Glasgow & Clyde, Glasgow, UK.

References

1. World Health Organisation. Antimicrobial resistance. http://www.who.int/antimicrobial-resistance/publications/global-action-plan/en/. Accessed 28 Aug 2018.
2. World Health Organisation. (2012). Action Plan for implementation of the European Strategy for the Prevention and Control of Noncommunicable Diseases 2012–2016 Retrieved from Copenhagen: http://www.euro.who.int/__data/assets/pdf_file/0019/170155/e96638.pdf?ua=1 Accessed 28 Aug 2018.
3. Nordmann P, Naas T, Poirel L. Global spread of Carbapenemase-producing Enterobacteriaceae. Emerg Infect Dis. 2011;17:1791–8.
4. National Center for Emerging and Zoonotic Infectious Diseases. Making Health Care Safer. https://www.cdc.gov/vitalsigns/hai/cre/index.html Accessed 28 Aug 2018.
5. Albiger B, Glasner C, Struelens MJ, Grundmann H, Monnet DL. Group. TESoC-PEW Carbapenemase-producing Enterobacteriaceae in Europe: assessment by national experts from 38 countries, May 2015. Eurosurveillance. 2015;20:30062.
6. Poole K, George R, Decraene V, et al. Active case finding for carbapenemase-producing Enterobacteriaceae in a teaching hospital: prevalence and risk factors for colonization. J Hosp Infect. 2016;94:125–9.
7. Falagas ME, Tansarli GS, Karageorgopoulos DE, Vardakas KZ. Deaths attributable to Carbapenem-resistant Enterobacteriaceae infections. Emerg Infect Dis. 2014;20:1170–5.
8. European Centre for Disease Prevention & Control. (2011). Risk assessment on the spread of carbapenemase-producing Enterobacteriaceae (CPE) through patient transfer between healthcare facilities, with special emphasis

on cross-border transfer. Retrieved from Stockholm: https://ecdc.europa.eu/sites/portal/files/media/en/publications/Publications/110913_Risk_assessment_resistant_CPE.pdf Accessed 28 Aug 2018.
9. Public Health England. (2014). Carbapenemase-producing Enterobacteriaceae: early detection, management and control toolkit for acute trusts. Retrieved from https://www.gov.uk/government/uploads/system/uploads/attachment_data/file/329227/Acute_trust_toolkit_for_the_early_detection.pdf Accessed 28 Aug 2018.
10. Center for Disease Control. (2015). Facility Guidance for Control of Carbapenem-resistant Enterobacteriaceae (CRE) (update). Retrieved from https://www.cdc.gov/hai/pdfs/cre/CRE-guidance-508.pdf Accessed 28 Aug 2018.
11. Health Protection Scotland. (2016). Toolkit for the early detection, management and control of carbapenemase-producing Enterobacteriaceae in Scottish acute settings. Retrieved from https://www.hps.scot.nhs.uk/resourcedocument.aspx?id=6633 Accessed 28 Aug 2018.
12. Wilson JMG, Jungner G. (1968). Principles and practice of screening for disease. Retrieved from Geneva: http://apps.who.int/iris/bitstream/10665/37650/17/WHO_PHP_34.pdf. Accessed 28 Aug 2018.
13. Proctor EK, Powell BJ, McMillen JC. Implementation strategies: recommendations for specifying and reporting. Implement Sci. 2013;8:139.
14. Dyakova E, Bisnauthsing KN, Querol-Rubiera A, et al. Efficacy and acceptability of rectal and perineal sampling for identifying gastrointestinal colonization with extended spectrum beta-lactamase Enterobacteriaceae. Clin Microbiol Infect. 2017;23:577.e1–3.
15. Francis JJ, O'Connor D, Curran J. Theories of behaviour change synthesised into a set of theoretical groupings: introducing a thematic series on the theoretical domains framework. Implement Sci. 2012;7:35.
16. Cane J, O'Connor D, Michie S. Validation of the theoretical domains framework for use in behaviour change and implementation research. Implement Sci. 2012;7:37.
17. Sinclair M, O'Toole J, Malawaraarachchi M, Leder K. Comparison of response rates and cost-effectiveness for a community-based survey: postal, internet and telephone modes with generic or personalised recruitment approaches. BMC Med Res Methodol. 2012;12:132.
18. Peduzzi P, Concato J, Kemper E, Holford TR, Feinstein AR. A simulation study of the number of events per variable in logistic regression analysis. J Clin Epidemiol. 1996;49:1373–9.
19. Faul F, Erdfelder E, Lang A-G, Buchner A. G*power 3: a flexible statistical power analysis program for the social, behavioral, and biomedical sciences. Behav Res Methods. 2007;39:175–91.
20. Parker V, Logan C, Currie B. (2014). Assessing ICU Staff-Perceived Barriers to Implementation of an Enhanced Carbapenem-Resistant Enterbacteriaceae Control Intervention. Retrieved from http://www.ahrq.gov/professionals/quality-patient-safety/patient-safety-resources/resources/advances-in-hai/hai-article4.html. Accessed 28 Aug 2018.
21. O'Neill J. (2016). Tackling drug-resistant infections globally: final report and recommendations. https://amrrevieworg/sites/default/files/160525_Final%20paper_with%20coverpdf. Accessed 28 Aug 2018.
22. McCullough AR, Parekh S, Rathbone J, Del Mar CB, Hoffmann TC. A systematic review of the public's knowledge and beliefs about antibiotic resistance–authors' response. J Antimicrob Chemother. 2016;71:2366.
23. Price L, Gozdzielewska L, Young M, et al. Effectiveness of interventions to improve the public's antimicrobial resistance awareness and behaviours associated with prudent use of antimicrobials: a systematic review. J Antimicrob Chemother. 2018. https://doi.org/10.1093/jac/dky076.
24. Lee C-R, Lee JH, Kang L-W, Jeong BC, Lee SH. Educational effectiveness, target, and content for prudent antibiotic use. Biomed Res Int. 2015;2015:13.
25. Manning M. The effects of subjective norms on behaviour in the theory of planned behaviour: a meta-analysis. Br J Soc Psychol. 2009;48:649–705.
26. Michie S, Richardson M, Johnston M, et al. The behavior change technique taxonomy (v1) of 93 hierarchically clustered techniques: building an international consensus for the reporting of behavior change interventions. Ann Behav Med. 2013;46:81–95.
27. Cole TJ. Setting number of decimal places for reporting risk ratios: rule of four. BMJ : British Medical Journal. 2015;350:h1845.
28. Cole TJ. Too many digits: the presentation of numerical data. Arch Dis Child. 2015;100:608–9.

Collateral damage of using colistin in hospitalized patients on emergence of colistin-resistant *Escherichia coli* and *Klebsiella pneumoniae* colonization and infection

W. Wangchinda[1], N. Pati[1], N. Maknakhon[1], C. Seenama[1], S. Tiengrim[2] and V. Thamlikitkul[1*]

Abstract

Background: Colistin has been used for therapy of carbapenem-resistant Gram-negative infections in Thailand, especially carbapenem-resistant *A. baumannii* and *P. aeruginosa*, for more than 10 years. However, the prevalence of colistin-resistant *A. baumannii* or *P. aeruginosa* is still less than 5%. Colistin-resistant Enterobacteriaceae has been increasingly reported globally over the past few years and the use of colistin in food animals might be associated with an emergence of colistin resistance in Enterobacteriaceae. This study aimed to determine the effect of colistin exposure in hospitalized patients who received colistin on development of colistin-resistant (CoR) *Escherichia coli* (EC) or *Klebsiella pneumoniae* (KP) colonization and infection.

Methods: A prospective observational study was performed in adult hospitalized patients at Siriraj Hospital who received colistin for treatment of infections during December 2016 and November 2017. The surveillance culture samples were collected from the stool and the site of infection of each patient who received colistin at the study enrollment, days 3 and 7 after the study enrollment, and once a week thereafter for determination of CoR EC and CoR KP. CoR EC and CoR KP were also tested for a presence of mcr-1 gene.

Results: One hundred thirty-nine patients were included. Overall prevalence of CoR EC or CoR KP colonization was 47.5% among 139 subjects. Prevalence of CoR EC or CoR KP colonization was 17.3% of subjects at study enrollment, and 30.2% after study enrollment. Use of fluoroquinolones, aminoglycosides, and colistin was found to be significantly associated with CoR EC or CoR KP colonization. The mcr-1 gene was detected in 13.0% of CoR EC or CoR KP isolates, and in 27.3% of subjects with CoR EC or CoR KP colonization. CoR EC or CoR KP colonization persisted in 65.2% of the subjects at the end of the study. Five patients with CoR KP infections received combination antibiotics and they were alive at hospital discharge.

Conclusions: Prevalence of CoR EC or CoR KP colonization in hospitalized patients receiving colistin was high and it was associated with the use of colistin. Therefore, patients who receive colistin are at risk of developing CoR EC or CoR KP colonization and infection.

Keywords: Thailand, Prevalence, Colonization, Colistin-resistant *Escherichia coli*, Colistin-resistant *Klebsiella pneumoniae*, Colistin, Hospitalization

* Correspondence: visanu.tha@mahidol.ac.th
[1]Division of Infectious Diseases and Tropical Medicine, Department of Medicine, Faculty of Medicine Siriraj Hospital, Mahidol University, 2 Wanglang Road, Bangkoknoi, Bangkok 10700, Thailand

Background

Colistin is one of the last-resort antibiotics available for treatment of infections caused by multidrug-resistant Gram-negative bacteria, including carbapenem-resistant *Acinetobacter baumannii*, carbapenem-resistant *Pseudomonas aeruginosa*, and carbapenem-resistant Enterobacteriaceae (CRE) [1]. Colistin is currently in wide use as a result of the increasing prevalence of infections caused by these bacteria. Moreover, colistin is widely used in livestock for prevention, control, and treatment of infections [2]. The prior use of colistin in humans and animals is associated with colistin resistance and/or increased colistin minimal inhibitory concentration (MIC) in Gram-negative bacteria [3–5]. A main mechanism of resistance to colistin in Gram-negative bacteria is mediated by modification of lipid A, which results in a reduction in colistin affinity for Gram-negative bacteria. Colistin resistance mechanisms are usually mediated by chromosome-encoded mutations in the PmrAB and PhoPQ two-component regulatory systems, or by MgrB inactivation [6]. The emergence of a plasmid-mediated gene (mcr-1) that encodes a protein conferring resistance to colistin in Enterobacteriaceae isolated from foods, animals, and patients was reported from China in 2015 [7]. Subsequently, mcr-1-producing colistin-resistant Enterobacteriaceae have been reported from many countries around the World [8]. Colistin use in food animals is suspected as the major driver of the emergence of this plasmid-mediated colistin-resistant gene [7]. Association between colistin use for therapy of carbapenem-resistant *A. baumannii* and *P. aeruginosa* infections in humans and the emergence of colistin-resistance in these bacteria has been reported [9–13]. However, the prevalence of and association between colistin use for therapy of carbapenem-resistant Gram-negative bacterial infections in humans and the emergence of colistin resistance in Enterobacteriaceae in individuals who receive colistin are not well-understood.

Accordingly, the aim of this study was to determine the effect of colistin use in hospitalized patients on emergence of colistin-resistant (CoR) *E. coli* (EC) and *K. pneumoniae* (KP) colonization and infection.

Methods

This prospective observational study was conducted at Siriraj Hospital, a 2300-bed university-based tertiary care hospital in Bangkok, Thailand, during December 2016 to November 2017. The study protocol was approved by the Siriraj Institutional Review Board, and written informed consent was obtained from all subjects.

Adult patients hospitalized in the medical wards or medical intensive care units at Siriraj Hospital who received colistin were included in this study. The decision to prescribe colistin treatment was made by each patient's attending physician. Each enrolled subject had a first surveillance stool or rectal swab culture sample collected as soon as possible within several days after receiving colistin. Subsequent stool or rectal swab samples were collected on days 3 and 7 after colistin treatment, and once a week thereafter until the patient left the hospital, died, or up to 4 weeks after receiving colistin if the previously collected samples did not reveal colistin-resistant (CoR) *E. coli* (EC) or *K. pneumoniae* (KP). Surveillance culture samples from the site of infection that precipitated the use of colistin therapy were also periodically collected if they were available. Collected surveillance culture samples were grown on a MacConkey agar plate. The lactose-fermenter bacterial colonies grown on primary MacConkey agar plate after overnight incubation at 35 °C with different morphology were subcultured. Identification of the targeted bacteria (EC and KP) was made by using traditional biochemical tests including growth on MacConkey agar, Kovac's oxidase, triple sugar iron agar reaction, indole production, methyl red, Voges-Proskauer, citrate utilization, production of hydrogen sulfide, urea hydrolysis, phenylalanine deaminase, lysine decarboxylase, ornithine decarboxylase, motility, malonate utilization, gas from glucose fermentation, lactose fermentation, manitol fermentation [14]. The minimum inhibitory concentration (MIC) of colistin was performed by broth microdilution method, and a colistin MIC ≥4 mg/L was considered colistin resistance. The susceptibility of isolated CoR EC and CoR KP to ceftriaxone and ertapenem was also assessed by disk diffusion method. Determination of presence of the mcr-1 gene was performed in CoR EC and CoR KP isolates using polymerase chain reaction (PCR) amplification [7]. Screening for the mcr-1 gene was performed by PCR with forward (5′-GTGTGGTACCGACGCTCGG-3′) and reverse (5′-CAAGCCCAATCGGCGCATC-3′) primers. PCR amplification was performed using i-Taq DNA polymerase under the following cycling conditions: 34 cycles of 94 °C for 20 s, 50 °C for 20 s, and 72 °C for 30 s, followed by 1 cycle of 72 °C for 5 min. PCR products were separated on a 1% agarose gel. The PCR amplicon size was approximately 460 bp.

Data collected from each subject included demographics, underlying diseases and conditions, type of isolated bacteria (true pathogen or colonizer), type of infection, previous antimicrobial treatment received during the 3-month period prior to study enrollment, antimicrobial treatment during the study period, and the outcome of colistin treatment. The dose, frequency and duration of colistin were also recorded.

The primary outcomes of this study were prevalence of colonization with CoR EC or CoR KP in subjects who received colistin during the study period, and the factors associated with CoR EC or CoR KP colonization. Colonization of CoR EC or CoR KP was defined as detection of CoR EC or CoR KP in surveillance culture samples in the absence of clinical features of infection at the site of the sample collection. CoR EC or CoR KP infection was defined according to the diagnosis of the patient's attending physician. The secondary outcomes were the clinical courses of colonization with CoR EC or CoR KP in patients who received colistin during the study period, the prevalence of the mcr-1 gene in isolated CoR EC and CoR KP, and the clinical courses of subjects with CoR EC or CoR KP colonization and infection.

Sample size calculation and data analysis

An overall colonization and infection rate of colistin-resistant Gram-negative bacteria in a cohort of critically-ill patients in intensive care units was 27% [3]. Therefore, it was estimated that at least 30% of subjects who received colistin would develop colonization with CoR EC or CoR KP during the study period. Using a variation in prevalence of developing CoR EC or CoR KP colonization during the study period of 8% and an acceptable type 1 two-sided error of 5%, a minimum sample size of 127 subjects was needed.

All data analyses were performed using SPSS Statistics version 16.0 (SPSS, Inc., Chicago, IL, USA). Demographics and clinical characteristics of patients were summarized using descriptive statistics. Categorical data are presented as frequency and percentage, and continuous data are shown as mean ± standard deviation or median and range. Comparison of categorical data was performed using chi-square test or Fisher's exact test, with Student's t-test used to compare continuous data. A *p*-value less than or equal to 0.05 was considered statistically significant.

Results

Study population

A total of 139 subjects were included. All enrolled patients received colistin, all had ≥2 stool or rectal swab samples collected, and all had their first sample collected within 5 days after the start of colistin treatment. The demographics and clinical characteristics of subjects are summarized in Table 1.

The mean age of subjects was 67.2 years, and the distribution between genders was not different. Most subjects had chronic underlying diseases or healthcare-associated conditions. Previous hospitalization within 3 months was observed in 52.5% of subjects. Lower respiratory tract infection was the most common site of infection, followed by blood stream infection and urinary tract infection. Colistin therapy was given to 79.1% of subjects with documented bacterial infections, and in 77.1% of episodes of documented bacterial infection. *A. baumannii* was the most common cause of documented infection, followed by *K. pneumoniae* and *P. aeruginosa*. *E. coli* and *Enterobacter cloacae* were found in only 4% of subjects. Most subjects received mechanical ventilation (84.2%) or central venous catheterization (61.2%). The mean APACHE II score was 21.8. Most patients received various antibiotics within 3 months prior to study enrollment, including carbapenems, cephalosporins, beta-lactam/beta-lactamase inhibitors, fluoroquinolones, vancomycin, aminoglycosides and colistin. The subjects received 166 courses of colistin during the study period. Colistin was given to 110 subjects (79.1%) with documented infections, with 29 patients (20.9%) being prescribed colistin as empirical therapy. The most frequent indication for colistin use was *A. baumannii* ventilator-associated pneumonia. The median duration of all colistin treatment courses was 9 days (range: 1–55).

Colistin-resistant *E. coli* or *K. pneumoniae*

The surveillance culture samples collected included 673 stool or rectal swab samples, 465 sputum samples, 103 urine samples, 2 percutaneous drainage samples, and 1 wound swab sample. Colistin resistance was observed in 246 isolates of EC and KP, of which 26 were EC and 220 were KP. One hundred and sixty-six isolates (67.5%) of CoR EC or CoR KP were recovered from stool or rectal swab samples, while 70 isolates (28.5%) and 10 isolates (4.1%) were recovered from sputum samples and urine samples, respectively. The MIC_{50}, MIC_{90}, and MIC range of all CoR EC and CoR KP isolates was 64, 128, and 4 to > 128 mg/L, respectively. The MIC_{50}, MIC_{90}, and MIC range of all CoR EC isolates was 8, 64, and 4 to 128 mg/L, respectively. The MIC_{50}, MIC_{90}, and MIC range of all CoR KP isolates was 64, 128, and 4 to > 128 mg/L, respectively. Among the 26 CoR EC isolates, 80.8% were resistant to ceftriaxone, and 11.5% were resistant to carbapenems. Ceftriaxone resistance and carbapenems resistance was observed in 96.8 and 75.5% of 220 CoR KP isolates, respectively.

Colistin-resistant *E. coli* or *K. pneumoniae* colonization in all collected clinical samples

The number of subjects colonized with CoR EC or CoR KP in the first surveillance culture samples at study enrollment, and the number of patients colonized with CoR EC or CoR KP in subsequent surveillance culture samples during the study period are shown in Fig. 1.

CoR EC or CoR KP colonization was detected in 66 of 139 subjects (47.5%). Sixty of those patients (43.2%) were colonized with CoR KP, and 13 subjects (9.4%) were colonized with CoR EC. CoR EC or CoR KP colonization was detected in 24 subjects (17.3%) at study enrollment, with 22 subjects (15.8%) colonized by CoR KP and 2 subjects (1.4%) colonized by CoR EC. Of the 115 subjects with no colonization of CoR EC or CoR KP at study enrollment, 42 subjects (36.5%) subsequently developed colonization with CoR EC or CoR KP. Of those,

Table 1 Demographics and clinical characteristics of 139 subjects

Variables	Values
Female gender, n (%)	70 (50.4%)
Age (yrs), mean ± SD	67.2 ± 15.9
Comorbid conditions, n (%)	131 (94.2%)
Diabetes mellitus	53 (38.1%)
Cardiovascular diseases	41 (29.5%)
Renal diseases	37 (26.6%)
Cerebrovascular diseases	35 (25.2%)
Solid malignancy	21 (15.1%)
Chronic pulmonary diseases	20 (14.3%)
Hematologic malignancy	16 (11.5%)
Liver diseases	10 (7.2%)
Organ transplantation	4 (2.9%)
HIV infection	2 (1.4%)
Previous hospitalization within 3 months, n (%)	73 (52.5%)
Site of infection in 139 patients at enrollment, n (%)	
Lower respiratory tract infection	93 (66.9%)
Blood stream infection	40 (28.8%)
Urinary tract infection	18 (12.9%)
Gastrointestinal tract infection	11 (7.9%)
Skin and soft tissue infection	8 (5.8%)
Surgical site infection	1 (0.7%)
Bone and joint infection	1 (0.7%)
Documented bacteria-caused infections in 110 patients that required colistin therapy, n (%)	
A. baumannii	79 (71.8%)
K. pneumoniae	18 (16.4%)
P. aeruginosa	9 (8.2%)
E. coli	2 (1.8%)
E. cloacae	2 (1.8%)
Medical procedure, n (%)	
Mechanical ventilation	117 (84.2%)
Central venous catheterization	85 (61.2%)
Chronic intermittent hemodialysis	53 (38.1%)
Severity of patient illness, mean ± SD	
APACHE II score at enrollment	21.8 ± 7.4
Antibiotic use for the current hospitalization prior to study enrollment, n (%)	134 (96.4%)
Carbapenems	112 (80.6%)
Cephalosporins	56 (40.3%)
Beta-lactam/beta-lactamase inhibitors	75 (54.0%)
Fluoroquinolones	39 (28.1%)
Vancomycin	43 (30.9%)
Aminoglycosides	6 (4.3%)
Colistin	9 (6.8%)
Colistin use within 3 months prior to study enrollment, n (%)	15 (10.8%)

39 subjects (33.9%) were colonized with CoR KP, and 8 (7.0%) were colonized with CoR EC.

Comparison of subjects with and without colistin-resistant *E. coli* or *K. pneumoniae* colonization during the study period

Comparison of subjects with (66 patients) and without (73 patients) CoR EC or CoR KP colonization during the study period is shown in Table 2.

The duration from hospital admission to the first surveillance culture sample collection, and the duration from study enrollment to the first surveillance culture sample collection during the study period were not significantly different between groups. The use of fluoroquinolones, aminoglycosides, or colistin within 3 months prior to study enrollment, and the amount, duration, and courses of colistin were all significantly greater in subjects with CoR EC or CoR KP colonization than in those without CoR EC or CoR KP colonization (all $p < 0.05$). The median and range of duration of the presence of CoR EC or CoR KP colonization was 13 days and 1–68 days, respectively. Neither CoR EC nor CoR KP was isolated from 23 subjects (34.8%) at the end of the study period, whereas 43 patients (65.2%) had persistent CoR EC or CoR KP colonization at the end of the study period. The median and range of duration of colistin use in subjects that had no CoR EC or CoR KP colonization at the end of the study was 11 days and 2–57 days, respectively. The corresponding values for patients who had persistent CoR EC or CoR KP colonization at the end of the study were 14 days and 3–65 days, respectively ($p = 0.43$). The length of hospital stay in subjects with CoR EC or CoR KP colonization was significantly longer than in subjects without CoR EC or CoR KP colonization. The rates of all-cause mortality at hospital discharge were similar between subjects with and without CoR EC or CoR KP colonization.

Comparison of subjects with and without colistin-resistant *E. coli* or *K. pneumoniae* colonization at study enrollment

CoR EC or CoR KP colonization was detected in 24 subjects (17.3%) at study enrollment. Twenty-two subjects (15.8%) were colonized with CoR KP, and 2 patients (1.4%) were colonized with CoR EC. Comparison of

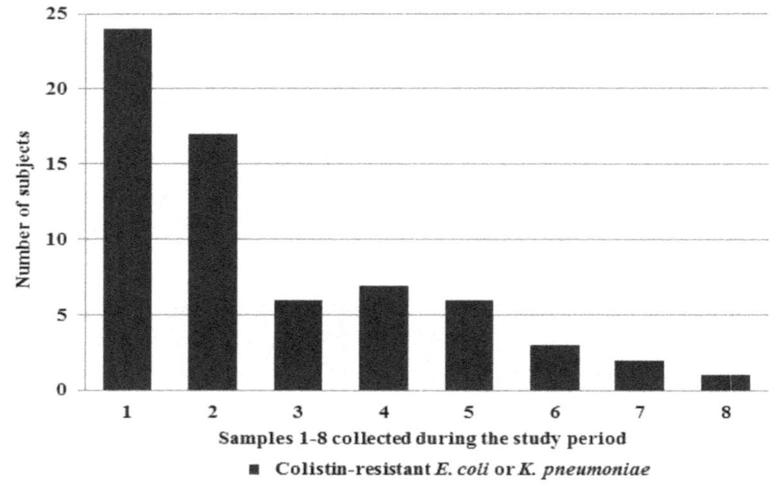

Fig. 1 Number of subjects colonized with colistin-resistant *E. coli* or *K. pneumoniae* in surveillance culture samples at each of 8 sample collections during the study period

subjects with and without CoR EC or CoR KP colonization at study enrollment is shown in Table 3.

Duration from hospital admission to study enrollment, and duration from study enrollment to first surveillance culture sample collection between subjects with and without CoR EC or CoR KP colonization were not significantly different between groups. The use of fluoroquinolones or vancomycin for the current hospitalization prior to study enrollment and surgery were significantly more prevalent in subjects with CoR EC or CoR KP colonization at study enrollment than in those without CoR EC or CoR KP colonization at study enrollment. The use of aminoglycosides for the current hospitalization prior to study enrollment and colistin use within 3 months prior to study enrollment were observed more often in subjects with CoR EC or CoR KP colonization at study enrollment. The median and range of the duration of the presence of CoR EC or CoR KP colonization were 18.5 days and 2–68 days, respectively. CoR EC or CoR KP was not isolated from 25.0% of 24 subjects at the end of the study period. In contrast, the remaining 75.0% of those subjects had persistent CoR EC or CoR KP colonization at the end of the study period. Length of hospital stay and the rate of all-cause mortality at hospital discharge in subjects with CoR EC or CoR KP colonization at study enrollment were both greater than in patients without CoR EC or CoR KP colonization at study enrollment.

Comparison of subjects with and without colistin-resistant *E. coli* or *K. pneumoniae* colonization after study enrollment among subjects without colonization by colistin-resistant *E. coli* or *K. pneumoniae* at study enrollment

Of the 115 subjects without colonization of CoR EC or CoR KP at study enrollment, 42 patients (36.5%) subsequently developed colonization with CoR EC or CoR KP. Comparison of subjects with and without CoR EC or CoR KP colonization after study enrollment among subjects without colonization by CoR EC or CoR KP at study enrollment is shown in Table 4.

Duration from hospital admission to the first surveillance culture sample collection, and duration from study enrollment to the first surveillance culture sample collection in patients with and without CoR EC or CoR KP colonization after study enrollment were not significantly different between groups. The use of colistin within 3 months prior to study enrollment, and the amount, duration, and courses of colistin were all significantly greater in patients with CoR EC or CoR KP colonization after study enrollment than in those without CoR EC or CoR KP colonization after study enrollment. The median and range of the time from study enrollment to the first detection of CoR EC or CoR KP colonization were 10 days and 3–42 days, respectively, and the mean duration was 14 days for CoR KP and 14 days for CoR EC. The median and range of the duration of the presence of CoR EC or CoR KP colonization was 7 days and 1–57 days, respectively. At the end of the study, CoR EC or CoR KP was and was not isolated from 59.5 and 40.5% of 42 subjects, respectively. Length of hospital stay in subjects with CoR EC or CoR KP colonization after study enrollment was significantly longer than in subjects without CoR EC or CoR KP colonization after study enrollment. The rate of all-cause mortality at hospital discharge was similar between subjects with and without CoR EC or CoR KP colonization after study enrollment.

Presence of mcr-1 gene among colistin-resistant *E. coli* and *K. pneumoniae* isolates

The mcr-1 gene was detected in 13.0% of 246 isolates of CoR EC or CoR KP. It was detected in 57.7% of 26 CoR

Table 2 Comparison of subjects with and without colistin-resistant *E. coli* or *K. pneumoniae* colonization during the study period

Variables	Colonization (*n* = 66)	No Colonization (*n* = 73)	*p*-value
Female gender (yrs), n (%)	33 (50.0%)	37 (50.7%)	0.94
Age (yrs), mean ± SD	65.7 ± 16.7	68.5 ± 15.1	0.32
Duration from hospital admission to first sample collection (days), median (range)	16 (1–106)	16 (2–81)	0.37
Duration from enrollment to first sample collection (days), median (range)	1 (1–4)	1 (1–5)	0.54
ICU admission, n (%)	24 (36.4%)	24 (32.9%)	0.67
Previous hospitalization, n (%)	36 (54.5%)	37 (50.7%)	0.65
APACHE II score at study enrollment, mean ± SD	21.6 ± 7.1	21.9 ± 7.6	0.77
Mechanical ventilation, n (%)	59 (89.4%)	58 (79.5%)	0.11
Indwelling central venous catheter, n (%)	45 (68.2%)	40 (54.8%)	0.11
Surgery, n (%)	45 (68.2%)	39 (53.4%)	0.08
Chronic intermittent hemodialysis, n (%)	8 (12.1%)	10 (13.7%)	0.78
Antibiotic use for the current hospitalization prior to study enrollment and during study period, n (%)			
Carbapenems	57 (86.4%)	66 (90.4%)	0.46
Cephalosporins	31 (47.0%)	31 (42.5%)	0.59
Beta-lactam/ beta-lactamase inhibitors	54 (81.8%)	52 (71.2%)	0.14
Fluoroquinolones	42 (63.6%)	33 (45.2%)	0.03
Vancomycin	40 (60.6%)	38 (52.1%)	0.31
Aminoglycosides	10 (15.2%)	2 (2.7%)	< 0.001
Antibiotic use for the current hospitalization prior to study enrollment, n (%)			
Carbapenems	52 (78.8%)	60 (82.2%)	0.61
Cephalosporins	26 (39.4%)	30 (41.1%)	0.84
Beta-lactam/beta-lactamase inhibitors	37 (56.1%)	38 (52.1%)	0.64
Fluoroquinolones	24 (36.4%)	15 (20.5%)	0.04
Vancomycin	22 (33.3%)	21 (28.8%)	0.56
Aminoglycosides	5 (7.6%)	1 (1.4%)	0.10
Colistin use within 3 months prior to study enrollment, n (%)	13 (19.7%)	2 (2.7%)	0.001
Total amount of colistin (mg), median (range)	3550 (400–12,550)	2000 (500–10,650)	< 0.001
Total duration of colistin use (days), median (range)	13.5 (2–58)	9 (2–32)	< 0.001
Total courses of colistin therapy, mean ± SD	1.4 ± 0.8	1.1 ± 0.4	0.003
Total courses of colistin therapy, range	1–4	1–3	
Patients who received more than 1 course of colistin therapy, n (%)	19 (28.8%)	7 (9.6%)	0.004
Length of hospital stay (days), median (range)	46.5 (12–246)	32 (6–192)	0.01
All-cause mortality at hospital discharge, n (%)	35 (53.0%)	35 (47.9%)	0.55

EC isolates, while only 7.7% of 220 CoR KP isolates showed presence of mcr-1. The colistin MIC of CoR EC isolates with the mcr-1 gene ranged from 4 to 16 mg/L (median: 8 mg/L), whereas the colistin MIC of CoR KP isolates with the mcr-1 gene ranged from 4 to > 128 mg/L (median: 32 mg/L). All isolates of CoR EC or CoR KP with the mcr-1 gene were colonizers. Presence of the mcr-1 gene was observed in 27.3% of the 66 subjects that had CoR EC or CoR KP. The mcr-1 gene was detected in 12.5% of 24 subjects with CoR EC or CoR KP at study enrollment, and in 35.7% of 42 subjects with colonization with CoR EC or CoR KP after study enrollment.

Colistin-resistant *E. coli* or *K. pneumoniae* infection

Five subjects had infections caused by CoR KP. Of those, three had infections at study enrollment, and 2 developed

Table 3 Comparison of subjects with and without colistin-resistant *E. coli* or *K. pneumoniae* colonization at study enrollment

Variables	Colonization at enrollment (n = 24)	No colonization at enrollment (n = 115)	p-value
Female gender	13 (54.2%)	57 (49.6%)	0.68
Age (yrs), mean ± SD	64.3 ± 18.8	67.8 ± 15.2	0.33
ICU admission, n (%)	9 (37.5%)	39 (33.9%)	0.77
Previous hospitalization, n (%)	15 (62.5%)	58 (50.4%)	0.28
Duration from hospital admission to enrollment (days), median (range)	19.5 (4–106)	15 (1–86)	0.10
Duration from enrollment to first sample collection (days), median (range)	1.5 (1–4)	1 (1–5)	0.48
APACHE II score at study enrollment, mean ± SD	20.6 ± 7.2	21.9 ± 7.4	0.65
Mechanical ventilation, n (%)	20 (83.3%)	97 (84.3%)	1.0
Indwelling central venous catheter, n (%)	17 (70.8%)	68 (59.1%)	0.29
Surgery, n (%)	19 (79.2%)	65 (56.5%)	0.04
Chronic intermittent hemodialysis, n (%)	4 (16.7%)	14 (12.2%)	0.74
Colistin use within 3 months prior to study enrollment, n (%)	4 (16.7%)	11 (9.6%)	0.47
Antibiotic use for the current hospitalization prior to study enrollment, n (%)			
Carbapenems	20 (83.3%)	92 (80.0%)	0.79
Cephalosporins	9 (37.5%)	47 (40.9%)	0.76
Beta-lactam/beta-lactamase inhibitors	16 (66.7%)	59 (51.3%)	0.17
Fluoroquinolones	13 (54.2%)	26 (22.6%)	0.002
Vancomycin	13 (54.2%)	30 (26.1%)	0.007
Aminoglycosides	3 (12.5%)	3 (2.6%)	0.06
Colistin	3 (13.6%)	6 (5.5%)	0.36
Length of hospital stay (days), median (range)	49.5 (13–138)	36 (6–246)	0.17
All-cause mortality at hospital discharge, n (%)	16 (66.7%)	54 (47.0%)	0.08

infections after the start of the study. Of the 3 subjects with infections caused by CoR KP at study enrollment, 2 had concurrent CoR KP colonization. Of the 2 subjects with infections caused by CoR KP after study enrollment, 1 had concurrent CoR KP colonization and the other had concurrent CoR EC colonization. The sites of infections were urinary tract infections (3 patients), ventilator-associated pneumonia (1 patient) and bacteremia (1 patient). All subjects received colistin in combination with either fosfomycin or aminoglycoside, and they were alive at hospital discharge. There was no infection caused by CoR EC among subjects who had CoR EC colonization throughout the study period.

Discussion

The overall CoR EC or CoR KP colonization rate of 47.5% among subjects who received colistin in the present study was relatively high, especially the development of CoR EC or CoR KP colonization after study enrollment when compared with data from previous reports [15–17]. However, the study populations in those previous reports were general hospitalized patients, and they did not limit their studies to only patients who received colistin. To the best of our knowledge, the present study is the first to examine the prevalence of CoR EC or CoR KP colonization among hospitalized patients who received colistin. The prevalence of CoR EC or CoR KP in surveillance culture samples collected from these subjects was also high. It should be noted that a much larger number of CoR KP isolates than CoR EC isolates was recovered from subjects in this study (220 isolates vs. 26 isolates, respectively).

Many factors may have contributed to the development of CoR EC and CoR KP colonization observed in this study. The subjects with CoR EC or CoR KP colonization at study enrollment may have acquired colistin-resistant bacteria from the community prior to hospitalization. The probability of community-acquired CoR EC or CoR KP is low, however, because it is extremely rare for individuals, foods, and the environment in the community in Thailand to harbor CoR EC or CoR KP [18, 19]. CoR EC and CoR KP have been detected at food animal farms in Thailand (especially swine farms) that use colistin extensively in the feed given to the swine to prevent and treat infection (V. Thamlikitkul. unpublished data). Most of the colistin-resistant Enterobacteriaceae found at swine farms in Thailand was *E. coli* while the prevalence of CoR EC isolates observed in

Table 4 Comparison of subjects with and without colistin-resistant *E. coli* or *K. pneumoniae* colonization after study enrollment among subjects without colonization with colistin-resistant *E. coli* or *K. pneumoniae* at study enrollment

Variables	Colonization after enrollment ($n = 42$)	No Colonization after enrollment ($n = 73$)	*p*-value
Female gender (yrs), n (%)	20 (47.6%)	37 (50.7%)	0.75
Age (yrs), mean ± SD	66.6 ± 15.6	68.5 ± 15.1	0.54
ICU admission, n (%)	15 (35.7%)	24 (32.9%)	0.76
Previous hospitalization, n (%)	21 (50.0%)	37 (50.7%)	0.94
APACHE II score at study enrollment, mean ± SD	21.8 ± 7.2	21.9 ± 7.6	0.92
Mechanical ventilation, n (%)	39 (92.9%)	58 (79.5%)	0.06
Indwelling central venous catheter, n (%)	28 (66.7%)	40 (54.8%)	0.21
Surgery, n (%)	26 (61.9%)	39 (53.4%)	0.38
Chronic intermittent hemodialysis, n (%)	4 (9.5%)	10 (13.7%)	0.51
Antibiotic use for current hospitalization prior to study enrollment and during study period, n (%)			
Carbapenems	35 (83.3%)	66 (90.4%)	0.26
Cephalosporins	20 (47.6%)	31 (42.5%)	0.59
Beta-lactam/beta-lactamase inhibitors	33 (78.6%)	52 (71.2%)	0.39
Fluoroquinolones	25 (59.5%)	33 (45.2%)	0.14
Vancomycin	23 (54.8%)	38 (52.1%)	0.78
Aminoglycosides	5 (11.9%)	2 (2.7%)	0.10
Antibiotic use for the current hospitalization after study enrollment, n (%)			
Carbapenems	19 (45.2%)	34 (46.6%)	0.89
Cephalosporins	6 (14.3%)	4 (5.5%)	0.17
Beta-lactam/beta-lactamase inhibitors	25 (59.5%)	36 (49.3%)	0.29
Fluoroquinolones	19 (45.2%)	25 (34.2%)	0.24
Vancomycin	17 (40.5%)	27 (37.0%)	0.71
Aminoglycosides	4 (9.5%)	2 (2.7%)	0.19
Colistin use within 3 months prior to study enrollment, n (%)	9 (21.4%)	2 (2.7%)	0.002
Total amount of colistin (mg), median (range)	2800 (400–9350)	2000 (300–10,650)	0.03
Total duration of colistin use (days), median (range)	13 (2–55)	9 (1–32)	0.03
Total courses of colistin therapy, mean ± SD	1.3 ± 0.6	1.1 ± 0.34	0.02
Total courses of colistin therapy, range	1–3	1–3	
Patients who received more than 1 course of colistin therapy, n (%)	10 (23.8%)	6 (8.2%)	0.02
Length of hospital stay (days), median (range)	46.5 (12–246)	32 (6–192)	0.04
All-cause mortality at hospital discharge, n (%)	35 (47.9%)	19 (45.2%)	0.78

this study was much lower than that of CoR KP isolates. A study from China reported the presence of colistin-resistant Enterobacteriaceae in healthy adults [20]. Subjects with CoR EC or CoR KP colonization at study enrollment in the present study may have had colonized CoR EC or CoR KP in their guts from prior hospitalizations. The transmission of CoR EC or CoR KP from other hospitalized patients with colonization or infections caused by these bacteria and/or from the hospital environment to subjects during hospitalization prior to study enrollment could not be excluded. The use of fluoroquinolones, vancomycin, or aminoglycosides, all of which are non-beta-lactam antibiotics, for the current hospitalization prior to study enrollment may have contributed to the development of CoR EC or CoR KP colonization at study enrollment, because these antibiotics were found to be or tended to be associated with subjects who had CoR EC or CoR KP colonization at study enrollment. Interestingly, the use of beta-lactams during the current hospitalization prior to study enrollment was not found to be significantly associated with CoR EC or CoR KP colonization at study enrollment. Colistin use within 3 months prior to study enrollment may also have contributed to the development of CoR EC or CoR KP colonization at study enrollment, although potential statistical significance could not be achieved due to the small size of our study population. CoR EC or CoR KP colonization could have developed in some subjects in the present study after exposure to colistin for only 3 days, which would be consistent with our previous observations in swine that showed colistin-resistant Enterobacteriaceae colonization in the guts of piglets that received colistin for only several days. Association between the emergence of CoR EC or CoR KP and the use of broad-spectrum antibiotics and colistin was previously reported [3, 11, 17, 21]. Colistin-resistant bacteria in patients with no history of colistin use was also reported [22–24].

In patients with no CoR EC or CoR KP colonization at study enrollment that developed CoR EC or CoR KP colonization after study enrollment, it appears evident that colistin use was the main contributing factor, because colistin use within 3 months prior to study enrollment and a larger total dose of colistin, longer duration of colistin, and multiple courses of colistin were all significantly associated with subjects who developed CoR EC or CoR KP colonization after study enrollment. In addition to the use of colistin, transmission of CoR EC or CoR KP from other hospitalized patients with colonization or infection with these colistin-resistant bacteria and/or from the hospital environment during hospitalization could also be potential causes of CoR EC or CoR KP colonization. Since the present study did not have a concurrent cohort of hospitalized patients who did not receive colistin, the effect and magnitude of these other potential causes of CoR EC or CoR KP colonization (in addition to colistin exposure) could not be quantified. Our previous study in CRE colonization and infections in hospitalized patients at our center revealed that approximately 10% of patients had colistin-resistant Enterobacteriaceae during their hospitalization (V. Thamlikitkul. unpublished data). Therefore, colistin use should still be considered a major contributing driver of CoR EC or CoR KP colonization in subjects who receive colistin. Two previous studies reported emergence of colistin resistance in *K. pneumoniae* after the use of colistin for digestive tract decontamination [25, 26]. Selective pressure of colistin use in these patients is likely to be one of the contributing factors for this emergence of colistin resistance.

CoR EC or CoR KP was not isolated from 34.8% of subjects with CoR EC or KP colonization at the end of the study period. The median and range of the duration of CoR EC or CoR KP colonization in these subjects were 18.5 days and 2–68 days, respectively. It should be kept in mind that collection of surveillance culture samples was not performed on a daily basis, but they were collected at enrollment, on days 3 and 7 after the start of colistin treatment, and once a week thereafter. As such, the reported duration from the first sample collection until the disappearance of CoR EC or CoR KP does not represent the real duration of colonization. The duration of colonization could be shorter than the reported duration since CoR EC or CoR KP could disappear between the sample collection times. These observations indicate that colistin resistance could be disappeared, which is similar to colistin resistance findings in Enterobacteriaceae studies in piglets that rapidly developed resistance when colistin was given, but the resistance was usually disappeared once colistin was discontinued (V. Thamlikitkul. unpublished data). Regarding subjects with persistent CoR EC or CoR KP colonization at the end of the study period, colonization duration data was not available since these patients were not followed beyond the end of the study period. The duration of colistin exposure in patients with persistent CoR EC or CoR KP colonization at the end of the study seemed to be longer than in those with no observable CoR EC or CoR KP colonization at the end of the study.

The mechanisms of colistin resistance in Enterobacteriaceae should be different from those in non-fermentative Gram-negative bacteria, especially *A. baumannii* and *P. aeruginosa*. *A. baumannii* and *P. aeruginosa* are far less likely to develop colistin resistance during exposure to colistin, because the prevalence of colistin-resistant *A. baumannii*-caused and *P. aeruginosa*-caused infections in hospitalized patients at Siriraj Hospital has been less than 5% even though colistin has been widely used for treatment of carbapenem-resistant *A. baumannii* and *P. aeruginosa* infections at Siriraj Hospital for longer than 10 years [27]. In contrast, brief exposure by *E. coli* and *K. pneumoniae* to colistin in hospitalized patients was associated with colistin resistance in *E. coli* and *K. pneumoniae*, as was observed in the present study and in the previous study that investigated colistin use in swine.

Although the number of CoR KP isolates was far larger than the number of CoR EC isolates in our study population, the prevalence of the mcr-1 gene in CoR KP isolates (7.7%) was much lower than in CoR EC isolates (57.7%). This observation was similar to observations from our previous study that the mcr-1 gene was detected in only 1.4% of 280 suspected CoR KP isolates, whereas it was detected in 29.7% of 37 suspected CoR EC isolates [28]. Again, similar to data from our previous study, the MICs of colistin in CoR EC isolates with the mcr-1 gene were lower than the colistin MICs in CoR KP isolates with the mcr-1 gene [28]. Since the mcr-1 gene was detected in only some isolates of CoR EC and in only a small portion of CoR KP isolates, CoR EC and CoR KP without the mcr-1 gene isolated from subjects in our study could be resistant to colistin via other types of plasmid-mediated mcr genes (including mcr-2, mcr-3, mcr-4, mcr-5), or other resistance mechanisms, or combined mechanisms of resistance [29–33]. We are currently investigating the mechanisms of colistin resistance among CoR EC and KP isolates without the mcr-1 gene.

CoR EC or CoR KP colonization in hospitalized patients could pose multiple threats to their own wellbeing and the wellbeing of others. Although this study found only 3 subjects who had CoR KP colonization and infection, hospitalized patients with CoR EC or CoR KP colonization should be considered to be at risk of developing infections due to CoR EC or CoR KP at a later time point. This later risk of infection was observed in neutropenic patients, in other immunocompromized patients or critically-ill patients who developed subsequent multidrug-resistant infections after colonization with the same multidrug-resistant bacteria, and surveillance culture collected from such patients to determine the presence of multidrug-resistant colonization was suggested because intestinal colonization with multidrug-resistant bacteria was found to be associated with subsequent infections caused by the same colonized multidrug-resistant bacteria [34–37]. Hospitalized patients with CoR EC or CoR KP colonization could transmit these colistin-resistant bacteria to other hospitalized patients, healthcare personnel, their relatives, and into the hospital environment. Patients with an antibiotic-resistant plasmid-mediated gene, such as mcr-1, in colonized bacteria could transfer this genetic mobile element to other bacteria residing in their body, other patients, or the hospital environment, which could result in further emergence and spread of colistin-resistant pathogens. Patients with persistent colonization of CoR EC or CoR KP could transmit these bacteria to others living in their home and into the environment in their community when they return home from the hospital, and these colistin-resistant bacteria may cause community-acquired infection in the future. The length of hospital stay in subjects with CoR EC or CoR KP colonization was significantly longer than the length of stay among subjects without CoR EC or CoR KP colonization; however, the all-cause mortality rate at hospital discharge was similar between subjects with and without CoR EC or CoR KP colonization.

The outcomes of infections caused by CoR EC or CoR KP are not always unfavorable or fatal. Many isolates of CoR EC and some isolates of CoR KP recovered from subjects in this study were still susceptible to carbapenems. Although all 5 subjects infected with CoR KP had infections caused by carbapenem-resistant isolates, all of them received combination of colistin and fosfomycin or aminoglycosides and they were alive at hospital discharge. Infection caused by CoR EC was not observed in this study. This may be mostly and simply due to the fact that there was only a small number of subjects who had colonization with CoR EC compared to a much more number of subjects with CoR KP colonization.

Polymyxins will continue to be a mainstay antimicrobial group for therapy of carbapenem-resistant *A. baumannii* and *P. aeruginosa* infections, both of which are very prevalent in hospital-acquired infections in many countries, including Thailand. Polymyxins will also be the treatment of choice for CRE infection, which has been an emerging hospital-acquired infection in Thailand over the past 5 years, since more effective, more efficient, and safer agents for treatment of these carbapenem-resistant Gram-negative infections are not yet available. The responsible physician should prescribe colistin for therapy of documented carbapenem-resistant Gram-negative infections that are susceptible to colistin at the shortest duration of treatment. Colistin should not be used in patients with carbapenem-resistant Gram-negative colonization, and it should be used as empirical antimicrobial therapy as rarely as possible. These strategies for the use of colistin may minimize collateral damage caused by the use of colistin regarding the development and transmission of CoR EC or CoR KP in both healthcare and community settings. However, even appropriate use of colistin is still a key driver of the inevitable emergence of CoR EC or CoR KP. The high prevalence of CoR EC or CoR KP colonization observed in this study is worrisome, and it may predict an increase in CoR EC or CoR KP infections in the future. The heavy use of colistin in hospitalized patients may result in infections caused by CoR EC or CoR KP becoming endemic in healthcare facilities in the near future.

Conclusions

Prevalence of CoR EC or CoR KP colonization in hospitalized patients receiving colistin was high and it was associated with the use of colistin. Therefore, patients who receive colistin are at risk of developing CoR EC or CoR KP colonization and infection.

Acknowledgements

The authors gratefully acknowledge Chulaluk Komoltri for assistance with statistical analysis.

Funding

This study was funded by grants from the Health Systems Research Institute, Thailand and the Faculty of Medicine Siriraj Hospital, Mahidol University.

Authors' contributions

WW and VT contributed to conception and design of the article. NP, NM CS and ST were responsible for microbiological tests. WW, NP, NM CS, ST and VT collected and analysed data. WW and VT wrote the first version of the manuscript. All authors critically revised the manuscript, and read and approved the final manuscript.

Consent for publication

Not applicable.

Competing interests

The authors declare that they have no competing interests

Author details

[1]Division of Infectious Diseases and Tropical Medicine, Department of Medicine, Faculty of Medicine Siriraj Hospital, Mahidol University, 2 Wanglang Road, Bangkoknoi, Bangkok 10700, Thailand. [2]Department of Clinical Microbiology and Applied Technology, Faculty of Medical Technology, Mahidol University, Bangkok, Thailand.

References

1. Biswas S, Brunel JM, Dubus JC, Reynaud-Gaubert M, Rolain JM. Colistin: an update on the antibiotic of the 21st century. Expert Rev Anti-Infect Ther. 2012;10:917–34.
2. Catry B, Cavaleri M, Baptiste K, Grave K, Grein K, Holm A, Jukes H, Liebana E, et al. Use of colistin-containing products within the European Union and European economic area (EU/EEA): development of resistance in animals and possible impact on human and animal health. Int J Antimicrob Agents. 2015;46:297–306.
3. Kontopidou F, Plachouras D, Papadomichelakis E, Koukos G, Galani I, Poulakou G, et al. Colonization and infection by colistin-resistant gram-negative bacteria in a cohort of critically ill patients. Clin Microbiol Infect. 2011;17:E9–e11.
4. Rhouma M, Beaudry F, Theriault W, Letellier A. Colistin in pig production: chemistry, mechanism of antibacterial action, microbial resistance emergence, and one health perspectives. Front Microbiol. 2016;7:1789.
5. Antoniadou A, Kontopidou F, Poulakou G, Koratzanis E, Galani I, Papadomichelakis E, et al. Colistin-resistant isolates of *Klebsiella pneumoniae* emerging in intensive care unit patients: first report of a multiclonal cluster. J Antimicrob Chemother. 2007;59:786–90.
6. Olaitan AO, Morand S, Rolain JM. Mechanisms of polymyxin resistance: acquired and intrinsic resistance in bacteria. Front Microbiol. 2014;5:643.
7. Liu YY, Wang Y, Walsh TR, Yi LX, Zhang R, Spencer J, et al. Emergence of plasmid-mediated colistin resistance mechanism MCR-1 in animals and human beings in China: a microbiological and molecular biological study. Lancet Infect Dis. 2016;16:161–8.
8. Wang R, van Dorp L, Shaw LP, Bradley P, Wang Q, Wang X, Jin L, Zhang Q, Liu Y, Rieux A, Dorai-Schneiders T, Weinert LA, Iqbal Z, Didelot X, Wang H, Balloux F. The global distribution and spread of the mobilized colistin resistance gene mcr-1. Nat Commun. 2018;9:1179.
9. Qureshi ZA, Hittle LE, O'Hara JA, Rivera JI, Syed A, Shields RK, et al. Colistin-resistant *Acinetobacter baumannii*: beyond carbapenem resistance. Clin Infect Dis. 2015;60:1295–303.
10. Inchai J, Liwsrisakun C, Theerakittikul T, Chaiwarith R, Khositsakulchai W, Pothirat C. Risk factors of multidrug-resistant, extensively drug-resistant and pandrug-resistant *Acinetobacter baumannii* ventilator-associated pneumonia in a medical intensive care unit of University Hospital in Thailand. J Infect Chemother. 2015;21:570–4.
11. Matthaiou DK, Michalopoulos A, Rafailidis PI, Karageorgopoulos DE, Papaioannou V, Ntani G, et al. Risk factors associated with the isolation of colistin-resistant gram-negative bacteria: a matched case-control study. Crit Care Med. 2008;36:807–11.
12. Durante-Mangoni E, Del Franco M, Andini R, Bernardo M, Giannouli M, Zarrilli R. Emergence of colistin resistance without loss of fitness and virulence after prolonged colistin administration in a patient with extensively drug-resistant *Acinetobacter baumannii*. Diagn Microbiol Infect Dis. 2015;82:222–6.
13. Kim Y, Bae IK, Jeong SH, Yong D, Lee K. In vivo selection of pan-drug resistant *Acinetobacter baumannii* during antibiotic treatment. Yonsei Med J. 2015;56:928–34.
14. Farmer JJ 3rd, Davis BR, Hickman-Brenner FW, McWhorter A, Huntley-Carter GP, Asbury MA, et al. Biochemical identification of new species and biogroups of Enterobacteriaceae isolated from clinical specimens. J Clin Microbiol. 1985;21:46–76.
15. Juhasz E, Ivan M, Pinter E, Pongracz J, Kristof K. Colistin resistance among blood culture isolates at a tertiary care Centre in Hungary. J Glob Antimicrob Resist. 2017;11:167–70.
16. Prim N, Turbau M, Rivera A, Rodriguez-Navarro J, Coll P, Mirelis B. Prevalence of colistin resistance in clinical isolates of Enterobacteriaceae: a four-year cross-sectional study. J Inf Secur. 2017;75:493–8.
17. Papadimitriou-Olivgeris M, Christofidou M, Fligou F, Bartzavali C, Vrettos T, Filos KS, et al. The role of colonization pressure in the dissemination of colistin or tigecycline resistant KPC-producing *Klebsiella pneumoniae* in critically ill patients. Infection. 2014;42:883–90.
18. Boonyasiri A, Tangkoskul T, Seenama C, Saiyarin J, Tiengrim S, Thamlikitkul V. Prevalence of antibiotic resistant bacteria in healthy adults, foods, food animals, and the environment in selected areas in Thailand. Pathog Glob Health. 2014;108:235–45.
19. Khamsarn S, Nampoonsak Y, Busamaro S, Tangkoskul T, Seenama C, Rattanaumpawan P, Boonyasiri A, Thamlikitkul V. Epidemiology of antibiotic use and antimicrobial resistance in selected communities in Thailand. J Med Assoc Thail. 2016;99:270–5.
20. Wang Y, Tian GB, Zhang R, Shen Y, Tyrrell JM, Huang X, et al. Prevalence, risk factors, outcomes, and molecular epidemiology of mcr-1-positive Enterobacteriaceae in patients and healthy adults from China: an epidemiological and clinical study. Lancet Infect Dis. 2017;17:390–9.
21. Giacobbe DR, Del Bono V, Trecarichi EM, De Rosa FG, Giannella M, Bassetti M, et al. Risk factors for bloodstream infections due to colistin-resistant KPC-producing *Klebsiella pneumoniae*: results from a multicenter case-control-control study. Clin Microbiol Infect. 2015;21:1106.e1–8.
22. Olaitan AO, Morand S, Rolain JM. Emergence of colistin-resistant bacteria in humans without colistin usage: a new worry and cause for vigilance. Int J Antimicrob Agents. 2016;47:1–3.
23. Chen S, Hu F, Zhang X, Xu X, Liu Y, Zhu D, et al. Independent emergence of colistin-resistant Enterobacteriaceae clinical isolates without colistin treatment. J Clin Microbiol. 2011;49:4022–3.
24. Nordmann P, Lienhard R, Kieffer N, Clerc O, Poirel L. Plasmid-mediated colistin-resistant *Escherichia coli* in bacteremia in Switzerland. Clin Infect Dis. 2016;62:1322–3.
25. Lubbert C, Faucheux S, Becker-Rux D, Laudi S, Durrbeck A, Busch T, et al. Rapid emergence of secondary resistance to gentamicin and colistin following selective digestive decontamination in patients with KPC-2-producing *Klebsiella pneumoniae*: a single-Centre experience. Int J Antimicrob Agents. 2013;42:565–70.
26. Halaby T, Al Naiemi N, Kluytmans J, van der Palen J, Vandenbroucke-Grauls CM. Emergence of colistin resistance in Enterobacteriaceae after the introduction of selective digestive tract decontamination in an intensive care unit. Antimicrob Agents Chemother. 2013;57:3224–9.
27. Thamlikitkul V, Popum S. Monitoring of effectiveness and safety of Colistin for therapy in resistant gram-negative bacterial infections in hospitalized patients at Siriraj hospital. J Med Assoc Thail. 2016;99:301–7.
28. Eiamphungporn W, Yainoy S, Jumderm C, Tan-arsuwongkul R, Tiengrim S, Thamlikitkul V. Prevalence of colistin resistance gene mcr-1 in colistin-resistant *Escherichia coli* and *Klebsiella pneumoniae* isolated from humans in Thailand. J Glob Antimicrob Resist. 2018; (In press)
29. Quan J, Li X, Chen Y, Jiang Y, Zhou Z, Zhang H, et al. Prevalence of mcr-1 in *Escherichia coli* and *Klebsiella pneumoniae* recovered from bloodstream infections in China: a multicentre longitudinal study. Lancet Infect Dis. 2017; 17:400–10.
30. Xavier BB, Lammens C, Ruhal R, Kumar-Singh S, Butaye P, Goossens H, et al. Identification of a novel plasmid-mediated colistin-resistance gene, mcr-2, in *Escherichia coli*, Belgium, June 2016. Euro Surveill. 2016;21:27.
31. Yin W, Li H, Shen Y, Liu Z, Wang S, Shen Z, et al. Novel plasmid-mediated colistin resistance gene mcr-3 in *Escherichia coli*. MBio. 2017;8(4)
32. Carattoli A, Villa L, Feudi C, Curcio L, Orsini S, Luppi A, et al. Novel plasmid-mediated colistin resistance mcr-4 gene in *Salmonella* and *Escherichia coli*, Italy 2013, Spain and Belgium, 2015 to 2016. Euro Surveill. 2017;22(31)
33. Borowiak M, Fischer J, Hammerl JA, Hendriksen RS, Szabo I, Malorny B. Identification of a novel transposon-associated phosphoethanolamine transferase gene, mcr-5, conferring colistin resistance in d-tartrate fermenting *Salmonella enterica* subsp. enterica serovar Paratyphi B. J Antimicrob Chemother. 2017;72:3317–24.
34. Schimpff SC, Young VM, Greene WH, Vermeulen GD, Moody MR, Wiernik PH. Origin of infection in acute nonlymphocytic leukemia. Significance of hospital acquisition of potential pathogens. Ann Intern Med. 1972;77:707–14.
35. Wingard JR, Dick J, Charache P, Saral R. Antibiotic-resistant bacteria in surveillance stool cultures of patients with prolonged neutropenia. Antimicrob Agents Chemother. 1986;30:435–9.
36. Pena C, Pujol M, Ardanuy C, Ricart A, Pallares R, Linares J, et al. Epidemiology and successful control of a large outbreak due to *Klebsiella pneumoniae* producing extended-spectrum beta-lactamases. Antimicrob Agents Chemother. 1998;42:53–8.
37. Tancrede CH, Andremont AO. Bacterial translocation and gram-negative bacteremia in patients with hematological malignancies. J Infect Dis. 1985; 152:99–103.

23

Attitude and perception of medical interns about antimicrobial resistance

Amanual Getnet Mersha

Abstract

Background: Antibiotic resistance is a global burden and reduction of antimicrobial resistance requires change in antimicrobial prescribing behavior of health workers. The current study aimed to evaluate the attitude and perception of Ethiopian medical interns towards antimicrobials resistance.

Methods: A multi center cross-sectional institutional based survey was conducted from August 2016 to October 2016 among medical interns in Ethiopia. Data entered and analyzed using Statistical Package for Social Sciences program (SPSS) software version 21.0 for Windows. Descriptive statistics, chi-square test and binary logistic regression analysis were used and statistical significance was set at *P-value* < 0.05 as a cut of point.

Results: Out of the 278 questionnaires distributed, 270 were returned completed giving a response rate of 97.1%. Most of the participants 256 (94.8%) wants to receive further education about antimicrobial stewardship. Chi-square test showed a significant difference between institutions about interns' attitude and perception concerning over usage of antimicrobials in their institutions; description of correct antimicrobial coverage; handling patients who demands antimicrobial therapy that is not indicated and finding reliable sources of information to treat infections (*P-value* < 0.05). Attaching at internal medicine wards during the survey and receiving antimicrobial stewardship training during the past 6 months were found to improve their attitude significantly by 2.68 and 3.48 times respectively.

Conclusions: The current study demonstrates an enormous desire of medical interns for further education about antimicrobial stewardship. Hence, it is strongly recommended to provide a comprehensive, regular, standard and up to date educational training in all medical institutions for our future prescribers. Medical institutions and stakeholders are recommended to advocate curriculums and policies that build up antimicrobial stewardship programs.

Keywords: Antimicrobial, Antimicrobial resistance, Medical intern, Education, Ethiopia

Background

Antimicrobials are the most commonly prescribed drugs in developing as well as many developed countries to treat and control infectious disease [1, 2]. Inappropriate use of antibiotics results in bacteria resistant to antibiotics in the community and hospital [3]. Antibiotic resistance is a worldwide problem, with a negative consequence on patient treatment outcomes [4]. Furthermore, patients infected with drug resistant bacterial infection need more expensive intervention, so antimicrobial resistance results in increased health care costs to families and societies [5].

Correspondence: amanuelget16@gmail.com
School of Medicine, College of Medicine and Health Sciences, University of Gondar, P.O. Box: 196, Gondar, Ethiopia

Reducing the burden of antimicrobial resistance is highly challenging in low-income countries than developed countries due to high prevalence of infection, irrational uses of antimicrobials, over-the-counter availability of antibiotics and lack of clinical microbiology laboratories for antimicrobial susceptibility testing in the developing countries [6].

In most countries health care system physicians are responsible for prescribing antibiotics. However, junior medical doctors feel unprepared for the complexity of antibiotic prescribing in their daily practice [7]. Several international studies have identified areas of lack of confidence and gaps in antibiotic prescribing knowledge, and have shown that medical students perceive a need for further education and training on antibiotic prescribing and antimicrobial stewardship program [8]. Education can influence prescribing behavior and can provide knowledge that will enhance the acceptance of stewardship strategies among health care practitioners [9]. In most countries education system, there are no enough antimicrobial resistance education programs at undergraduate level and are still being conducted at the postgraduate level in healthcare institutions [10]. Evidence suggests that a multifaceted approach is favored at improving the organization of the healthcare system and changing physicians' prescribing behavior and practice [11].

Reduction of antimicrobial resistance requires change in antimicrobial prescribing behavior of health workers, antimicrobial prescribing patterns and physicians' behavior towards the magnitude of antimicrobial resistance problem [12]. The World Health Organization has recommended training for medical undergraduates students regarding appropriate prescription of antimicrobials [13]. It is necessary that our future doctors are better equipped with better knowledge, attitude towards antimicrobial use and resistance [14]. Unlike the senior physicians or infectious specialists who have a large amount of experience and knowledge in infection treatment, the junior doctors usually have limited knowledge and skills to reduce the potential risk of antimicrobial resistance [15]. Therefore, antimicrobial stewardship efforts should be made to standardize the prescribing behaviors of medical inters [16].

In Ethiopia, few studies were conducted concerning the prevalence and associated factors of inappropriate use of antibiotic [17, 18]. However, there is no study conducted in Ethiopia to assess the attitude and perception of medical inters towards antimicrobial resistance. Hence, the purpose of this study is to assess the attitude and perception of medical inters on antimicrobial resistance at teaching hospitals in Ethiopia. The information generated in this study would be instrumental in planning and implementing preventive and control interventions on antimicrobial resistance and applying antimicrobial stewardship program at regional and national levels.

Methods

Study design and setting

A multi center cross-sectional institutional based survey was conducted from August 2016 to October 2016 among interns working in three teaching hospitals (hospitals that provide medical education to future health professionals) in Ethiopia. All of the three medical institutes included in the study are tertiary level teaching hospitals with a graduate and post graduate residency programs.

Sample size determination and procedure

A two-stage sampling procedure was employed to select participants of the study. In the first stage, all 11 institutions with practicing interns in Ethiopia were listed and three institutions were randomly selected. In the second stage, the list of practicing interns were taken and participants selected by using a random selection method. To determine the sample size, a single population proportion formula was used with the assumption of 95% confidence interval, 5% margin of error, 50% estimated perceived need of further training about antimicrobial stewardship, and 10% for possible non-response was taken to determine a final sample size of 278. The total sample was proportionally allocated based on the number of interns in each institution (Institution A - 148, Institution B - 151, and Institution C - 145).

Data collection and management

After a thorough review of relevant literatures a structured questionnaire validated to our setting was prepared and reviewed by subject experts [19–22]. The questionnaire is divided into three parts. The first part assesses participants' characteristics including gender, age, AMS training in the last 6 months (trainings that focus on antimicrobial prescribing, appropriate use of antimicrobials, and antimicrobial resistance), and ward distribution during filling the questionnaire. The second part assesses interns' attitude and perception about antimicrobial prescribing and antimicrobial resistance. A 5-point Likert scale, whose responses range from 'strongly agree' to 'strongly disagree' was used to assess their attitude and perception. The third section assessed interns' attitudes and perceptions about their education level about appropriate antimicrobial use and antimicrobial stewardship. In this section also a 5-point Likert scale, whose responses ranged from 'very good' to 'very poor' was used. The questionnaire was pretested on 5% of the sample size prior to the real data collection, which was excluded from the final study, and appropriate modifications were also done.

Statistical analysis

After checking the completeness, the three institutions were de-identified and recoded as "A", "B", and "C". Answer to questions that used a five point Likert scale was condensed in to two classes (agree/strongly agree and neutral/disagree/strongly disagree) and (good/very good and neutral/poor/very poor). Data entered and analyzed using Statistical Package for Social Sciences program (SPSS) software version 21.0 for Windows. The analysis of answers for other questions involved descriptive quantitative statistics described using frequency and percentage. Chi-square tests were applied to compare between sites and statistical significance was set at $P < 0.05$ as a cut of point. Binary logistic regression analysis was employed to assess possible associations between different variables and intern's attitude and perception. To investigate possible associated factors with attitude towards antimicrobial stewardship, agree or strongly agree to four or more of the following six attitude questions (inappropriate use of antimicrobials causes antimicrobial resistance; strong knowledge of antimicrobials is important in my medical career; appropriate use of antimicrobials will reduce problems with antimicrobial-resistant organisms; inappropriate use of antimicrobials can harm patients; poor infection-control practices cause spread of antimicrobial resistance; prescribing broad-spectrum antimicrobials when equally effective narrower-spectrum antimicrobials are available increases antimicrobial resistance) were used as a cut-off point to say "good attitude". Analysis was done by a person who was not involved in the coding process of institutes.

Ethical consideration

This study was approved by the ethical review board of University of Gondar. Written informed consent from the participants was also received before conducting this study. The obtained information from the participants was kept confidential.

Results

Characteristics of the participants

Out of the 278 questionnaires distributed to three centers (Institution A - 93, Institution B – 94, and Institution C - 91), 270 were returned completed giving a response rate of 97.1%. The mean age of participants was 25.21 ± 3.74 years old. Almost one-third of participants 89(32.9%) were female and the remaining 181(67.1%) of respondents were male. Among the participants 31(11.5%) had received antimicrobial stewardship training in the past 6 months before the study. Among the participants 71(26.3%) are working at internal medicine wards; 66(24.4%) are working at pediatrics wards; 64(23.7%) are working at gynecology and obstetrics wards and 69(25.6%) are working at surgical wards.

Attitudes and perceptions about antimicrobial prescribing and resistance

As illustrated in Table 1, 266 (98.5%) of participants perceived that acquiring strong knowledge of antimicrobials is important in their future medical career. The majority of medical interns included in the current study 256 (94.8%) wants to obtain further education regarding antimicrobials resistance. Majority of medical interns believed there are over usage of antimicrobials nationally 245 (90.7%) and 252 (93.3%) of study participants perceive antimicrobials resistance as a national concern. Three-fourth of participants 197 (72.9%) perceived that antimicrobials are being overused in their hospital with differences between educational institutes range from 53 to 89%. Chi-square test was performed to evaluate whether these proportion differences among centers are significance and it was found to be significant (*P - value* of 0.032). About one-third of the interns 82 (30.4%) have a perception that new antimicrobials will be developed that will alleviate the problem of antibiotics resistance with a significant group differences among educational institutions that ranges between 19.3 and 39.8% (*P - value* of 0.021) (Table 1).

Perceptions of medical interns about their educational level towards antimicrobial stewardship

As demonstrates in Table 2, 71 (26.3%) of medical interns believe they can describe the correct range of coverage for antimicrobials. Chi-square test performed among the three institutional groups included in this

Table 1 Medical Interns' attitudes and perceptions about antimicrobial prescribing and resistance

Variables	Agree/strongly Agree N (%)	*P - value*
Inappropriate use of antimicrobials causes antimicrobial resistance	261 (96.6%)	0.071
Strong knowledge of antimicrobials is important in my medical career	266 (98.5%)	0.321
I would like more education on antimicrobials resistance	256 (94.8%)	0.092
Appropriate use of antimicrobials will reduce problems with antimicrobial-resistant organisms	258 (95.5%)	0.135
I would like more education on the appropriate use of antimicrobials	254 (94.0%)	0.219
Antimicrobials are overused nationally	245 (90.7%)	0.319
Inappropriate use of antimicrobials can harm patients	261 (96.6%)	0.424
New antimicrobials will be developed in the future that will keep up with the problem of antibiotics resistance	82 (30.4%)	0.021*
Poor infection-control practices cause spread of antimicrobial resistance	244 (90.4%)	0.950
Antimicrobials are overused in our hospitals	197 (72.9%)	0.032*
Prescribing broad-spectrum antimicrobials when equally effective, narrower-spectrum antimicrobials are available increases antimicrobial resistance	258 (95.5%)	0.670
Antimicrobial resistance is a significant problem in our hospitals	258 (95.5%)	0.561
Antimicrobial resistance is a significant problem nationally	252 (93.3%)	0.862

*Refers to statistically significant differences (*p-value* < 0.05) in the percentages of different teaching hospitals using χ^2 test

Table 2 Medical Interns' perceptions of their education regarding antimicrobial stewardship

Variables	Good/Very Good (%)	*P- value*
Describe the correct range of coverage for antimicrobials	71 (26.3%)	0.014*
Change from intravenous to oral antimicrobials and vice verse	62 (22.9%)	0.821
Handle a patient who demands antimicrobial therapy that is not indicated	80 (29.6%)	0.033*
Escalate antimicrobial therapy	98 (36.3%)	0.662
Select the best antimicrobial for a specific infection	95 (35.2%)	0.431
Find reliable sources of information to treat infections	119 (44.1%)	0.039*
When to start antimicrobial therapy	133 (49.3%)	0.652
Basic mechanisms of antimicrobial resistance	195 (72.2%)	0.238

*Refers to statistically significant differences (*p-value* < 0.05) in the percentages of different teaching hospitals using $\chi2$ test

multicenter study to evaluate whether these proportion differences among centers are significance and was found to be significant (*P - value* of 0.014, range 18.2–31.1%). Among all participants 190(70.4%) interns feel incompetent to handle a patient who demands antimicrobial therapy while it is not indicated with a significant group differences (*P - value* of 0.033, range 56.9–81.2%). Among the participants 119 (44.1%) of interns believe they can found reliable sources of information to treat infections with significant differences between institutes (*P - value* of 0.039, range 31.9–50.9%) (Table 2).

Factors associated with better attitudes and perceptions towards antimicrobial stewardship

Logistic regression analysis was employed to assess possible associations between different variables and intern's attitude and perception. According to the results from bivariate logistic regression, there were statistically significant differences in age, sex, ward attachment during the study period and receiving antimicrobial stewardship training. Variables that were significantly associated with the intern's attitude and perception in the bivariate analysis (*p*-value < 0.2) were further examined in multivariate logistic regression. Accordingly, ward attachment during the study period and receiving antimicrobial stewardship training in the past 6 months remained to be significant in the multivariate logistic model. The odds of having good attitude and perception about antimicrobial stewardship was found to have 2.68 times higher among interns attached at internal medicine wards during the data collection than interns attached at surgical wards (AOR = 2.68, 95% CI = 1.73–7.19, *p*-value - 0.032). Receiving antimicrobial stewardship training during the past 6 months was found to be 3.48 folds associated with good attitude towards antimicrobial stewardship(AOR = 3.48, 95% CI = 2.97–5.31, *p*-value - 0.006) (Table 3).

Discussion

Antimicrobial resistance imposes a substantial public health burden all around the globe [1]. In the current study, the vast majority of medical interns believed that antimicrobial resistance is a main concern in their hospitals as well as in the nation at large. A considerable number of participants reported over usage of antimicrobials nationally. Interestingly, a quarter of participants reported absence of antimicrobial over usage in their hospitals with a statistically significant difference between the participating institutions (*p-value,* 0.032). This result is in line with a study conducted in seven European medical schools which reported that majority of the participants (92%) believe antimicrobial resistance as a national concern [23]. Similarly, a study done at three US medical schools also reported majority (94%) of participants believe presence of antimicrobial usage nationally and 65% believe over usage in their hospital with substantial difference among medical schools [19].

Substantial number of participants perceived that strong knowledge of antimicrobials is important in their

Table 3 Factors Associated with better attitudes and perceptions about Antimicrobial stewardship

Variable	N (%)	AOR(95% CI)	*P-value*
Age (25.21 ± 3.74 years old)			0.091
Sex			0.280
Male	181(67.1%)		
Female	89 (32.9%)		
Ward attachments during the study		2.68 (1.73–7.19)	0.032*
Internal Medicine	71 (26.3%)		
Pediatrics	66 (24.4%)		
Gynecology and Obstetrics	64 (23.7%)		
Surgery	69 (25.6%)		
Interns who received AMS training during the past 6 months		3.48 (2.97–5.31)	0.006*
Yes	31 (11.5%)		
No	239 (88.5%)		

* Refers to statistically significant association

medical career and they would like to gain further education on antimicrobials use and resistance. Other studies conducted among medical students and junior physicians in china, USA, and Europe also come up with similar findings [14, 19, 23]. Less than one third of interns believed new antimicrobials will be developed that will alleviate the problem of antibiotics resistance with significant differences among educational institutes (*p-value,* 0.021). A multi-center study done in central China also reported a significant difference among participating medical schools regarding development of new antimicrobials [14]. .This could be due to lack of a standardized, comprehensive, and up to date training concerning antimicrobial stewardship.

One of the main components of reducing antibiotic resistance is administering a specific antimicrobial to cover a specific organism. This study demonstrated that only a quarter of interns believe they can describe the correct range of coverage for antimicrobials with a significant difference between institutions (*p-value,* 0.014). This finding is comparable with study done in other countries [14, 19]. Furthermore, less than a quarter believes they know when to switch from intravenous to oral antimicrobials and vice verse. Proportionally higher number of participants lacks confidence selecting the best antimicrobial for a specific infection. Medical schools are recommended to develop a locally validated protocols concerning switching from intravenous to oral antimicrobials and vice verse [24–26].

.Having a basic understanding of the mechanisms for the development of antimicrobial resistance and finding a reliable source of information to treat infections is vital to challenge the evolving issue of antimicrobial resistance. In the current study, almost three fourth of participants believe they have basic knowledge of mechanisms of antimicrobial resistance. Less than half of the interns believe they can find reliable sources of information to treat infections with statistically significant variation among the different sites (*p-value,* 0.039). This difference may be partially explained by variation in internet access and difference in curriculum interpretation between institutions.

Handling patients who demands antimicrobial therapy without any indication is also vital to reduce the inappropriate use of antimicrobials. Substantial number of participants lacks confidence on how to handle a patient who demands antimicrobial treatment while it is not indicated with a statistically significant difference among study institutions (*p-value,* 0.033). The significant difference between institutions may be due to differences in type of clients visiting the institutions [9, 27]. In Ethiopia medical students receive a detailed lectures and seminars concerning antibiotics, mechanisms of antibiotic resistance and preventing strategies of resistance as part of Pharmacology course in their pre-clinical year. A multi center survey conducted in South Africa illustrated the existence of a huge training gap among final year medical students [28]. The odds of having good attitudes and perceptions about antimicrobial resistance among interns attached at internal medicine wards were found to have 2.68 times better attitudes and perceptions about antimicrobial resistance than interns attached at surgical wards. It could be due to differences in the types of patients admitted at medical and surgical wards. Most of the patients admitted at medical wards in developed countries have infectious disease. Hence, interns at medical wards tend to know more about antimicrobial resistance. Interns who received antimicrobial stewardship training during the past 6 months tends to have better attitudes and perceptions about antimicrobial resistance then those interns who didn't receive training in the 6 month period before the study. This result is in line with other studies conducted among a Varity of communities. In one randomized controlled trial conducted among general practitioners of France, standardized educational seminar on antibiotic improve the irrational prescription of antimicrobials [29, 30].

Strength and limitation of the study

This study highlights an area of antimicrobial stewardship where there is lack of literature in Ethiopia. Yet, the survey has some limitations that should be taken into account while interpreting the results. As the study was a cross-sectional survey conducted in only three institutions, caution should be exercised when generalizing the findings. Even with the above limitations, this survey has significant implications for combating antimicrobial resistance.

Conclusion and Recommendation

The current study demonstrates an enormous desire of medical interns for further education about antimicrobials stewardship. Medical interns believe the gained education concerning appropriate antimicrobial use and antimicrobial stewardship is not enough. Based on our finding we recommend that medical interns should acquire a comprehensive, regular, scheduled and up to date educational training on antimicrobial stewardship so as to answer their educational demand and to combat the issue of antimicrobial resistance by endowing the young physicians with sufficient knowledge. It is recommended to medical institutions and other stakeholders to advocate curriculums and policies that build up antimicrobial stewardship programs in the country. An arrangement should be made that can prepare and disseminate locally validated antimicrobial use guidelines with commonly available antimicrobials in the institution.

Abbreviations
AM: Antimicrobial; AMR: Antimicrobial Resistance

Acknowledgements
The author acknowledges the Support of University of Gondar and all the study participants.

Funding
No financial support was gained to conduct this study.

Author's contribution
AGM the principal investigator of the study involved in conceptualization, study design, data collection, design, and writing the manuscript. The author read and approved the final manuscript.

Consent for publication
Not applicable.

Competing interests
The author declares that he has no competing interests.

References
1. van Bijnen EM, den Heijer CD, Paget WJ, Stobberingh EE, Verheij RA, Bruggeman CA, et al. The appropriateness of prescribing antibiotics in the community in Europe: study design. BMC Infect Dis. 2011;11:293. https://doi.org/10.1186/1471-2334-11-293.
2. Cagri Buke A, Ermertcan S, Hosgor-Limoncu M, Ciceklioglu M, Eren S. Rational antibiotic use and academic staff. Int J Antimicrob Agents. 2003; 21(1):63–6.
3. Costelloe C, Metcalfe C, Lovering A, Mant D, Hay AD. Effect of antibiotic prescribing in primary care on antimicrobial resistance in individual patients: systematic review and meta-analysis. Bmj. 2010;340:c2096. https://doi.org/10.1136/bmj.c2096.
4. Cosgrove SE. The relationship between antimicrobial resistance and patient outcomes: mortality, length of hospital stay, and health care costs. Clin Infect Dis. 2006;42(Suppl 2):S82–9. https://doi.org/10.1086/499406.
5. Coast J, Smith RD, Millar MR. Superbugs: should antimicrobial resistance be included as a cost in economic evaluation? Health Econ. 1996;5(3):217–26. https://doi.org/10.1002/(sici)1099-1050(199605)5:3<217::aid-hec200>3.0.co;2-s.
6. Vila J, Pal T. Update on antibacterial resistance in low-income countries: factors favoring the emergence of resistance. Open Infec Dis J. 2010;4:38–54. https://doi.org/10.2174/1874279301004020038.
7. Mattick K, Kelly N, Rees C. A window into the lives of junior doctors: narrative interviews exploring antimicrobial prescribing experiences. J Antimicrob Chemother. 2014;69(8):2274–83. https://doi.org/10.1093/jac/dku093.
8. Pulcini C, Gyssens IC. How to educate prescribers in antimicrobial stewardship practices. Virulence. 2013;4(2):192–202. https://doi.org/10.4161/viru.23706.
9. Dellit TH, Owens RC, McGowan JE Jr, Gerding DN, Weinstein RA, Burke JP, et al. Infectious Diseases Society of America and the Society for Healthcare Epidemiology of America guidelines for developing an institutional program to enhance antimicrobial stewardship. Clin Infect Dis. 2007;44(2): 159–77. https://doi.org/10.1086/510393.
10. Ohl CA, Luther VP. Health care provider education as a tool to enhance antibiotic stewardship practices. Infect Dis Clin N Am. 2014;28(2):177–93. https://doi.org/10.1016/j.idc.2014.02.001.
11. Davey P, Marwick CA, Scott CL, Charani E, McNeil K, Brown E, et al. Interventions to improve antibiotic prescribing practices for hospital inpatients. Cochrane Database Syst Rev. 2017;2:Cd003543. https://doi.org/10.1002/14651858.CD003543.pub4.
12. Pulcini C, Williams F, Molinari N, Davey P, Nathwani D. Junior doctors' knowledge and perceptions of antibiotic resistance and prescribing: a survey in France and Scotland. Clin Microbiol Infect. 2011;17(1):80–7. https://doi.org/10.1111/j.1469-0691.2010.03179.x.
13. World Health Organization. The evolving threat of antimicrobial resistance: options for action: executive summary: World Health Organization; 2012. http://apps.who.int/iris/bitstream/handle/10665/44812/9789241503181_eng.pdf;sequence=1.
14. Yang K, Wu D, Tan F, Shi S, Guo X, Min Q, et al. Attitudes and perceptions regarding antimicrobial use and resistance among medical students in Central China. Springerplus. 2016;5(1):1779. https://doi.org/10.1186/s40064-016-3454-0.
15. Charani E, Cooke J, Holmes A. Antibiotic stewardship programmes--what's missing? J Antimicrob Chemother. 2010;65(11):2275–7. https://doi.org/10.1093/jac/dkq357.
16. Hecker MT, Aron DC, Patel NP, Lehmann MK, Donskey CJ. Unnecessary use of antimicrobials in hospitalized patients: current patterns of misuse with an emphasis on the antianaerobic spectrum of activity. Arch Intern Med. 2003; 163(8):972–8. https://doi.org/10.1001/archinte.163.8.972.
17. Erku DA, Mekuria AB, Belachew SA. Inappropriate use of antibiotics among communities of Gondar town, Ethiopia: a threat to the development of antimicrobial resistance. Antimicrob Resist Infect Control. 2017;6:112. https://doi.org/10.1186/s13756-017-0272-2.
18. Gebeyehu E, Bantie L, Azage M. Inappropriate use of antibiotics and its associated factors among urban and rural communities of Bahir Dar City Administration, Northwest Ethiopia. PLoS One. 2015;10(9):e0138179. https://doi.org/10.1371/journal.pone.0138179.
19. Abbo LM, Cosgrove SE, Pottinger PS, Pereyra M, Sinkowitz-Cochran R, Srinivasan A, Hooton TM. Medical students' perceptions and knowledge about antimicrobial stewardship: how are we educating our future prescribers? Clin Infect Dis. 2013;57(5):631–8. https://doi.org/10.1093/cid/cit370.
20. Justo JA, Gauthier TP, Scheetz MH, Chahine EB, Bookstaver PB, Gallagher JC, et al. Knowledge and attitudes of doctor of pharmacy students regarding the appropriate use of antimicrobials. Clin Infect Dis. 2014;59(Suppl 3):S162–9. https://doi.org/10.1093/cid/ciu537.
21. Khan AKA, Banu G, Reshma KK. Antibiotic resistance and usage-a survey on the knowledge, attitude, perceptions and practices among the medical students of a southern Indian teaching hospital. J Clin Diagn Res. 2013;7(8): 1613–6. https://doi.org/10.7860/jcdr/2013/6290.3230.
22. Andre M, Vernby A, Berg J, Lundborg CS. A survey of public knowledge and awareness related to antibiotic use and resistance in Sweden. J Antimicrob Chemother. 2010;65(6):1292–6. https://doi.org/10.1093/jac/dkq104.
23. Dyar OJ, Pulcini C, Howard P, Nathwani D. European medical students: a first multicentre study of knowledge, attitudes and perceptions of antibiotic prescribing and antibiotic resistance. J Antimicrob Chemother. 2014;69(3): 842–6. https://doi.org/10.1093/jac/dkt440.
24. Subramanian A, Adhimoolam M, Kannan S. Study of drug-drug interactions among the hypertensive patients in a tertiary care teaching hospital. Perspect Clin Res. 2018;9(1):9–14. https://doi.org/10.4103/picr.PICR_145_16.
25. Davey P, Garner S. Professional education on antimicrobial prescribing: a report from the specialist advisory committee on antimicrobial resistance (SACAR) professional education subgroup. J Antimicrob Chemother. 2007; 60(Suppl 1):i27–32. https://doi.org/10.1093/jac/dkm154.
26. Brink A, Schoeman J, Muntingh G. Undergraduate antibiotic stewardship training: are we leaving our future prescribers 'flapping in the wind. S Afr Med J. 2017;107(5):357–8. https://doi.org/10.7196/SAMJ.2017.v107i5.12496.
27. Gauthier TP, Lantz E, Heyliger A, Francis SM, Smith L. Internet-based institutional antimicrobial stewardship program resources in leading US academic medical centers. Clin Infect Dis. 2014;58(3):445–6. https://doi.org/10.1093/cid/cit705.
28. Wasserman S, Potgieter S, Shoul E, Constant D, Stewart A, Mendelson M, Boyles TH. South African medical students' perceptions and knowledge about antibiotic resistance and appropriate prescribing: are we providing adequate training to future prescribers? S Afr Med J. 2017;107(5):405–10. https://doi.org/10.7196/SAMJ.2017.v107i5.12370.
29. Little P, Stuart B, Francis N, Douglas E, Tonkin-Crine S, Anthierens S, Yardley L. Effects of internet-based training on antibiotic prescribing rates for acute respiratory-tract infections: a multinational, cluster, randomised, factorial, controlled trial. Lancet. 2013;382(9899):1175–82. https://doi.org/10.1016/s0140-6736(13)60994-0.
30. Le Corvoisier P, Renard V, Roudot-Thoraval F, Cazalens T, Veerabudun K, Canoui-Poitrine F, Attali C. Long-term effects of an educational seminar on antibiotic prescribing by GPs: a randomised controlled trial. Br J Gen Pract. 2013;63(612):e455–64. https://doi.org/10.3399/bjgp13X669176.

24

Travel to Asia is a strong predictor for carriage of cephalosporin resistant *E. coli* and *Klebsiella spp.* but does not explain everything; prevalence study at a Norwegian hospital 2014–2016

Laura Espenhain[1,2*], Silje Bakken Jørgensen[3], Truls Michael Leegaard[3,4], Michaela Marie Lelek[3], Siri Haug Hänsgen[3], Britt Nakstad[4,5], Marianne Sunde[6,7] and Martin Steinbakk[1]

Abstract

Background: We aimed to estimate the prevalence of faecal carriage of extended-spectrum cephalosporin (ESC) resistant *E. coli* and *K. pneumoniae* (ESCr-EK) and vancomycin resistant enterococci (VRE) in patients upon hospital admission and identify factors associated with carriage to better target interventions and to guide empirical antibiotic treatment.

Methods: Between October 2014 and December 2016, we recruited patients admitted to a Norwegian university hospital. A rectal swab and questionnaire covering possible risk factors for colonisation were collected upon admission. Isolates were characterized by phenotypic methods. ESCr-EK isolates were subject to whole genome sequencing. We calculated prevalence and adjusted prevalence ratios (aPR) using binomial regression.

Results: Of 747 patients, 45 (6.0%) were colonised with ESCr-EK, none with VRE. The ESCr-EK isolates in 41 patients were multidrug resistant; no isolates were non-suceptible to meropenem. Prevalence of ESCr-EK was higher among travellers to Asia (aPR = 6.6; 95%CI 3.6–12; $p < 0.001$). No statistical significant difference in carriage was observed between departments, age or any other factors in the univariable analyses.

Conclusions: The observed prevalence of ESCr-EK colonisation upon admission was in the same range but lower than that reported in similar studies from Europe. Travel to Asia was a strong predictor for colonisation of ESCr-EK to be considered when administering empirical antimicrobial treatment. As less than one third of colonised patients had travelled to Asia, and no other factors investigated were found to be strongly associated with carriage, these findings underscore that healthcare personnel must apply standard infection control precautions for all patients.

Keywords: Prevalence, Beta-lactam resistance, Hospitals, university, Cross-sectional, Studies, Enterobacteriaceae, Epidemiology, Drug resistance, multiple

* Correspondence: laura_espenhain@hotmail.com
[1]Department of Antibiotic Resistance and Infection Prevention, Norwegian Institute of Public Health, PO Box 222 Skøyen, 0213 Oslo, NO, Norway
[2]European Programme for Intervention Epidemiology Training (EPIET), European Centre for Disease Prevention and Control, (ECDC), Stockholm, Sweden
Full list of author information is available at the end of the article

Background

Escherichia coli and other *Enterobacteriaceae* frequently cause nosocomial and community acquired infections [1] and the burden due to infection with *Enterobacteriaceae* resistant to extended-spectrum cephalosporins (ESC) is increasing worldwide [2]. Infections are often preceded by colonisation of the gut with these bacteria. Among *Enterobacteriaceae*, resistance to ESC is often caused by production of extended-spectrum beta-lactamases (ESBLs) or plasmid mediated AmpC (pAmpC) [2]. In a hospital setting, carriage of *Enterobacteriaceae* resistant to ESC (ESCr-E) is not only a concern for the individual patient, but also for the surrounding patients as these bacteria can spread via the faecal-oral route between patients within the hospital [3]. In addition, plasmids conferring ESC resistance can be transferred between different bacterial strains and species. Outbreaks of ESBL-producing *E. coli* and *Klebsiella spp.* have been reported in healthcare institutions in Norway [4–6]. Yet another concern is that ESC-resistance often occurs along with co-resistance to important non-beta-lactam antibiotic classes [7], significantly limiting treatment options for these patients.

Enterobacteriaceae are part of the normal gut flora and pose a complex challenge as eradication is problematic [8]. If introduced within a hospital, infection prevention and control rely on strict compliance to standard precautions [3, 9]. The Norwegian Institute of Public Health (NIPH) recommends isolation of patients in general hospital wards if they carry carbapenemase producing *Enterobacteriaceae* or vancomycin resistant enterococci. Patients who carry ESC resistant *Enterobacteriaceae* should be isolated if admitted to departments with particularly vulnerable patients (neonatal, cancer or intensive care units) [10]. Even though the Nordic countries have a low prevalence of antimicrobial resistance among *Enterobacteriaceae*, resistance to ESC in *E. coli* and *Klebsiella ssp* in urine and blood specimens is increasing [11]. In order to better target interventions to prevent spread between patients and to guide empirical antibiotic treatment we aimed to estimate the prevalence of faecal carriage of ESC resistant *E. coli* and *K. pneumoniae* (ESCr-EK) and vancomycin resistant enterococci (VRE) in patients upon hospital admission, and to identify factors associated with carriage. Additionally we aimed to explore the diversity of ESCr-EK and determine the genetic background for resistance to ESC.

Methods

Design, setting and study population

The cross-sectional study was carried out at Akershus University Hospital, a secondary care facility located in a mixed urban and rural area east of the Norwegian capital Oslo. The catchment area covers around 10% (500,000 persons) of the Norwegian population. Trained nurses recruited patients upon admission. In the adult's emergency department, recruitment took place on selected weekdays between October 2014 and July 2015, all patients presenting between 8 am and 11 am were invited to participate. In the children's emergency department, all patients/parents admitted during selected weeks in the period between January 2015and July 2016 were invited to participate. From October 2015 to December 2016 recruitment was expanded to three surgical units (thoracic, urology, and orthopaedic) where all patients presenting for pre-surgical examination prior to elective surgery were invited to participate.

Patients with suspected acute coronary disease, in need of immediate intensive care, and adult patients unable to give informed consent were not recruited.

Data collection

Consenting patients or parents of patients below 16 years of age completed a questionnaire with 26 questions, including demographics and possible risk factors for colonisation with ESCr-EK such as travel outside of the Nordic countries, antibiotic consumption, health care and medical devices within the 12 months prior to recruitment. Only information about risk factors prior to admission was collected. One rectal swab was collected at admission or maximum 24 h after admission.

Microbiology

Rectal swabs were collected and transported in liquid medium (eSwab, Copan, Italy). The samples were stored at 4 °C for maximum 14 h, with subsequent plating on blood agar for growth control, and on two selective lactose agar plates with the addition of either 1 mg/ml cefotaxime or 1 mg/ml ceftazidime for detection of ESCr-EK, produced in-house. For the detection of vancomycin resistant Enterococci, we used Brilliance VRE plates (Oxoid, ThermoFisher Scientific, MA, USA). Morphologically distinct colonies from each selective plate were subcultured, and identified by MALDI-TOF mass spectrometry (MALDI-TOF, Bruker Daltonics, Bremen, Germany). Isolates of *E. coli* or *Klebsiella* spp. were frozen at -80 °C for later analysis. We did susceptibility disk testing and interpretation of clinical breakpoints according to EUCAST methodology (http://www.eucast.org/fileadmin/src/media/PDFs/EUCAST_files/Breakpoint_tables/Breakpoint_table_v_4.0.xls, 2017), and divided the antibacterial agents into six classes: Penicillins (Ampicillin), cephalosporins and penicillins in combination with betalactam-inhibitors (cefoxitin, cefotaxime, ceftazidime and piperacillin-tazobactam), carbapenems (meropenem), (fluoro)quinolones (ciprofloxacine and nalidixin), aminoglycosides (gentamicin), and folate-pathway inhibitors (trimethoprim-sulphamethoxazole). We defined multidrug resistance as non-susceptibility (i.e. resistant or intermediate susceptible) to three or more of the above antibiotic classes.

From each patient positive for ESCr-EK, one isolate was selected for whole genome sequencing (WGS). If the patient carried both ESC resistant *E. coli* and *Klebsiella spp.*, one isolate per species was included for WGS. Furthermore, if a patient carried several morphologically different strains of the same species, and if the strains had different antimicrobial susceptibility patterns (indicative of polyclonal carriage), one representative isolate for each pattern was included for WGS. WGS was done with Illumina technology (Illumina, San-Diego, USA), and data were analysed on the publicly available platform at the Center for Genomic Epidemiology [12]. Default threshold settings were used for MLST and ResFinder [13, 14].

Statistical analysis

We expressed the prevalence of ESCr-EK upon admission as the number of patients positive for ESCr-EK per 100 patients enrolled in the study. For the descriptive analysis, and to evaluate independent factors associated with colonisation we performed uni- and multivariable binominal regression analyses. We grouped countries into five regions (Europe, Asia, Americas, Africa and Australia). The category "Asia" included countries in the Middle-East as well as Central and East Asia (listed in Additional file 1). In the multivariable analyses variables with a p-value of < 0.2 were included in the model one by one starting with the factor with the highest prevalence ratio. Model fit was evaluated using the likelihood-ratio test. P-values < 0.05 were considered significant. Health care outside of the Nordic countries, included in the national screening guidelines, was included in the final model irrespective of level of significance.

Human subject protection

Informed consent was obtained from each patient or parents of patients below 16 years of age. The Regional Committees for Medical and Health Research Ethics (REC 2012/2234) and the hospital's privacy protection officer approved the study protocol. The study was funded by the NIPH.

Results

Participation

In total, 747 rectal swabs accompanied by a completed questionnaire were collected from patients upon admission. Among the participants, 391 (52%) participants were male, ranging from 43% in the orthopaedic unit to 62% in the urology unit. Twenty per cent were below three years of age and 39% were 65 years or older. An estimate of 84% of patients invited to participate accepted.

Microbiology

Patients

Of the 747 rectal swabs, 45 (6.0%) contained one or more isolate resistant to cefotaxime and/or ceftazidime. *E. coli* was found in 43 of the 45 samples and *K. pneumoniae* in five, i.e. both ESC resistant *E. coli* and *K. pneumoniae* were identified in three samples. Co-resistance to fluoroquinolones, piperacillin-tazobactam and gentamicin was observed in ESCr-EK isolates from 39, 11 and 10 patients, respectively. The ESCr-EK isolates in 41 patients were multidrug resistant. No patients carried isolates non-susceptible to meropenem. Carriage of vancomycin resistant enterococci was not detected in any of the participants.

Isolates

In total, 57 ESCr-EK isolates from the 45 ESCr-EK carriers were subject to WGS. Among these, 51 isolates from 42 patients harboured one or more ESBL genes of the bla_{CTX-M} groups (5.6% of all patients) and five isolates from four patients harboured pAmpC genes (bla_{DHA-1} or bla_{CMY-42}) (Table 1). In one patient both bla_{CTX-M} and bla_{DHA-1} were identified in different isolates. One isolate harboured both $bla_{CTX-M-15}$ and bla_{CMY-42}. In two isolates, one *E. coli* and one *K. pneumoniae*, ResFinder v3.0 (accessed July 27th 2018) did not detect any resistance mechanism to explain ESC resistance.

Among the 57 isolates that were subject to WGS, 25 different MLSTs were identified in *E.coli* and two in *K. pneumoniae*. One fourth of the *E. coli* [14] belonged to ST131 (Table 2). Three patients carried several *E. coli* strains with different MLSTs. Nine MLSTs (34, 83, 93, 99, 349, 398, 410, 485, and 617) were found only in patients who had solely travelled to Asia.

Epidemiology

In the univariable analyses (Table 3), we observed a significantly higher prevalence of ESCr-EK in patients who had travelled to Asia (33%) compared with those who had not travelled to Asia (4.5%), in patients who had travelled outside of the Nordic countries (11%) compared to patients who had not (3.9%), and in patients

Table 1 Genotypes of ESCr-EK isolates ($n = 52$ E.coli and 5 *K. pneumoniae*) from 45 ESCr-EK carriers

Enzyme	gene identified	*E. coli*	*K. pneumoniae*
ESBL	$bla_{CTX-M-15}$	28	1
	$bla_{CTX-M-55}$	6	
	$bla_{CTX-M-27}$	6	
	bla_{OXA-1}[a]	8	
	$bla_{CTX-M-14(+b)}$	5	
	$bla_{CTX-M-1}$	4	
	$bla_{CTX-M-3}$	1	1
	bla_{TEM-33}	1	
pAmpC	bla_{DHA-1}	2	2
	bla_{CMY-42}	1	
Uncertain	None detected	1	1

[a]bla_{-OXA-1} always occurring in isolates also harbouring $bla_{CTX-M-15}$

Table 2 Distribution of MLST types ESCr-EK isolates ($n = 52$ E.coli and 5 K. pneumoniae) from 45 ESCr-EK carriers

MLST type	*E. coli*	*K. pneumoniae*
131	14	
38	5	
405	4	
10	2	
34	2	
69	2	
83	2	
357	2	
648	2	
Unknown MLST[a]	2	3
Other MLST types[b]	15	2
Total	52	5

[a]MLST not resolved
b*E. coli*: MLST48, 73, 93, 99, 167, 394, 398, 410, 485, 617, 1163, 1193, 1611, 1722, 3036. *K. pneumoniae*: MLST37, 1427

who had received health care outside the Nordic countries (14%) compared to those who had not (5.6%). A higher, but non-significant, prevalence was observed in patients born outside Norway (11%) compared to patients born in Norway (5.9%), and in those who had travelled to Africa (18%) compared to those who had not (5.8%). No statistical significant difference in carriage was observed between departments of recruitment or age in years or age group or any other factors in the univariable analyses (Table 3).

In the multivariable analyses, travel to Asia was the only factor associated with carriage. Health care outside the Nordic countries was also included in the reported model as it is part of the national screening recommendations. The binominal regression analysis showed that travellers to Asia had a significantly higher prevalence of ESCr-EK carriage compared to those who had not travelled (PR 6.1; 95% CI 3.4–11; $p < 0.001$) (Table 4). Travel to Asia was primarily to Thailand ($n = 17$), Turkey ($n = 17$), and Pakistan ($n = 6$).

Discussion

In this study, including 747 patients from two emergency departments and three surgical units, we found no *E.coli* or *Klebsiella spp.* resistant to carbapenems, and no vancomycin resistant enterococci. The prevalence of colonisation of ESCr-EK upon admission was 6.0%. A major predictor for colonisation was travel to Asia. However, the majority of colonised patients had not been to Asia 12 months prior to admission.

The observed prevalence of ESCr-EK (6.0%) and ESBL-EK colonisation (5.6%) at admission was in the same range but lower than reported in similar studies from Germany (7.5–9.5%) [15], the Netherlands (8.2%) [16], and Israel (10.8%) [17] and slightly higher than previously reported in healthy individuals in Sweden (4.7%) [18] and Norway (4.9%) [19]. Varying methods and definitions challenge direct comparison between studies and this may, at least in part, explain these differences between countries. Other explanations may be differences in age, ethnicity, co-morbidity, previous hospital admissions or a true lower prevalence upon admission in the Norwegian population compared to the prevalence in the Netherlands, Germany or Israel. To our knowledge, there has been no previous Norwegian studies of ESBL prevalence in patients at admittance to hospital.

Self-reported use of antibiotics has been found to be a risk factor for ESC-E colonisation at admission in Germany [15]. We could not confirm this finding, nor could studies from the Netherlands [16] and Sweden [18]. Differing antibiotic-prescription policies may be one explanation for this. It was not possible to perform stratified analyses on antibiotics class as one third of participants who had used antibiotics 12 months prior to the admission did not indicate which class.

Consistent with other studies, visiting Asia within 12 months prior to faecal sampling, was associated with ESCr-EK colonisation (PR 6.8, $p < 0.001$). Prevalence ranging from 13 to 45% has been found in Swedish [18, 20] and Danish [21] travellers to Asia. In accordance with our study, none of these studies found carbapenem-resistant *Enterobacteriaceae*. However, the methods we used were not optimised to detect carbapenemases like OXA-48, which do not also confer resistance to cefotaxime or ceftazidime. The higher prevalence in patients who had travelled to Asia is also consistent with results from prevalence studies from Asia (Pakistan [22], Thailand [23–25], Turkey [26]) on different populations and types of specimens, where a prevalence of up to 40–77% has been reported even in healthy adults and food products.

This study covers a convenience sample of a population utilizing the hospital. We recruited patients from two emergency departments and three elective surgery units, and a wide range of ages from infancy to elderly patients. It was not practically feasible to recruit critically ill patients admitted to intensive care units in the hospital. Hence, we do not describe the prevalence of ESCr-EK in units with patients at the higher risk for a severe outcome if colonised with resistant bacteria. The prevalence tended to be higher amongst patients who reported having received health care outside of the Nordic countries. However, there were not enough patients in this category to give sufficient power to quantify a difference. The data collected was not detailed to a level allowing for stratification on type of health care (hospital admission, dental care, primary health care, etc.).

Table 3 Number of patients, carriers, percent carriers, crude prevalence ratio (PR) and *p*-values from the univariable binominal regressions by risk factors for ESCr-EK carriage up to 12 months prior to admission ($n = 747$)

		Total no. of patients	Carriage of ESCr-EK		Prevalence ratio (PR)	*p*-value
			No. of patients	(%)		
		747	45	(6.0%)		
Demography	Female	356	16	(4.5%)		
	Male	391	29	(7.4%)	1.65	0.10
	0-17 year	222	11	(4.9%)		
	18 - 64 years	233	18	(7.7%)	1.81	0.10
	65 + years	292	16	(5.5%)	1.17	0.67
	Born in Norway	675	40	(5.9%)		
	Not born in Norway	45	5	(11.1%)	1.88	0.16
	Parents born in Norway	593	35	(5.9%)		
	One or both parents not born in Norway	114	8	(7.0%)	1.19	0.65
Department of inclusion	Emergency department (adult)	122	11	(9.0%)		
	Emergency department (children)	222	11	(4.9%)	0.56	0.14
	Thoracic unit	194	11	(5.7%)	0.63	0.26
	Orthopaedic unit	141	7	(5.0%)	0.56	0.20
	Urology unit	68	5	(7.3%)	0.81	0.69
Exposures 12 months prior to admission	No travel outside of the Nordic countries[a]	512	20	(3.9%)	0.37	0.00
	Travel to Europe (vs. no travel to Europe)	175	11	(6.3%)	1.1	0.87
	Travel to America (vs. no travel to America)	22	1	(4.6%)	0.75	0.77
	Travel to Africa (vs. no travel to Africa)	11	2	(18.2%)	3.11	0.08
	Travel to Asia (vs. no travel to Asia)	51	15	(29.4%)	6.82	0.00
	No health care (vs. health care)	499	32	(6.4%)	0.82	0. 55
	Admitted to a Norwegian hospital[b]	224	11	(4.9%)	0.81	0.55
	Medical examination or treatment outside the Nordic countries[c]	28	4	(14.3%)	2.54	0.05
	Work in health care (vs. other type of job)	38	3	(7.9%)	0.95	0.94
	Work in farming	11	0	(0.0%)	-	-
	Other type of job	193	16	(8.3%)		
	No contact to animals at work	188	17	(9.0%)		
	Contact to animals at work	22	1	(4.5%)	0.50	0.49
	No permanent urinary catheter	668	40	(6.0%)		
	Permanent urinary catheter	10	0	(0.0%)	-	-
	No medical devices put through skin/mucosa before admission	639	39	(6.1%)		
	Medical devices put through skin/mucosa	46	2	(4.3%)	0.71	0.63
	No wound or skin infections	616	34	(5.5%)		
	Wound or skin infections	76	6	(7.9%)	1.43	0.40
	No antibiotic consumption	515	28	(5.4%)		
	Antibiotic consumption	232	17	(7.3%)	1.35	0.31

[a](vs. travel outside of the Nordic countries)
[b](vs. not admitted to a Norwegian hospital)
[c](vs. no medical examination or treatment outside the Nordic countries)

Table 4 Number of patients, carriers and adjusted prevalence ratio (aPR), 95% CI and *p*-values from the multivariable binominal regression model by risk factors for ESCr-EK carriage up to 12 months prior to admission ($n = 741$)

	Total	Number of ESCr-EK carriers	aPR	95% CI	*p*-value
Number of patients	741	44			
Travel to Asia the past 12 months	50	14	6.1	(3.43–11)	< 0.001
Medical examination or treatment outside the Nordic countries	28	4	1.7	(0.74–3.9)	0.212

aPR Adjusted prevalence ratio

The genetic mechanisms behind ESC resistance was mainly ESBL production due to $bla_{CTX\text{-}M}$. Only two ESCr-EK could not be explained by ESBL or pAmpC production. We found a large diversity of MLSTs in the 45 patients carrying ESCr-EK, making comparison with previous findings challenging. Sixteen different MLSTs were found in patients who had travelled to Asia, nine of these were found in travellers who had only been in Asia. However, many of these MLSTs represent well-known clones that have been found in various sources in several countries, including in Norway [7]. The dominant ESBL allele was $bla_{CTX\text{-}M\text{-}15}$ which has emerged and disseminated worldwide [27] and has previously been found in travellers returning from all over the world [20], and in environmental samples from our area [7]. The ESBL allele $bla_{CTX\text{-}M\text{-}55}$ has been found to be one of the most commonly encountered ESBL-encoding genes in *Enterobacteriaceae* from food animals in China and has also been found in food animals in Europe together with other CTX-M types [28, 29] suggesting the potential importance of animal-to-human spread via contaminated food [20].

In our study, travel to Asia was primarily to Thailand and Pakistan. We expect that travel to other high endemic areas in Asia like India, or to Africa as found in other studies [18, 20], might also be a risk factor for colonisation as also indicated in our study. All the ESCr-EK isolates from patients who had travelled to Asia were multidrug resistant.

Urinary tract infections and bacteraemia are often preceded by colonisation of the gut [17, 30]. As more than one third of patients who had travelled to Asia within the last 12 months carried ESCr-EK, we would recommend that these patients receive empiric antimicrobial treatment effective against ESCr-EK if they present with signs of serious infections of possible Gram-negative origin. According to findings in several studies, and repeated here, ESCr-EK are often multidrug resistant, and carbapenems is probably the safest choice for empirical treatment [31]. Treatment should always be adjusted and, if possible, de-escalated as soon as culture results are available [32, 33].

Certain ESCr-EK phylogroups or subclones have been linked to increased potential to cause severe infections because of higher virulence [18]. More knowledge of the more virulent phylogroups or subclones and risk factors for colonisation would allow targeted screening/treatment guidelines. As of today, the national guidelines for ESCr-EK infection control and prevention do not differentiate between MLSTs.

Conclusion

The prevalence of colonisation of ESCr-EK upon admission was 6.0%, none of the isolates identified from the patients produced carbapenemases and we did not identify any VRE, supporting other surveillance studies which indicate that carbapenemase-producing *E. coli* and *Klebsiella and* VRE are still very uncommon in the Norwegian population [11, 19]. Travel to Asia was a strong predictor for colonisation of ESCr-EK to be considered when administering empiric antimicrobial treatment. Less than one third of the colonised patients had travelled to Asia, and no other factors investigated were found to be strongly associated with carriage. For infection prevention and control, these findings underscore that health care personnel cannot rely solely on risk assessment and screening results but must apply standard infection control precautions for *all* patients.

Acknowledgements
Not applicable

Funding
The study was funded by the NIPH.

Authors' contributions
SBJ and MSt design the study, MML, BN and SBJ took part in the recruitment of participants and collection of questionnaires and swabs. SHH analysed the samples and interpreted the results. LE combined, analysed and interpreted the laboratory and epidemiological data. SBJ double checked and verified any discrepancy in the data. MSu analysed the wgs output. LE drafted the manuscript and SBJ, MSu and MSt revised it critically. TML and BN revised the advanced manuscript. All authors read and approved the final manuscript.

Consent for publication
Not applicable

Competing interests
The authors LE, SBJ, TML, MSu, SHH and MSt declare that they have no competing interests. BN has received funding from MSD as national lead invesgitator in Phamacokinetics Phase 1 study MK 1986 (Tedizolid) and 7655 (combination of imipenem, cilastatin and relebactam) for children outside of the submitted work.

Author details
[1]Department of Antibiotic Resistance and Infection Prevention, Norwegian Institute of Public Health, PO Box 222 Skøyen, 0213 Oslo, NO, Norway. [2]European Programme for Intervention Epidemiology Training (EPIET), European Centre for Disease Prevention and Control, (ECDC), Stockholm, Sweden. [3]Department of Clinical Microbiology and Infection Control, Akershus University Hospital, Lørenskog, Norway. [4]Institute for Clinical Medicine, Campus Ahus, University of Oslo, Nordbyhagen, Norway. [5]Department of Paediatrics and Adolescents Medicine, Akershus University Hospital, Lørenskog, Norway. [6]Department of Molecular Biology, Norwegian Institute of Public Health, Oslo, Norway. [7]Section for Food Safety and Emerging Health Threats, Norwegian Veterinary Institute, Nordbyhagen, Norway.

References

1. World Health Organisation. Antimicrobial resistance: global report on surveillance. World Health Organization. Geneva: WHO, 2014. ISBN 978 92 4 156474 8
2. de Kraker ME, Jarlier V, Monen JC, Heuer OE, van de Sande N, Grundmann H. The changing epidemiology of bacteraemias in Europe: trends from the European antimicrobial resistance surveillance system. Clin Microbiol Infect. 2013;19(9):860–8.
3. Tacconelli E, Cataldo MA, Dancer SJ, De Angelis G, Falcone M, Frank U, et al. ESCMID guidelines for the management of the infection control measures to reduce transmission of multidrug-resistant gram-negative bacteria in hospitalized patients. Clin Microbiol Infect. 2014;20(Suppl 1):1–55.
4. Naseer U, Natas OB, Haldorsen BC, Bue B, Grundt H, Walsh TR, et al. Nosocomial outbreak of CTX-M-15-producing E. coli in Norway. APMIS. 2007;115(2):120–6.
5. Jorgensen SB, Bojer MS, Boll EJ, Martin Y, Helmersen K, Skogstad M, et al. Heat-resistant, extended-spectrum beta-lactamase-producing Klebsiella pneumoniae in endoscope-mediated outbreak. J Hosp Infect. 2016;93(1):57–62.
6. Tofteland S, Naseer U, Lislevand JH, Sundsfjord A, Samuelsen O. A long-term low-frequency hospital outbreak of KPC-producing Klebsiella pneumoniae involving Intergenus plasmid diffusion and a persisting environmental reservoir. PLoS One. 2013;8(3):e59015.
7. Jorgensen SB, Soraas AV, Arnesen LS, Leegaard TM, Sundsfjord A, Jenum PA. A comparison of extended spectrum beta-lactamase producing Escherichia coli from clinical, recreational water and wastewater samples associated in time and location. PLoS one [internet]. 2017 PMC5645111]; 12(10):[e0186576 p.]. Available from: https://doi.org/10.1371/journal.pone.0186576.
8. Biehl LM, Schmidt-Hieber M, Liss B, Cornely OA, Vehreschild MJ. Colonization and infection with extended spectrum beta-lactamase producing Enterobacteriaceae in high-risk patients - review of the literature from a clinical perspective. Crit Rev Microbiol. 2016;42(1):1–16.
9. European Center for Disease Control and Prevention. Systematic review of the effectiveness of infection control measures to prevent the transmission of extended-spectrum beta-lactamase-producing Enterobacteriaceae through cross-border transfer of patients. Stockholm: European Centre for Disease Prevention and Control; 2014.
10. Folkehelseinstitutttet. ESBL-holdige gramnegative stavbakterier - smitteverntiltak i helseinstitusjoner2015.
11. NORM/NORM-VET2016. Usage of Antimicrobial Agents and Occurrence of Antimicrobial Resistance in Norway. Tromsø/Oslo: NORM/NORM-VET, 2017 1890–9965.
12. Center for Genomic Epidemiology. [cited 2018 27 July]. Available from: www.genomicepidemiology.org.
13. Zankari E, Hasman H, Cosentino S, Vestergaard M, Rasmussen S, Lund O, et al. Identification of acquired antimicrobial resistance genes. J Antimicrob Chemother. 2012;67(11):2640–4.
14. Larsen MV, Cosentino S, Rasmussen S, Friis C, Hasman H, Marvig RL, et al. Multilocus sequence typing of total-genome-sequenced bacteria. J Clin Microbiol. 2012;50(4):1355–61.
15. Hamprecht A, Rohde AM, Behnke M, Feihl S, Gastmeier P, Gebhardt F, et al. Colonization with third-generation cephalosporin-resistant Enterobacteriaceae on hospital admission: prevalence and risk factors. J Antimicrob Chemother. 2016;71(10):2957–63.
16. Platteel TN, Leverstein-van Hall MA, Cohen Stuart JW, Thijsen SF, Mascini EM, van Hees BC, et al. Predicting carriage with extended-spectrum beta-lactamase-producing bacteria at hospital admission: a cross-sectional study. Clin Microbiol Infect. 2015;21(2):141–6.
17. Ben-Ami R, Schwaber MJ, Navon-Venezia S, Schwartz D, Giladi M, Chmelnitsky I, et al. Influx of extended-spectrum beta-lactamase-producing enterobacteriaceae into the hospital. Clin Infect Dis. 2006;42(7):925–34.
18. Ny S, Lofmark S, Borjesson S, Englund S, Ringman M, Bergstrom J, et al. Community carriage of ESBL-producing Escherichia coli is associated with strains of low pathogenicity: a Swedish nationwide study. J Antimicrob Chemother. 2017;72(2):582–8.
19. Ulstad CR, Solheim M, Berg S, Lindbaek M, Dahle UR, Wester AL. Carriage of ESBL/AmpC-producing or ciprofloxacin non-susceptible Escherichia coli and Klebsiella spp in healthy people in Norway. Antimicrob Resist Infect Control. 2016;5:57.
20. Ostholm-Balkhed A, Tarnberg M, Nilsson M, Nilsson LE, Hanberger H, Hallgren A, et al. Travel-associated faecal colonization with ESBL-producing Enterobacteriaceae: incidence and risk factors. J Antimicrob Chemother [internet]. 2013;68(9):2144–53 pp.]. Available from: https://doi.org/10.1093/jac/dkt167.
21. Lausch KR, Fuursted K, Larsen CS, Storgaard M. Colonisation with multi-resistant Enterobacteriaceae in hospitalised Danish patients with a history of recent travel: a cross-sectional study. Travel Med Infect Dis. 2013;11(5):320–3.
22. Abrar S, Hussain S, Khan RA, Ul Ain N, Haider H, Riaz S. Prevalence of extended-spectrum-beta-lactamase-producing Enterobacteriaceae: first systematic meta-analysis report from Pakistan. Antimicrob Resist Infect Control. 2018;7:26.
23. Boonyasiri A, Tangkoskul T, Seenama C, Saiyarin J, Tiengrim S, Thamlikitkul V. Prevalence of antibiotic resistant bacteria in healthy adults, foods, food animals, and the environment in selected areas in Thailand. Pathogens and global health. 2014;108(5):235–45.
24. Luvsansharav UO, Hirai I, Nakata A, Imura K, Yamauchi K, Niki M, et al. Prevalence of and risk factors associated with faecal carriage of CTX-M beta-lactamase-producing Enterobacteriaceae in rural Thai communities. J Antimicrob Chemother. 2012;67(7):1769–74.
25. Sasaki T, Hirai I, Niki M, Nakamura T, Komalamisra C, Maipanich W, et al. High prevalence of CTX-M beta-lactamase-producing Enterobacteriaceae in stool specimens obtained from healthy individuals in Thailand. J Antimicrob Chemother. 2010;65(4):666–8.
26. Tekiner IH, Ozpinar H. Occurrence and characteristics of extended spectrum beta-lactamases-producing Enterobacteriaceae from foods of animal origin. Braz J Microbiol. 2016;47(2):444–51.
27. Oteo J, Perez-Vazquez M, Campos J. Extended-spectrum [beta]-lactamase producing Escherichia coli: changing epidemiology and clinical impact. Curr Opin Infect Dis. 2010;23(4):320–6.
28. Ma J, Liu JH, Lv L, Zong Z, Sun Y, Zheng H, et al. Characterization of extended-spectrum beta-lactamase genes found among Escherichia coli isolates from duck and environmental samples obtained on a duck farm. Appl Environ Microbiol. 2012;78(10):3668–73.
29. Snow LC, Warner RG, Cheney T, Wearing H, Stokes M, Harris K, et al. Risk factors associated with extended spectrum beta-lactamase Escherichia coli (CTX-M) on dairy farms in north West England and North Wales. Prev Vet Med. 2012;106(3–4):225–34.
30. Rodriguez-Bano J, Lopez-Cerero L, Navarro MD, Diaz de Alba P, Pascual A. Faecal carriage of extended-spectrum beta-lactamase-producing Escherichia coli: prevalence, risk factors and molecular epidemiology. J Antimicrob Chemother. 2008;62(5):1142–9.
31. Sheu CC, Lin SY, Chang YT, Lee CY, Chen YH, Hsueh PR. Management of infections caused by extended-spectrum beta-lactamase-producing Enterobacteriaceae: current evidence and future prospects. Expert Rev Anti-Infect Ther. 2018;16(3):205–18.
32. Helsedirektoratet. Nasjonal faglig retningslinje for bruk av antibiotika i sykehus. In: Helsedirektoratet, editor. Oslo 2017.
33. Healthcare Infection Control Practices Advisory Committee. Antibiotic stewardship statement for antibiotic guidelines – recommendations of the healthcare infection control practices advisory (HICPAC) committee 2016.

Alarming levels of antimicrobial resistance among sepsis patients admitted to ICU in a tertiary care hospital in India

D. Nagarjuna[1,4], Gajanand Mittal[2], Rakesh Singh Dhanda[3], Rajni Gaind[2] and Manisha Yadav[1,5*]

Abstract

Background: Hospital acquired infections (HAI) are principal threats to the patients of intensive care units. An increase in the antimicrobial resistance (AMR) observed in gram negative bacteria is a great challenge to deal with. HAI and AMR lead to prolonged hospitalization and additional doses of anti-microbial treatment affecting patient's fitness and finances. Present study was undertaken to determine the pathotypes, genetic diversity and the antimicrobial resistance of *E.coli* in isolates from the patients admitted to intensive care unit at a tertiary care hospital in Delhi, India.

Methods: *E.coli* isolates ($N = 77$) obtained from the blood culture of patients diagnosed with sepsis and the isolates ($N = 71$) from the stool culture of patients admitted in intensive care unit (ICU) but not diagnosed with sepsis were investigated for their pathotypes, adherence patterns and genetic diversity by Enterobacterial Repeated Intergenic Consensus-polymerase chain reaction (ERIC-PCR). A Kirby-Bauer Disc diffusion test and antimicrobial susceptibility assays were performed according to the Clinical and Laboratory Standards Institute (CLSI) guidelines. Extended-spectrum β-lactamase (ESBL) genes and sequence type 131 (ST131) clone were characterised genotypically by gene-specific PCRs.

Results: Pathotypes analysis revealed 46 and 16% of the blood *E.coli* isolates were ETEC and EAEC respectively, in contrast to the fecal isolates wherein 22% of the isolates were ETEC and 28.5% were EAEC. EPEC, STEC and EIEC pathotypes were not detected in blood or fecal isolates. Of all the isolates studied, more than 90% of the blood and 70% of the fecal isolates were found to be resistant to cephalosporins. On the other hand, 68% of blood and 44% of the fecal isolates were found to be ESBL producers. Interestingly 83% of the blood isolates contained CTX-M15, whereas only 21% of them contained CTX-M9 genes. On the other hand CTX-M15 genes were found in 90% and CTX-M9 genes were found in 63% of the fecal isolates.

(Continued on next page)

* Correspondence: manisha.dhanda@gmail.com; manisha.yadav@regionh.dk
[1]Dr. B. R. Ambedkar Centre for Biomedical Research (ACBR), University of Delhi (North Campus), Delhi 110007, India
[5]Current address: Department of Clinical Microbiology, Rigshospitalet, Copenhagen, Denmark
Full list of author information is available at the end of the article

(Continued from previous page)

Conclusion: The antimicrobial resistant profile found in this study is alarming and poses a great threat to public health. Apparently an increased antimicrobial resistance to the extensively used cephalosporins is affecting an optimal drug therapy for patients. In addition, the presence of catheters, prolonged duration of stay in the hospital and poor hygienic conditions due to infrequent urination of the patient can lead to an additional vulnerability. Therefore continuous surveillance and rational use of antibiotics along with effective hygienic measures are urgently recommended in such settings.

Keywords: *Escherichia coli*, Sepsis, Intensive care unit (ICU), Pathotypes, Enterobacterial repeated intergenic consensus (ERIC), Antimicrobial resistance (AMR)

Background

Health-care associated infections (HAIs) are a major public health concern throughout the world. Patients admitted in an intensive care unit (ICU) are at higher risk of developing bacteraemia and septicaemia [1] due to invasive procedures such as peripheral cannulation, central venous catheter placement, tracheal incubation and ventilation [2]. In addition, longer duration of stay in the hospital increases the risk of acquiring HAIs [3, 4]. The endogenous flora of the patient's mucous membranes or hollow viscera can be the source of pathogens causing infection. Incisions made near the perineum or groin, may result in contamination with faecal flora like *Escherichia coli* (*E.coli*). Being a harmless commensal as well as a pathogen, *E.coli* exhibits great genetic diversity. It causes a wide array of disease and is responsible for around 17–37% of both community and hospital acquired clinically significant blood stream infections (BSIs) [5] and a major cause of mortality from these infections [5–8].

The rapid evolution of extended-spectrum cephalosporin and carbapenem resistance in Enterobacteriaceae which has spread globally and rapidly in the last decade is one of the most prevalent areas of drug resistance [9]. Pathogenic *E.coli* developed resistance to every class of antibiotics introduced to treat human and animal infections. Resistance to the commonly used oral antibiotics like trimethoprim-sulphamethoxazole, amoxicillin increased steadily over time. Fluoroquinolone-resistant and extended-spectrum β-lactamase (ESBL)-producing *E.coli* have enormously increased in the past two decades. The ESBL genes are frequently encoded on transferable plasmids that encode resistance genes. Acquisition of such resistant genes by commensal or fecal isolates leads to multidrug resistant (MDR) pathogens. This increase in resistance is linked to a specific clone *E.coli* sequence type 131 (ST131) that had spread worldwide since 2008 [10–15].

Previously we reported fecal *E.coli* isolates to cause endogenous infection in immune-compromised hosts. Fecal *E.coli* from the patients admitted in ICU showed similar virulence profile as that of *E.coli* isolates from the blood of sepsis patients [16]. In the present paper, we report the pathotypes, adherence patterns, genetic relatedness and the antibiotic resistance profile among blood and fecal isolates. Even though similar studies were reported [17, 18], to the best of our knowledge studies on the population at risk like those admitted in ICU were not reported from India.

Methods

Clinical specimens and isolation of *E.coli* isolates

A total of 148 *E.coli* isolates previously collected and studied for their virulence profile and phylogroups [16] were used for this study. Samples were collected from February 2011 to August 2013 as described before [16]. Briefly, the first group of *E.coli* isolates ($N = 77$) were obtained from the blood culture of sepsis patients and the second group ($N = 71$) were obtained from the faeces of patients who were admitted in ICU for various reasons for example had undergone cardiovascular surgery, cases of road transport accident etc. but were not diagnosed with sepsis.

E.coli Pathotypes

Pathotyping was performed by a multiplex PCR using the primers *uidA*, *pic*, *bfp*, *invE*, *LT*, *escV*, *aggR*, *stx1a*, *stx2a*, *st1b*, *st1a*, *astA* corresponding to the genes defining the appropriate pathotypes as previously reported [19]. EAEC strains harbour *astA*, *aggR*, and *pic* genes and can be confirmed if found positive in a combination of *pic and aggR* or *aggR* and *astA*. Isolates found positive for either LT toxin (LT) or heat-stable toxin (ST) were designated as ETEC, whereas designated as EIEC if found positive for *invE*, and as EPEC if found positive for *escV and bfp*. STEC isolates were positive for *stx* and negative to *bfp* however in the presence or absence of *escV*. A primer pair for the detection of the *E.coli*-specific *uidA* gene was also included.

HeLa cells culture & adherence assays

HeLa cells were grown in Dulbecco's Modified Eagle Medium (DMEM) with 10% fetal bovine serum (FBS; Pan-Biotech, Germany) in the presence of 1% antibiotic mixture (penicillin and streptomycin; Life Technologies, USA) in an environment of 5% CO_2 at 37 °C. Adherence assay was performed on the monolayer of HeLa cells, which were upto 50% confluent [18]. Briefly, HeLa cells were first washed with phosphate buffered saline (PBS, pH 7.4). After washing, 1.0 ml of fresh medium (DMEM supplemented with 2% FBS) was added to the cell monolayers. The HeLa cells thereafter were inoculated with approximately 10^8 CFU/mL suspensions of *E.coli* grown in LB broth (overnight culture), diluted 1:50 and incubated at 37 °C. After 6 h of incubation, the cells were washed twice with PBS and thereafter fixed with methanol (Merck, Germany) for 1 h. The methanol-fixed cells were then stained with May Grünwald-Giemsa stain for 1 h and destained with 70% ethanol. Cells were observed under inverted microscope after fixation at 20X (Nikon, Eclipse TS100).

Analysis of Enterobacterial repeated intergenic consensus (ERIC) sequences

E.coli isolates were fingerprinted using ERIC-PCR. The primers used for the ERIC-PCR reaction were ERIC-F 5'-AAGTAAGTGACTGGGGTGAGCG-3' and ERIC-R 5'-ATGTAAGCTCCTGGGGATTCAC-3′ [20]. The gel images were captured using a Gel-documentation system. All the bands obtained were normalized using ImageLab software. Depending upon the molecular weight of the reference marker, a weighted matrix was generated. Using the PyELph v1.4 software, each band in each lane was analysed to obtain the band size with reference to the marker bands. All the band sizes so obtained were treated as an input for further analysis. A binary code of 1 or 0 was introduced to each band subjected to the presence and/or absence of the band respectively. On the basis of such generated binary matrix file, a phylogenetic tree and principle component analysis was constructed through NTSYS-pc 2.02 J software. Band intensity is an important characteristic for this analysis. The bands with very low resolutions were ignored by the ImageLab software as background noise after manually checking each band. The band profiles of the DNA fragments obtained after PCR amplification using specific primers for ERIC sequences were determined. The fingerprints obtained consisted of 5 to 15 bands ranging in size from 100 bp to 1 kb.

Antibiotic susceptibility assay

Individual antimicrobial disks of Amikacin 30mcg (AK), Cefepime 30mcg (CPM), Cefoperazone 75mcg (CPZ), Cefoxitin 30mcg (CX), Ceftazidime 30mcg (CAZ), Ciprofloxacin 5mcg (CIP), Gentamicin 10mcg (GEN) (HiMedia, India) were placed on the surface of the agar using sterile forceps. The disks were in complete contact with the agar surface by pressing down with forceps. 10 disks each were placed on a 150-mm plate and each had a gap of more than 24 mm between them. The plates were thereafter inverted and incubated at 37 °C for 18 h. Diameters of the inhibition zones were measured to the nearest millimetre using calibrated scale.

Screening of ESBL producers

An inert flat circular ring having a disk of Aztreonam (30 μg), Cefpodoxime (10 μg), Cefpodoxime/Clavulanic acid (10/5 μg), and Ceftazidime (30 μg) with a 6 mm diameter on its projections was used. According to the CLSI guidelines [21], isolates showing Cefpodoxime(10 μg) < 17 mm, Ceftazidime(30 μg) < 22 mm, Aztreonam (30 μg) < 27 mm, Cefotaxime (30 μg) < 27 mm, Ceftriaxone (30 μg) < 25 mm in the initial screening were considered as potential ESBL-producer. ESBL producer isolates were further screened with another set of discs having Cefpodoxime (10 μg), Cefpodoxime/Clavulanic acid (10/5 μg), Ceftazidime (30 μg), Ceftazidime/Clavulanic acid (30/10 μg), Cefotaxime (30 μg) and Cefotaxime/Clavulanic acid (30/10 μg). An increase of ≥2 mm in zone diameter for antimicrobial agent that were tested alone versus when tested in combination with Clavulanic acid confirmed the isolate as a potent ESBL producer.

Genotypic characterisation of ESBL genes

The presence of ESBL genes was tested by two multiplex PCRs, the first one detects TEM/SHV/ OXA-1 (Temoneira/ Sulfhydryl variable/ Oxacillin hydrolysing capabilities) group and the second one detects CTX-M groups 1, 2 and 9 [22].

Detection of ST131 gene and Fim H30 and H30-Rx sub-clones by PCR

Detection of the ST131-O16 and ST131-O25b clades was carried out by PCR using the primers previously described [23]. ST131 isolates were further characterized by screening them for ST131-associated SNPs in *mdh* (i.e., C288T and C525T) and *gyrB* (i.e., C621T, C729T, and T735C) [24]. Further, ST131-associated Fim H30 and H30-Rx sub-clone were identified by PCR. All ST131 positive isolates were tested for *fimH* 30 allele (encoding a variant of the type 1 fimbrial adhesin) corresponding with the main FQ resistance–associated subset within ST131, using the allele-specific primers as decribed before [24, 25]. The H30-Rx sub-clone was identified by detection of a specific single-nucleotide polymorphism (SNP) (G723A) within the allantoin-encoding gene, ybbW using the Primers AP63 and AP66 as described before [26].

Statistical analysis

Fishers Exact test was used to compare pathotypes between the blood and fecal *E.coli* isolates. Z-test was used to compare the prevalence of ESBL and ST131 clone between the blood and fecal *E.coli* isolates. *P* value of $p < 0.05$ was considered significant.

Results

Comparison of pathotypes between blood and fecal *E.coli* isolates

Our data showed that 62% of the blood *E.coli* isolates were designated to one of the pathotypes studied, among which 46% were ETEC and 16% were EAEC. While in case of fecal *E.coli* isolates (50.5%), 22% were ETEC and 28.5% were EAEC ((Fig. 1). 38% of the blood and 49.5% of the fecal isolates do not belong to any of the pathotypes investigated (Fig. 1). We did not find any of the blood or fecal *E.coli* isolates positive for EPEC, STEC and EIEC.

Adherence assays in HeLa cells

Localized adherence was observed among 32 and 21% of the blood and fecal isolates. Diffused adherence pattern was observed in 20% of both blood and fecal isolates. Aggregative adherence was observed among 10.5% of the fecal and only 1.5% of the blood isolates (Fig. 2a, b). A large proportion of the isolates showed localized adherence, which is characteristic of EPEC, but none of the isolates were found positive for *bfp*. Among the isolates designated as ETEC based on the PCR results, some of the isolates were locally adhered (38.46%) some were diffused (15.38%) and a few with aggregative adherence (5.1%). Among the isolates designated as EAEC, a large proportion showed diffused adherence (31.81%) and aggregative (15.9%) thereby correlating with the PCR results. (Fig. 2a, c).

ERIC analysis

The ERIC–PCR profiles allowed differentiation of all the *E.coli* isolates into six main clusters. Both analyses were reported under ~ 0.00 to 0.50 matrix distance evaluation. All the blood isolates analysed were found to be clustered into two groups at 0.25 SM with Cluster 1 comprising of 44 *E.coli* isolates and cluster 2 comprising 22 *E.coli* isolates (Fig. 3a). The fecal *E.coli* isolates were clustered into four groups at 0.25 SM with cluster 1 comprising of 22 *E.coli* isolates, followed by cluster 2 of 21 *E.coli* isolates, cluster 3 of 20 *E.coli* isolates and cluster 4 comprising of 11 *E.coli* isolates (Fig. 3a). We observed that blood isolates were more similar with respect to the banding pattern. The principal component analysis (PCA) showed the diversity among the blood and fecal *E.coli* isolates. The fecal *E.coli* isolates were found to be more diverse as observed by PCA analysis (Fig. 3b).

Antibiotic susceptibility assay

The fecal *E.coli* isolates were found to be resistant for Cefoxitin (70%), Cefpodxime (89%), Cefpodoxime/clavulanic acid (89%), Ceftazidime (69%), Ceftazidime/clavulanic acid (55%), Cefotaxime (87%), Cefotaxime/Clavulanic acid (81%), Ceftriaxone (87%), Cefaperazone (88%) and Cefipime (79%) (Fig. 4a). Among the blood *E.coli* isolates, 88% were found to be resistant for Cefoxitin, Cefpodxime (98.5%), Cefpodoxime/clavulanic acid (98.5%),

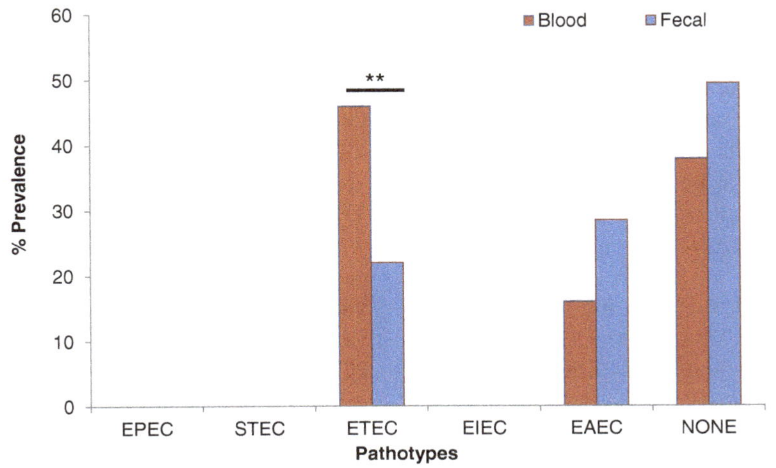

Fig. 1 Prevalence of pathotypes in blood and fecal *E.coli* isolates from sepsis and non-sepsis patients respectively. *p* value is $^{**}p \leq 0.01$. EPEC: Enteropathogenic *E.coli*; STEC: Shiga toxin-producing *E.coli*; ETEC: Entero-toxigenic *E. coli*; EIEC: entero-invasive *E.coli*; EAEC: Entero-aggregative *E.coli*

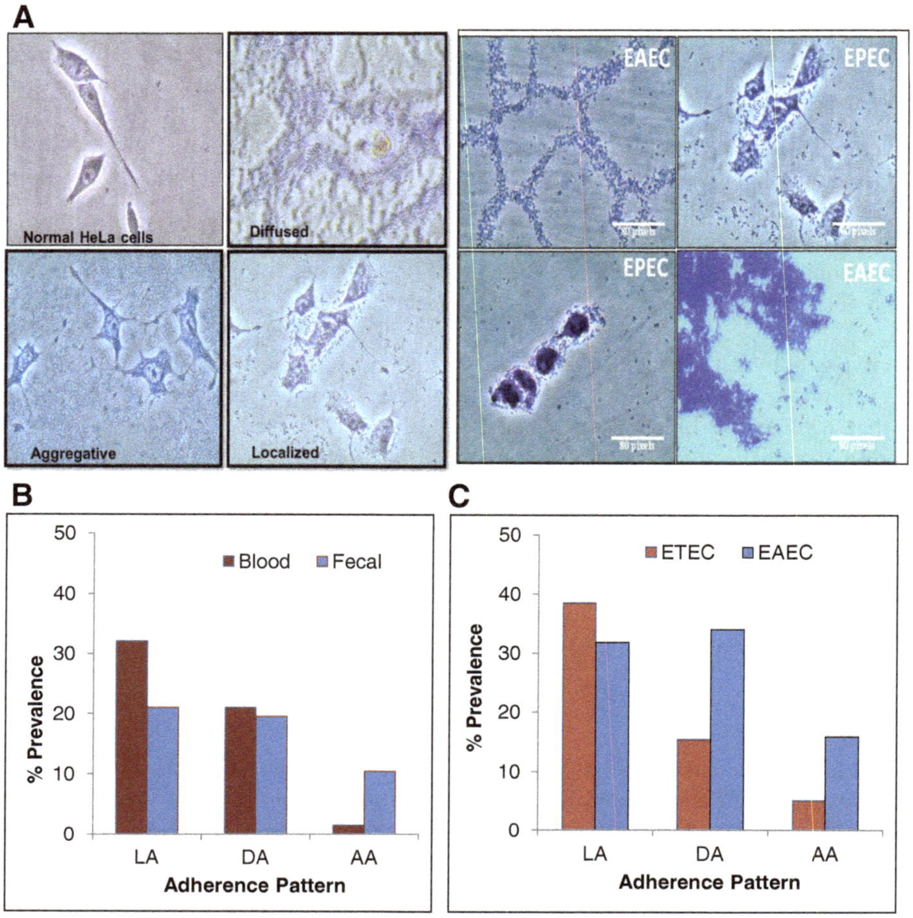

Fig. 2 a Representative characteristic adherence patterns of *E.coli* in EAEC and ETEC as seen in HeLa cells upon infection (L: Localized; D: Diffused and A: Aggregative pattern). Scale is 100 μM; **b** Overall prevalence of adherence patterns in blood and fecal *E.coli* isolates from sepsis and non-sepsis patients respectively; **c** Prevalence of adherence patterns among EAEC and ETEC

Ceftazidime (91%), Ceftazidime/clavulanic acid (69%), Cefotaxime (94%), Cefotaxime/clavulanic acid (90%), Ceftriaxone (92.5%), Cefaperazone (92.5%) and Cefepime (91%) (Fig. 4b). Fecal *E.coli* isolates were resistant to Piperacillin (75%), Aztreonam (72%), Amikacin (34%), Gentamicin (51%), Ciprofloxacin (85%). Whereas blood *E.coli* isolates were found to be resistant for Piperacillin (76%), Amikacin (63%), Gentamicin (70%), Ciprofloxacin (91%), and Aztreonam (88%) (Fig. 4a-b).

ESBL producers and identification of ESBL genes

ESBL producers confer resistance to third generation Cephalosporins (e.g., Ceftazidime, Cefotaxime, and Ceftriaxone) and monobactams (e.g., Aztreonam) but do not affect cephamycins (e.g., Cephoxitin and Cefotetan) or carbapenems (e.g., Meropenem or Imipenem) (Fig. 5a). According to the observed susceptibility patterns, it was found that 68% of blood *E.coli* isolates were found to be ESBL producers whereas 44% of the fecal isolates were confirmed as ESBL producers (Fig. 5b). ESBL genes were identified by ESBL gene specific PCR. Among the blood *E.coli* isolates, 83% of the isolates showed CTX-M15, while only 21% of them had CTX-M9, whereas TEM was observed in 74%, SHV in 17%, OXA-1 in 74% of the isolates. In case of fecal *E.coli* isolates, CTX-M15 was observed in 90%, CTX-M9 in 63%, of the isolates and TEM, SHV, and OXA-1 were observed in 88, 17, 96% respectively (Fig. 6).

Prevalence of ST131 clone

ST131 clone was identified using ST131 clone specific PCR method (Additional file 1: Figure S1). Our results showed that 80% of the fecal *E.coli* isolates were positive for ST131 clone while in 92% among the blood isolates (Fig. 7a). In addition, all the *E.coli* isolates were further used for identification of ST131 with associated SNPs i.e. *mdh*36 and *gyrB*47. We found that all ST131 positive isolates were also positive for both ST131 associated

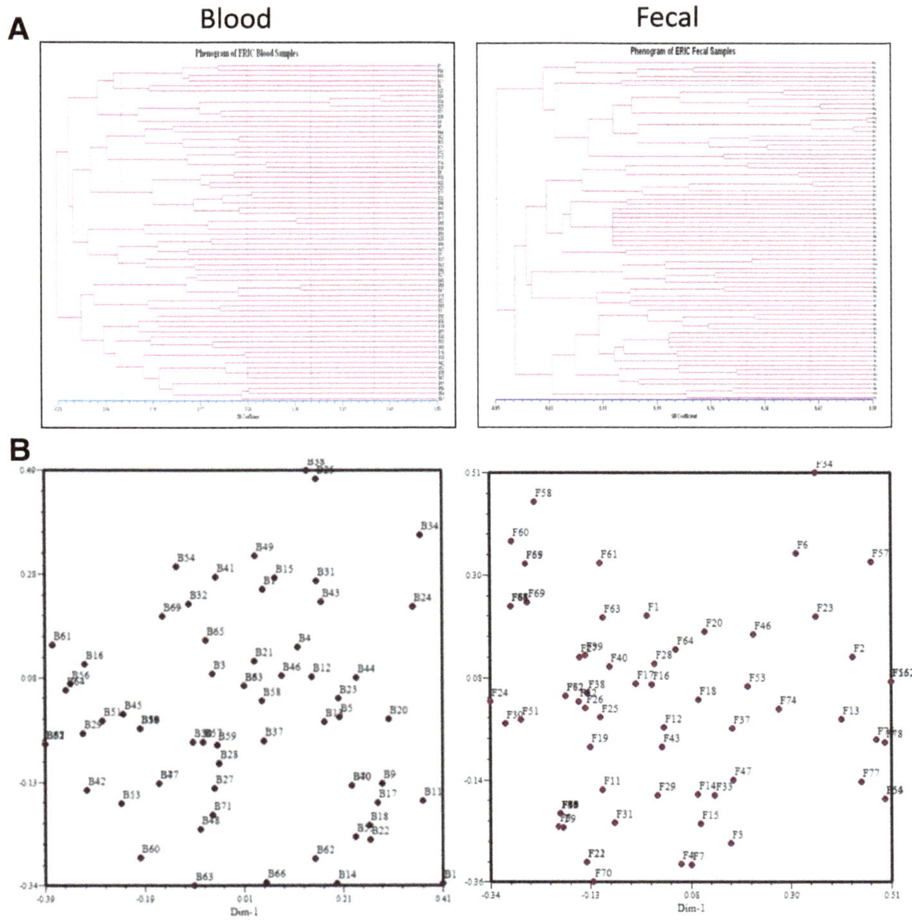

Fig. 3 a Phenogram and **b** Principal component analysis showing the genomic similarity among blood and the fecal *E.coli* isolates as carried out by computer-assisted ERIC-PCR DNA fingerprint analysis (see material and methods for detail)

SNPs. All the isolates that were positive for ST131 were tested and further confirmed for FimH 30 and FimH 30-Rx sub groups of ST131 clone (Additional file 2: Figure S2). We found that 91.5% of the blood *E.coli* isolates and 83% of the fecal isolates belong to the FimH 30 and FimH 30-Rx sub groups (Fig. 7b).

Discussion

Identification of *E. coli* pathotypes in association with blood stream infections is limited in many developing countries because routine diagnostic screens only the micro-organism, the conventional microbiological testing is unable to distinguish between normal flora and pathogenic strains of *E. coli* [27]. Entero pathogenic *E.coli* (EPEC) is a major etiological agent of infant diarrhea predominantly in developing countries [28–30]. ETEC defined by their production of the plasmid-encoded heat-labile (LT) and heat-stable (STIa/STIb) toxins is the leading cause of traveler's diarrhea [31]. ETEC & EAEC are the most commonly identified pathogens in our study. It was found that the proportion of ETEC was significantly higher among the blood isolates as compared to fecal *E.coli* isolates ($p = 0.029$). However, we did not find any significant difference in the proportion of EAEC between blood and fecal *E.coli* isolates. Our data showed a large proportion of the isolates with localized adherence, which is a known characteristic of EPEC however none of the isolates were found positive for EPEC by PCR.

All the blood isolates analysed by ERIC-PCR were found to be clustered into two groups while fecal *E.coli* isolates were clustered into four groups. The principal component analysis (PCA) of the blood *E.coli* isolates were more similar among themselves with respect to the ERIC band profiles while the fecal *E.coli* isolates were more diverse. We can correlate the observation of PCA and cluster analysis with the hypothesis that a single strain from the gut may be the source of endogenous infection which may prompt an "overspill" bacteraemia.

Antibiotic susceptibility results showed that more than 70% of the fecal *E.coli* isolates and more than 90% of the

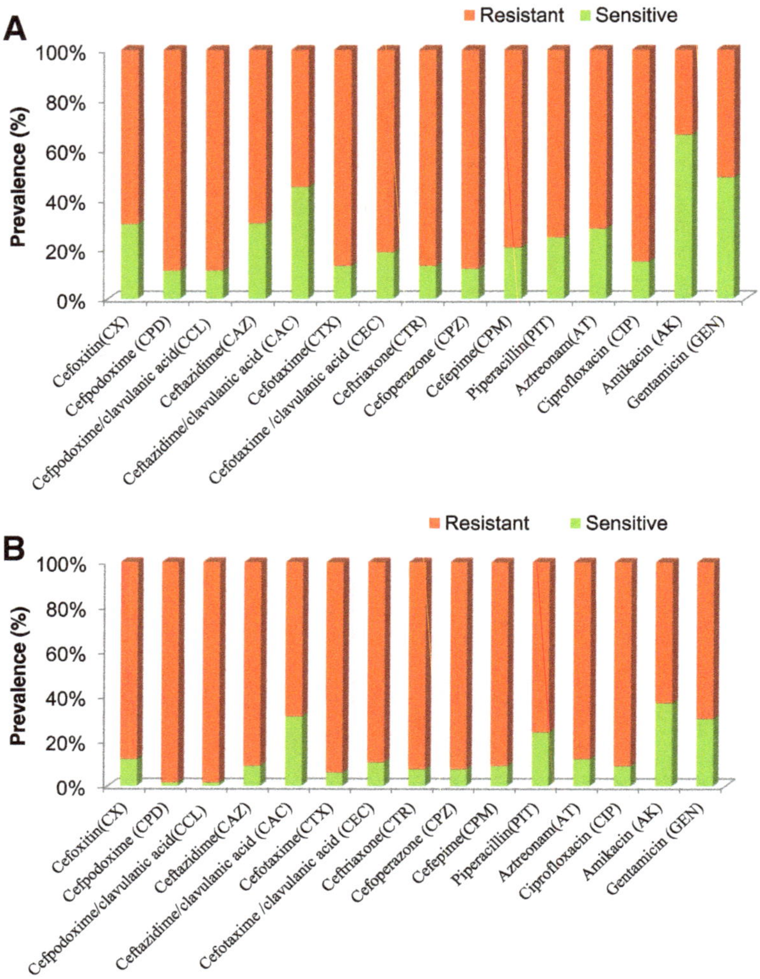

Fig. 4 Antibiotic susceptibility pattern of fecal (**a**) and blood (**b**) *E.coli* isolates from non-sepsis and sepsis patients respectively

blood isolates were resistant to all of the cephalosporins tested. Among the fecal isolates, we observed a slight decrease in susceptibility to cephalosporin in combination with an inhibitor clavulanic acid. Fecal *E.coli* isolates were resistant to Cefpodoxime/clavulanic acid (89%), Ceftazidime/clavulanic acid (55%) and Cefotaxime/clavulanic acid (81%). While blood *E.coli* isolates were resistant to Cefpodoxime/clavulanic acid (98.5%), Cefotaxime/clavulanic acid (90%), Ceftazidime (91%) and Ceftazidime/clavulanic acid (69%). A significant decrease in susceptibility to Ceftazidime in combination with clavulanic acid was observed as compared to Ceftazidime alone.

However, among the other classes of antibiotics aminoglycosides, fluoroquinolone, and monobactams studied, 85% of the fecal isolates were resistant to Ciprofloxacin, 75% were resistant to Piperacillin, 72% for Aztreonam, 34% for Amikacin and 51% for Gentamicin. Whereas, 91% of the blood isolates were resistant to Ciprofloxacin, 76% were resistant to Piperacillin, 88% for Aztreonam, 63% for Amikacin, and 70% for Gentamicin. In comparison to blood isolates, fecal isolates were more susceptible to amikacin (34% verses 63%) and gentamicin (51% verses 70%). Overall, 68% of the blood isolates were found to be ESBL producers whereas 44% of the fecal isolates were confirmed as ESBL producers by observing the susceptibility patterns in disc synergy tests with clavulanic acid.

Antibiotic resistance in *E.coli* can be conferred by both chromosomal and plasmid-encoded genes. Resistance to ciprofloxacin was observed in concurrence with cephalosporin resistance. ESBLs degrade the β-lactam moiety of penicillin derivatives, cephalosporins, monobactams, and Carbapenems. The ESBL genes are frequently encoded on transferable plasmids that encode resistance genes. Acquisition of such resistant genes by commensal or fecal isolates leads to MDR pathogens. The three major groups of ESBL enzymes are TEM, SHV and CTX-M. Among the CTX-M-type ESBLs, CTX-M-15 is widely

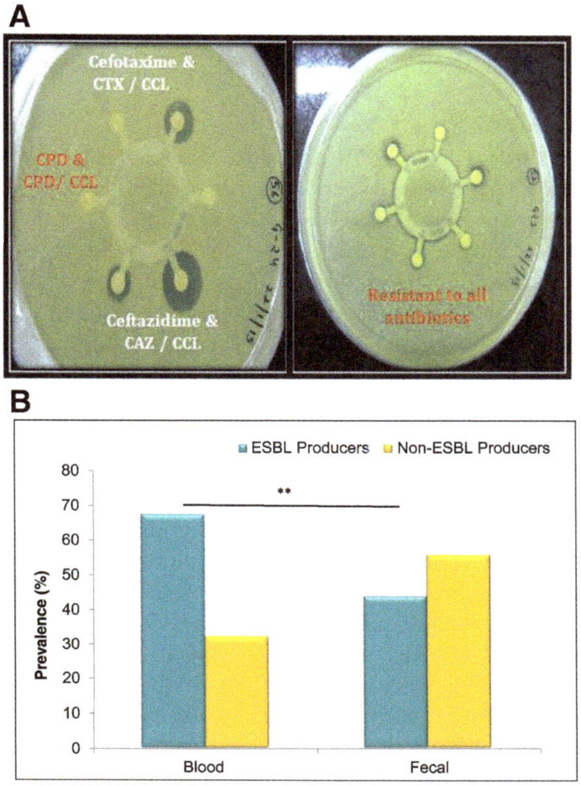

Fig. 5 a Picture representing the antibiotic disc diffusion test for extended spectrum Beta-Lactamase (ESBL) producers. Each circular disc contains the antibiotic of specific concentration. Clear zone around the disc indicates zone of Inhibition. **b** Prevalence of ESBL producers between blood and fecal *E.coli* isolates from sepsis and non-sepsis patients respectively. *P* value is $^{**}p = 0.001$

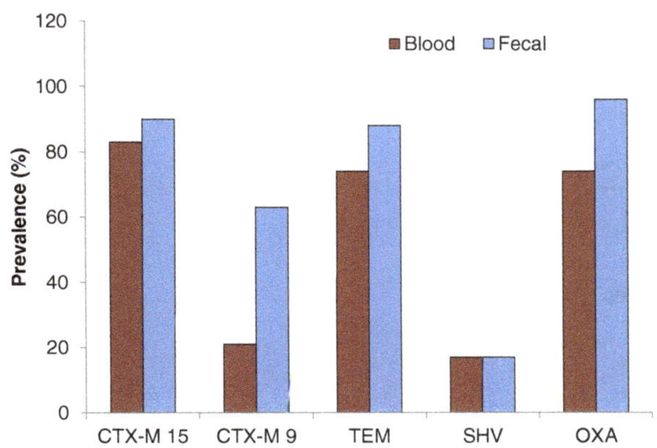

Fig. 6 Comparision of different ESBL genes in blood and fecal *E.coli* isolates from sepsis and non-sepsis patients respectively using gene specific PCR

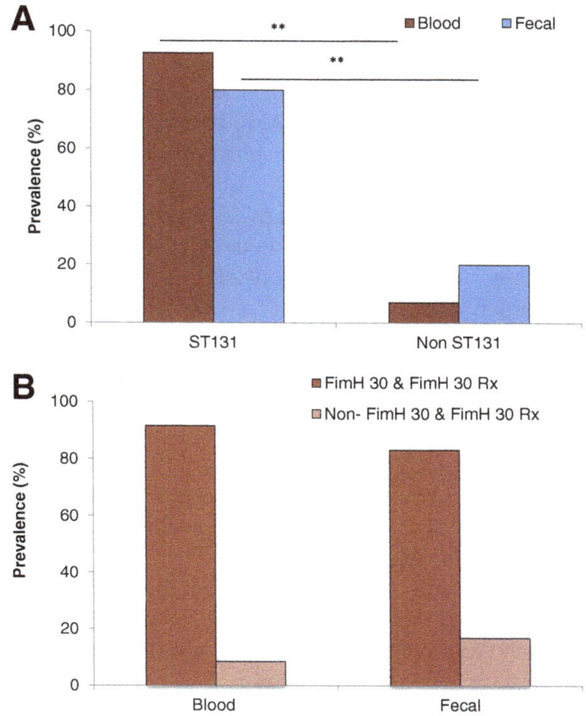

Fig. 7 a Prevalence of ST131 clone **b** Prevalence of FimH30 and FimH30-Rx sub groups of ST131 clone among blood and fecal *E.coli* isolates from sepsis and non-sepsis patients respectively. $^{**}p = 0.0119$

distributed worldwide [32], and are the most prevalent in India [33]. In our study, we found that 83% of the blood *E.coli* isolates whereas 90% of the fecal isolates showed CTX-M15; CTXM-15 producing isolates were reported to have reduced susceptibility to Cefepime [34]. Our results are in line with the observation since 91 and 79% of the blood and fecal isolates respectively are resistant to Cefepime. Therefore, Cefepime which is a fourth generation cephalosporin is administered intravenously and used primarily for treatment of pneumonia, UTIs, and intra-abdominal infections, can no longer be a choice of drug.

The gut has been thought to be a repository of pathogens and an incredible source for the development of antibiotic resistance [35]. Overall the carriage of ESBL genes is more in fecal isolates than that of the blood isolates CTX-M9 (63% verses 21%), CTX-M15 (90% verses 83%), TEM (88% verses 74%), and OXA-1 (96% verses 74%). Previously, it was demonstrated as an intestinal colonization by gram-negative organisms before the onset of the disease [36]. We propose a similar scenario since we have found CTX-M15 as a predominant ESBL gene among the fecal isolates in our study. There is a significant increase in the prevalence of CTX-M enzyme producing *E.coli* worldwide. We report the detection of CTX-M group 9 genes and the CTX-M15 as a predominant ESBL gene among fecal isolates. Our results also highlight the importance of studying gut flora in assessing the changing repertoire of organisms to investigate the pattern of antibiotic susceptibilities. We found prevalence of ESBL -producers more among the blood isolates whereas the isolates showing the ESBL genes were found predominantly among fecal isolates.

The high resistance patterns against all of the 15 antibiotics we studied compelled us to further analyse the isolates for the ST131 clone. *E.coli* ST131 clone is well known affiliated with the worldwide spread of CTX-M15 enzyme. ST131 isolates were associated with extra-intestinal infections, frequently in UTI and bacteraemia. Initially detected in a community, later ST131 isolates were also obtained from health care settings [13]. ST131 strains are MDR and patients with such infections are at high risk of having constrained treatment choices with a prolonged duration of disease. We observed that 80% of the fecal isolates and 92% of the blood isolates belonged to ST131 clone, a sub-clonal lineage of *E.coli* ST131 that contains the type 1 fimbriae fimH30 (H30) allele and is termed as FimH 30 sub group. Isolates of this sub group were reported resistant to fluoro-quinolones (FQ) with only < 1% of FQ-susceptible isolates. The abrupt expansion and genetic similarity among the H30 strains clue that the emergence of FQ-resistant ST131 strains was driven by clonal expansion and dissemination. Isolates of H30 ST131 sub-clone were found to be resistant for more than 3 antibiotic classes and with CTX-M1. Within the H30 lineage, Price et al., identified a close distinct sub lineage with more extensive antimicrobial resistance profile called H30-Rx. This sub lineage was formed from H30 strains that carried CTX-M15 distinguished from ESBL-negative H30 strains by 3 core genome SNPs [26]. Interestingly, in association with the high resistance to Ciprofloxacin (85% fecal and 91% blood isolates), we found 83% of the fecal and 91.5% of the blood *E.coli* isolates belonged to FimH 30 and FimH 30-Rx sub groups.

A few studies reported the prevalence of ST131 clone from India. Among them is a study from neonatal isolates, which reported 9% prevalence of ST131 [37]. Another study reported 70% prevalence of ST131 among the ESBL producing strains [38]. MLST is the most accurate and competent method for detection of ST131 clones. But it is tedious and costly. Especially, its application for investigating the MDR clone for clinical diagnosis is not possible. ST131 clone rapid detection assays were previously reported [23, 39]. Even though those methods may validate ST131, the results usually vary and need a confirmation by MLST. It is alarming to find a higher prevalence of ST131 clone isolates in our study evidenced by extreme antibiotic resistant and carriage of ESBL genes.

Conclusion

This study emphasizes the need for the differential identification of specific pathotypes in order to facilitate appropriate counter measures. The genomic diversity analysed by ERIC-PCR portrayed the diversity of *E.coli* strains in the gut. There are more outliers among the fecal isolates. A large extent of blood isolates studied were ESBL-producers and resistant to Cephalosporins. Even though the resistant profiles of fecal isolates are lower in comparison to blood isolates, the isolates lodging the antibiotic resistant genes were more among the fecal isolates. ST131 strains are MDR and linked to spread of the antibiotic resistance. We observed a higher prevalence of ST131 isolates. Patients with such infections are at risk of constrained treatment choices and prolonged duration of disease. The antimicrobial resistance profiles found in this study pose a great threat to public health. Increasing anti-microbial resistance among *E.coli* to the commonly used cephalosporins hinders the decision of the optimal drug therapy for patients. Continuous surveillance and rational use of antibiotics along with effective hygienic measures are urgently needed in our setting.

Study bias and weakness/limitations

There may be selection bias as a fraction of cases were selected for the study from a large group of patients in the ICU. The controls samples may be more biased as they were selected based on a few inclusive criteria that they are admitted in ICU and not having sepsis.

Abbreviations

AMR: Antimicrobial resistance; CLSI: Clinical and laboratory standards institute; DMEM: Dulbecco's modification of eagle medium; ERIC: Enterobacterial repeated intergenic consensus; ESBL: Extended-spectrum β-lactamase; HAI: Hospital acquired infections; ICU: Intensive care unit; OXA: Oxacillin hydrolysing capabilities; PCA: Principal component analysis; PCR: Polymerase chain reaction; SHV: Sulfhydryl variable; ST131: Sequence type 131; TEM: Temoneira

Acknowledgements

We acknowledge Ms. Jannat and Ms. Anupama for technical help during this study.

Funding

This study was funded by the Research & Development grant (RC/2015/9677), University of Delhi, Delhi, India.

Authors' contributions

DN, RSD and MY designed experiments and analysed the data. DN and GM collected samples and performed experiments. RG contributed to experimental design and helped to write the manuscript. RSD and MY conceptualized directed the study and wrote the manuscript. All authors read and approved the final manuscript.

Consent for publication
Not applicable.

Competing interests
The authors declare that they have no competing interests.

Author details
[1]Dr. B. R. Ambedkar Centre for Biomedical Research (ACBR), University of Delhi (North Campus), Delhi 110007, India. [2]Department of Microbiology, Vardhman Mahavir Medical College (VMMC) and Safdarjung Hospital, Delhi 110029, India. [3]Stem Cell Laboratory, Longboat Explorers AB, SMiLE Incubator, Scheelevägen 2, 22381 Lund, Sweden. [4]Current address: Department of Biotechnology, Indian Institute of Technology, Roorkee 247667, India. [5]Current address: Department of Clinical Microbiology, Rigshospitalet, Copenhagen, Denmark.

References
1. Timsit JF, Laupland KB. Update on bloodstream infections in ICUs. Curr Opin Crit Care. 2012;18(5):479–86.
2. Al-Zahrani A, Alsulaimani EEA, Abbadi S. Healthcare Associated Infection in the Neonatal Intensive Care Unit of King Abdl Azz Specialist Hospital, Taif, KSA. Adv Infect Dis. 2013;3(4):300–5.
3. Sheng WH, et al. Impact of nosocomial infections on medical costs, hospital stay, and outcome in hospitalized patients. J Formos Med Assoc. 2005;104(5):318–26.
4. Sheng WH, et al. Comparative impact of hospital-acquired infections on medical costs, length of hospital stay and outcome between community hospitals and medical centres. J Hosp Infect. 2005;59(3):205–14.
5. Russo TA, Johnson JR. Medical and economic impact of extraintestinal infections due to Escherichia coli: focus on an increasingly important endemic problem. Microbes Infect. 2003;5(5):449–56.
6. Laupland KB, et al. Incidence, risk factors and outcomes of Escherichia coli bloodstream infections in a large Canadian region. Clin Microbiol Infect. 2008;14(11):1041–7.
7. Olesen B, et al. A comparative study of nosocomial and community-acquired strains of Escherichia coli causing bacteraemia in a Danish University hospital. J Hosp Infect. 1995;31(4):295–304.
8. Ron EZ. Distribution and evolution of virulence factors in septicemic Escherichia coli. Int J Med Microbiol. 2010;300(6):367–70.
9. World Health Organization., Antimicrobial resistance: 2014 global report on surveillance. 2014.
10. Nicolas-Chanoine MH, et al. Intercontinental emergence of Escherichia coli clone O25:H4-ST131 producing CTX-M-15. J Antimicrob Chemother. 2008; 61(2):273–81.
11. Yumuk Z, et al. Turkey: a further country concerned by community-acquired Escherichia coli clone O25-ST131 producing CTX-M-15. J Antimicrob Chemother. 2008;62(2):284–8.
12. Johnson JR, et al. Escherichia coli sequence type ST131 as the major cause of serious multidrug-resistant E. coli infections in the United States. Clin Infect Dis. 2010;51(3):286–94.
13. Mathers AJ, Peirano G, Pitout JD. Escherichia coli ST131: the quintessential example of an international multiresistant high-risk clone. Adv Appl Microbiol. 2015;90:109–54.
14. Peirano G, Pitout JD. Molecular epidemiology of Escherichia coli producing CTX-M beta-lactamases: the worldwide emergence of clone ST131 O25:H4. Int J Antimicrob Agents. 2010;35(4):316–21.
15. Peirano G, et al. High prevalence of ST131 isolates producing CTX-M-15 and CTX-M-14 among extended-spectrum-beta-lactamase-producing Escherichia coli isolates from Canada. Antimicrob Agents Chemother. 2010;54(3):1327–30.
16. Nagarjuna D, et al. Faecal Escherichia coli isolates show potential to cause endogenous infection in patients admitted to the ICU in a tertiary care hospital. New Microbes New Infect. 2015;7:57–66.
17. Toval F, et al. Characterization of Escherichia coli isolates from hospital inpatients or outpatients with urinary tract infection. J Clin Microbiol. 2014;52(2):407–18.
18. Riveros M, et al. Adhesion patterns in diffusely adherent Escherichia coli (DAEC) strains isolated from children with and without diarrhea. Rev Peru Med Exp Salud Publica. 2011;28(1):21–8.
19. Muller D, et al. Identification of unconventional intestinal pathogenic Escherichia coli isolates expressing intermediate virulence factor profiles by using a novel single-step multiplex PCR. Appl Environ Microbiol. 2007;73(10):3380–90.
20. Versalovic J, Koeuth T, Lupski JR. Distribution of repetitive DNA sequences in eubacteria and application to fingerprinting of bacterial genomes. Nucleic Acids Res. 1991;19(24):6823–31.
21. CLSI, Performance standards of Antimicrobial Disc Susceptibility Tests, Twenty Seventh Informational Supplement. 2017. Clinical and Laboratory Standard Institute M100-S27 CLSI (Jan 2017).
22. Dallenne C, et al. Development of a set of multiplex PCR assays for the detection of genes encoding important beta-lactamases in Enterobacteriaceae. J Antimicrob Chemother. 2010;65(3):490–5.
23. Clermont O, et al. Rapid detection of the O25b-ST131 clone of Escherichia coli encompassing the CTX-M-15-producing strains. J Antimicrob Chemother. 2009;64(2):274–7.
24. Johnson JR, et al. Epidemic clonal groups of Escherichia coli as a cause of antimicrobial-resistant urinary tract infections in Canada, 2002 to 2004. Antimicrob Agents Chemother. 2009;53(7):2733–9.
25. Johnson JR, et al. Abrupt emergence of a single dominant multidrug-resistant strain of Escherichia coli. J Infect Dis. 2013;207(6):919–28.
26. Price LB, et al. The epidemic of extended-spectrum-beta-lactamase-producing Escherichia coli ST131 is driven by a single highly pathogenic subclone, H30-Rx. MBio. 2013;4(6):e00377–13.
27. Vieira N, et al. High prevalence of enteroinvasive Escherichia coli isolated in a remote region of northern coastal Ecuador. Am J Trop Med Hyg. 2007; 76(3):528–33.
28. Kaper JB, Nataro JP, Mobley HL. Pathogenic Escherichia coli. Nat Rev Microbiol. 2004;2(2):123–40.
29. Chen HD, Frankel G. Enteropathogenic Escherichia coli: unravelling pathogenesis. FEMS Microbiol Rev. 2005;29(1):83–98.
30. Dean P, Maresca M, Kenny B. EPEC's weapons of mass subversion. Curr Opin Microbiol. 2005;8(1):28–34.
31. Nataro JP, Kaper JB. Diarrheagenic *Escherichia coli*. Clin Microbiol Rev. 1998; 11(1):142–201 Erratum in Clin Microbiol Rev 1998 Apr;11(2):403.
32. Pitout JD, Laupland KB. Extended-spectrum beta-lactamase-producing Enterobacteriaceae: an emerging public-health concern. Lancet Infect Dis. 2008;8(3):159–66.
33. Ensor VM, et al. Occurrence, prevalence and genetic environment of CTX-M beta-lactamases in Enterobacteriaceae from Indian hospitals. J Antimicrob Chemother. 2006;58(6):1260–3.
34. Park YS, et al. Clinical and microbiologic characteristics of cephalosporin-resistant Escherichia coli at three centers in the United States. Antimicrob Agents Chemother. 2012;56(4):1870–6.
35. Salyers AA, Gupta A, Wang Y. Human intestinal bacteria as reservoirs for antibiotic resistance genes. Trends Microbiol. 2004;12(9):412–6.
36. Donskey CJ. Antibiotic regimens and intestinal colonization with antibiotic-resistant gram-negative bacilli. Clin Infect Dis. 2006;43(Suppl 2):S62–9.
37. Roy S, et al. Insight into neonatal septicaemic Escherichia coli from India with respect to phylogroups, serotypes, virulence, extended-spectrum-beta-lactamases and association of ST131 clonal group. Epidemiol Infect. 2015; 143(15):3266–76.
38. Hussain A, et al. Multiresistant Uropathogenic Escherichia coli from a region in India where urinary tract infections are endemic: genotypic and phenotypic characteristics of sequence type 131 isolates of the CTX-M-15 extended-Spectrum-β-lactamase-producing lineage. Antimicrob Agents Chemother. 2012;56(12):6358–65.
39. Johnson JR, et al. Rapid and specific detection, molecular epidemiology, and experimental virulence of the O16 subgroup within Escherichia coli sequence type 131. J Clin Microbiol. 2014;52(5):1358–65.

Permissions

All chapters in this book were first published in AR&IC, by BioMed Central; hereby published with permission under the Creative Commons Attribution License or equivalent. Every chapter published in this book has been scrutinized by our experts. Their significance has been extensively debated. The topics covered herein carry significant findings which will fuel the growth of the discipline. They may even be implemented as practical applications or may be referred to as a beginning point for another development.

The contributors of this book come from diverse backgrounds, making this book a truly international effort. This book will bring forth new frontiers with its revolutionizing research information and detailed analysis of the nascent developments around the world.

We would like to thank all the contributing authors for lending their expertise to make the book truly unique. They have played a crucial role in the development of this book. Without their invaluable contributions this book wouldn't have been possible. They have made vital efforts to compile up to date information on the varied aspects of this subject to make this book a valuable addition to the collection of many professionals and students.

This book was conceptualized with the vision of imparting up-to-date information and advanced data in this field. To ensure the same, a matchless editorial board was set up. Every individual on the board went through rigorous rounds of assessment to prove their worth. After which they invested a large part of their time researching and compiling the most relevant data for our readers.

The editorial board has been involved in producing this book since its inception. They have spent rigorous hours researching and exploring the diverse topics which have resulted in the successful publishing of this book. They have passed on their knowledge of decades through this book. To expedite this challenging task, the publisher supported the team at every step. A small team of assistant editors was also appointed to further simplify the editing procedure and attain best results for the readers.

Apart from the editorial board, the designing team has also invested a significant amount of their time in understanding the subject and creating the most relevant covers. They scrutinized every image to scout for the most suitable representation of the subject and create an appropriate cover for the book.

The publishing team has been an ardent support to the editorial, designing and production team. Their endless efforts to recruit the best for this project, has resulted in the accomplishment of this book. They are a veteran in the field of academics and their pool of knowledge is as vast as their experience in printing. Their expertise and guidance has proved useful at every step. Their uncompromising quality standards have made this book an exceptional effort. Their encouragement from time to time has been an inspiration for everyone.

The publisher and the editorial board hope that this book will prove to be a valuable piece of knowledge for researchers, students, practitioners and scholars across the globe.

List of Contributors

Reza Ranjbar
Molecular Biology Research Center, Baqiyatallah University of Medical Sciences, Tehran, Iran

Mojtaba Masoudimanesh
Doctor Veterinary Medicine, College of Veterinary Medicine, Islamic Azad University, Shahrekord Branch, Shahrekord, Iran

Farhad Safarpoor Dehkordi
Young Researchers and Elites Club, Shahrekord Branch, Islamic Azad University, Shahrekord, Iran

Nematollah Jonaidi-Jafari
Health Research Center, Baqiyatallah University of Medical Sciences, Tehran, Iran

Ebrahim Rahimi
Department of Food Hygiene and Public Health, College of Veterinary Medicine, Shahrekord Branch, Shahrekord, Iran

Aida Bianco, Maria Simona Capano, Valentina Mascaro, Claudia Pileggi and Maria Pavia
Department of Health Sciences, University of Catanzaro "Magna Græcia", Via T. Campanella, 115, 88100 Catanzaro, Italy

Lok Bahadur Shrestha, Narayan Raj Bhattarai and Basudha Khanal
Microbiology and Infectious Diseases, B. P. Koirala Institute of Health Sciences (BPKIHS), Dharan, Nepal

Nguyen Van Vinh Chau and Nguyen Huu Hien
The Hospital for Tropical Diseases, 764 Vo Van Kiet, Quan 5, Ho Chi Minh City, Vietnam

Nguyen Phu Huong Lan
The Hospital for Tropical Diseases, 764 Vo Van Kiet, Quan 5, Ho Chi Minh City, Vietnam
Oxford University Clinical Research Unit, The Hospital for Tropical Diseases, Wellcome Trust Major Overseas Programme, Ho Chi Minh City, Vietnam

Christine J. Boinett
The Hospital for Tropical Diseases, 764 Vo Van Kiet, Quan 5, Ho Chi Minh City, Vietnam
Oxford University Clinical Research Unit, The Hospital for Tropical Diseases, Wellcome Trust Major Overseas Programme, Ho Chi Minh City, Vietnam
Centre for Tropical Medicine and Global Health, Nuffield Department of Clinical Medicine, Oxford University, Oxford, UK

Tu Le Thi Phuong, Duy Pham Thanh, Nga Tran Vu Thieu, Dung Tran Thi Ngoc, Ha Thanh Tuyen and Phat Voong Vinh
Oxford University Clinical Research Unit, The Hospital for Tropical Diseases, Wellcome Trust Major Overseas Programme, Ho Chi Minh City, Vietnam

Guy E. Thwaites
Oxford University Clinical Research Unit, The Hospital for Tropical Diseases, Wellcome Trust Major Overseas Programme, Ho Chi Minh City, Vietnam
Centre for Tropical Medicine and Global Health, Nuffield Department of Clinical Medicine, Oxford University, Oxford, UK

Stephen Baker
Oxford University Clinical Research Unit, The Hospital for Tropical Diseases, Wellcome Trust Major Overseas Programme, Ho Chi Minh City, Vietnam
Centre for Tropical Medicine and Global Health, Nuffield Department of Clinical Medicine, Oxford University, Oxford, UK
The Department of Medicine, Cambridge University, Cambridge, UK

Matthew J. Ellington
Antimicrobial Resistance and Healthcare Associated Infection Unit, National Infection Service, Public Health England, Public Health England, London, UK

Silje Bakken Jørgensen
Department of Microbiology and Infection Control, Akershus University Hospital, Lørenskog, Norway

Øyvind Andreas Fladberg
Department of Microbiology and Infection Control, Akershus University Hospital, Lørenskog, Norway
Department of Medical Biochemistry and Microbiology, Uppsala University, Uppsala, Sweden

Hege Vangstein Aamot
Department of Microbiology and Infection Control, Akershus University Hospital, Lørenskog, Norway
Department of Clinical Molecular Biology (EpiGen), Division of Medicine, Akershus University Hospital and University of Oslo, Lørenskog, Norway

Japheth Awuletey Opintan and Mercy Jemima Newman
Medical Microbiology Department, School of Biomedical and Allied Health Sciences, Korle-Bu, Accra, Ghana

Matt Smith, Caroline King, Adele Dickson, Jeni Park, Fraser Smith, Kay Currie and Paul Flowers
Institute for Applied Health Research, Glasgow Caledonian University, Glasgow, Scotland G4 0BA, UK

Mark Davis
School of Social Sciences, Monash University, Melbourne 3800, Australia

Sewunet Admasu Belachew
Department of Clinical Pharmacy, School of Pharmacy, University of Gondar Chechela Street, Lideta Sub city Kebele, 16 Gondar, Ethiopia

Daniel Asfaw Erku
Department of Clinical Pharmacy, School of Pharmacy, University of Gondar Chechela Street, Lideta Sub city Kebele, 16 Gondar, Ethiopia
Department of clinical pharmacy, School of Pharmacy, College of Medicine and Health Sciences, University of Gondar, Ethiopia

Abebe Basazn Mekuria
Department of Pharmacology, School of Pharmacy, University of Gondar Chechela Street, Lideta Sub city Kebele, 16 Gondar, Ethiopia

Reza Ranjbar
Molecular Biology Research Center, Systems Biology and Poisonings Institute, Baqiyatallah University of Medical Sciences, Tehran, Iran

Farhad Safarpoor Dehkordi
Young Researchers and Elites Club, Shahrekord Branch, Islamic Azad University, Shahrekord, Iran

Mohammad Hossein Sakhaei Shahreza
Doctor Veterinary Medicine, Faculty of Veterinary Medicine, Shahrekord Branch, Islamic Azad University, Shahrekord, Iran

Ebrahim Rahimi
Department of Food Hygiene and Public health, Faculty of Veterinary Medicine, Shahrekord Branch, Shahrekord, Iran
Department of Food Hygiene and Quality Control, Faculty of Veterinary Medicine, Shahrekord Branch, Islamic Azad University, Shahrekord, Iran

Cornelius Remschmidt, Michael Behnke, Axel Kola, Luis A. Peña Diaz, Anna M. Rohde, Petra Gastmeier and Frank Schwab
Institute of Hygiene and Environmental Medicine, Charité-Universitätsmedizin Berlin, Hindenburgdamm 27, 12203 Berlin, Germany

Prabhu Raj Joshi and Mahesh Acharya
Central Department of Microbiology, Tribhuvan University, Kirtipur, Kathmandu, Nepal

Trishna Kakshapati
Annapurna Neurological Institute and Allied Sciences, Maitighar, Kathmandu, Nepal

Udomluk Leungtongkam and Rapee Thummeepak
Department of Microbiology and Parasitology, Faculty of Medical Science, Naresuan University, Phitsanulok, Thailand

Sutthirat Sitthisak
Department of Microbiology and Parasitology, Faculty of Medical Science, Naresuan University, Phitsanulok, Thailand
Centre of Excellence in Medical Biotechnology, Faculty of Medical Science, Naresuan University, Phitsanulok, Thailand

Zhen Xu
National Demonstration Center for Experimental Preventive Medicine Education, Tianjin Medical University, Qixiang Road No. 22, Tianjin 300070, China
School of Biological and Chemical Sciences, Queen Mary University of London, London, UK

Ronald R. Cutler
School of Biological and Chemical Sciences, Queen Mary University of London, London, UK

Hermine V. Mkrtchyan
School of Biological and Chemical Sciences, Queen Mary University of London, London, UK
School of Health, Sport and Biosciences, University of East London, E1 4NS, London, UK

Haroun N. Shah
Department of Natural Sciences, Middlesex University, The Burroughs Hendon, Middlesex NW4 4BT, UK

Raju Misra
Natural History Museum, Cromwell Rd, London SW7 5BD, UK

Jiazhen Chen and Wenhong Zhang
Department of Infectious Diseases, Huashan Hospital, Fudan University, Shanghai 200040, China

Yuting Liu
Tianjin Xiqing hospital, Tianjin 300380, China

Rachael M. Tomb, Scott J. MacGregor and John G. Anderson
The Robertson Trust Laboratory for Electronic Sterilisation Technologies (ROLEST), Department of Electronic and Electrical Engineering, University of Strathclyde, Glasgow, UK

Michelle Maclean
The Robertson Trust Laboratory for Electronic Sterilisation Technologies (ROLEST), Department of Electronic and Electrical Engineering, University of Strathclyde, Glasgow, UK
Department of Biomedical Engineering, University of Strathclyde, Glasgow, UK

John E. Coia
Department of Clinical Microbiology, Glasgow Royal Infirmary, Glasgow, UK

Shyam Kumar Mishra, Keshab Parajuli, Basista Prasad Rijal and Bharat Mani Pokhrel
Department of Clinical Microbiology, Institute of Medicine, Tribhuvan University Teaching Hospital, Kathmandu, Nepal

Narayan Prasad Parajuli
Department of Clinical Microbiology, Institute of Medicine, Tribhuvan University Teaching Hospital, Kathmandu, Nepal
Department of Laboratory Medicine, Manmohan Memorial Institute of Health Sciences, Khola Pravesh Marg, Soalteemode, Kathmandu, Nepal

Subhash Prasad Acharya
Department of Anesthesiology and Critical Care, Institute of Medicine, Tribhuvan University Teaching Hospital, Kathmandu, Nepal

Andrew A. Mahony
Department of Infectious Diseases, Austin Health, 145 Studley Rd, Heidelberg, VIC 3084, Australia
Department of Medicine, The University of Melbourne, Heidelberg, VIC 3084, Australia

Andrew H. Buultjens
Department of Microbiology and Immunology, The University of Melbourne at The Peter Doherty Institute for Infection and Immunity, Melbourne, VIC 3000, Australia

Elizabeth A. Grabsch
Department of Microbiology, Austin Health, Heidelberg, VIC 3084, Australia

Torsten Seemann
Melbourne Bioinformatics, The University of Melbourne, Parkville, VIC 3010, Australia

John K. Ferguson
Division of Microbiology, Health Pathology, NSW
Department of Immunology and Infectious Diseases, John Hunter Hospital, University of Newcastle, Newcastle, NSW 2305, Australia

Anna Różańska, Agnieszka Chmielarczyk, Dorota Romaniszyn and Małgorzata Bulanda
Jagiellonian University Medical College, Faculty of Medicine, Chair of Microbiology, Czysta str. 18, 31-121 Kraków, Poland

Monika Walkowicz, Piotr Osuch and Tadeusz Knych
Faculty of Non-Ferrous Metals, Department of Metal Working and Physical Metallurgy of Non-Ferrous Metals, AGH University of Science and Technology, al. Mickiewicza 30, 30-059 Kraków, Poland

Peter Kreidl, Astrid Mayr, Guido Hinterberger, Michael Berktold, Ludwig Knabl, Stefan Fuchs, Wilfried Posch, Cornelia Lass-Flörl and Dorothea Orth-Höller
Department of Hygiene, Microbiology and Social Medicine, Division of Hygiene and Medical Microbiology, Medical University of Innsbruck, Innsbruck, Schoepfstr. 41, 6020 Innsbruck, Austria

Stephan Eschertzhuber
Department of Anesthesia and Critical Care, Centre of Operative Medicine, Medical University of Innsbruck, Anichstr. 35, 6020 Innsbruck, Austria

Alois Obwegeser
Department of Neurosurgery, University Hospital of Innsbruck, Anichstr. 35, 6020 Innsbruck, Austria

Wenxia Zhang
Institute of Antibiotics, Huashan Hospital, Fudan University, 12 M. Wulumuqi Rd, Shanghai 200040, China
Department of Clinical Laboratory, Shuguang Hospital Affiliated to Shanghai University of Traditional Chinese Medicine, 528 Zhangheng Rd, Shanghai 201203, China

Yan Guo, Yang Yang, Dong Dong, Demei Zhu and Fupin Hu
Institute of Antibiotics, Huashan Hospital, Fudan University, 12 M. Wulumuqi Rd, Shanghai 200040, China
Key Laboratory of Clinical Pharmacology of Antibiotics, Ministry of Health, Shanghai, China

Jiayin Li, Yiyuan Zhang and Ping He
Department of Medical Microbiology and Immunology, Shanghai Jiao Tong University School of Medicine, Shanghai 200025, China

Addisu Gize Yeshanew and Rozina Ambachew Geremew
Department of Microbiology, St. Paul's Hospital Millennium Medical College, Addis Ababa, Ethiopia

David Herren and Jonas Marschall
Department of Infectious Diseases and Hospital Epidemiology, Bern University Hospital and University of Bern, Bern, Switzerland

Andreas Kronenberg
Department of Infectious Diseases and Hospital Epidemiology, Bern University Hospital and University of Bern, Bern, Switzerland
Institute for Infectious Diseases, University of Bern, Bern, Switzerland

Alexia Cusini
Department of Infectious Diseases and Hospital Epidemiology, Bern University Hospital and University of Bern, Bern, Switzerland
Infectious Diseases Unit, Cantonal Hospital, 7000 Chur, Switzerland

Lukas Bütikofer
CTU Bern, and Institute of Social and Preventive Medicine (ISPM), University of Bern, Bern, Switzerland

Catherine Plüss-Suard
Service of Hospital Preventive Medicine, Lausanne University Hospital, Lausanne, Switzerland

Kay Currie, Caroline King, Kareena McAloney-Kocaman, Nicola J. Roberts, Jennifer MacDonald, Adele Dickson, Paul Flowers and Lesley Price
School of Health and Life Sciences, Glasgow Caledonian University, Cowcaddens Road, Glasgow, Scotland G4 0BA, UK

Jacqui Reilly
School of Health and Life Sciences, Glasgow Caledonian University, Cowcaddens Road, Glasgow, Scotland G4 0BA, UK
NHS Health Protection Scotland, Glasgow, UK

Shona Cairns
NHS Health Protection Scotland, Glasgow, UK

Nitish Khanna
NHS Greater Glasgow and Clyde, Glasgow, UK

W. Wangchinda, N. Pati, N. Maknakhon, C. Seenama and V. Thamlikitkul
Division of Infectious Diseases and Tropical Medicine, Department of Medicine, Faculty of Medicine Siriraj Hospital, Mahidol University, 2 Wanglang Road, Bangkoknoi, Bangkok 10700, Thailand

S. Tiengrim
Department of Clinical Microbiology and Applied Technology, Faculty of Medical Technology, Mahidol University, Bangkok, Thailand

Amanual Getnet Mersha
School of Medicine, College of Medicine and Health Sciences, University of Gondar, Gondar, Ethiopia

Martin Steinbakk
Department of Antibiotic Resistance and Infection Prevention, Norwegian Institute of Public Health, 0213 Oslo, NO, Norway

Laura Espenhain
Department of Antibiotic Resistance and Infection Prevention, Norwegian Institute of Public Health, 0213 Oslo, NO, Norway
European Programme for Intervention Epidemiology Training (EPIET), European Centre for Disease Prevention and Control, (ECDC), Stockholm, Sweden

Silje Bakken Jørgensen, Michaela Marie Lelek and Siri Haug Hänsgen
Department of Clinical Microbiology and Infection Control, Akershus University Hospital, Lørenskog, Norway

Truls Michael Leegaard
Department of Clinical Microbiology and Infection Control, Akershus University Hospital, Lørenskog, Norway
Institute for Clinical Medicine, Campus Ahus, University of Oslo, Nordbyhagen, Norway

Britt Nakstad
Institute for Clinical Medicine, Campus Ahus, University of Oslo, Nordbyhagen, Norway
Department of Paediatrics and Adolescents Medicine, Akershus University Hospital, Lørenskog, Norway

Marianne Sunde
Department of Molecular Biology, Norwegian Institute of Public Health, Oslo, Norway
Section for Food Safety and Emerging Health Threats, Norwegian Veterinary Institute, Nordbyhagen, Norway

D. Nagarjuna
Dr. B. R. Ambedkar Centre for Biomedical Research (ACBR), University of Delhi (North Campus), Delhi 110007, India
Current address: Department of Biotechnology, Indian Institute of Technology, Roorkee 247667, India

Manisha Yadav
Dr. B. R. Ambedkar Centre for Biomedical Research (ACBR), University of Delhi (North Campus), Delhi 110007, India
Current address: Department of Clinical Microbiology, Rigshospitalet, Copenhagen, Denmark

Gajanand Mittal and Rajni Gaind
Department of Microbiology, Vardhman Mahavir Medical College (VMMC) and Safdarjung Hospital, Delhi 110029, India

Rakesh Singh Dhanda
Stem Cell Laboratory, Longboat Explorers AB, SMiLE Incubator, Scheelevägen 2, 22381 Lund, Sweden

Index

www.ingramcontent.com/pod-product-compliance
Lightning Source LLC
LaVergne TN
LVHW080656210926
848485LV00003B/387